Alzheimer's Disease

Alzheimer's Disease

Edited by **Joshua Barnard**

FOSTER
ACADEMICS

New Jersey

Published by Foster Academics,
61 Van Reypen Street,
Jersey City, NJ 07306, USA
www.fosteracademics.com

Alzheimer's Disease
Edited by Joshua Barnard

International Standard Book Number: 978-1-63242-039-8 (Hardback)

Printed in the United States of America.

Contents

Preface

The main aim of this book is to educate learners and enhance their research focus by presenting diverse topics covering this vast field. This is an advanced book which compiles significant studies by distinguished experts in the area of analysis. This book addresses successive solutions to the challenges arising in the area of application, along with it; the book provides scope for future developments.

This book gives an extensive overview on the pathogenesis and diagnosis of Alzheimer's disease. Over 6 million Europeans, out of which more than a quarter of people who are over the age of 85 and 10% who are over the age of 65, have been affected by Alzheimer's Dementia (AD). Given the steady aging of European societies, cognitive decline and dementia have grown into a crucial health problem with a great socioeconomic effect on patients, their caregivers and families, society, and national health care policy. The amount of people with dementia is estimated to double by 2030 and further increase by 2050. There is a critical requirement for creative methods to boost understanding of pathological events that would transform into the establishment of successful prevention or new treatment techniques. Advancements in comprehending pathological events in AD have been achievable by employing cell cultures, genetically modified organisms and animal models that do not have the complexity of events happening in humans. It is necessary that we conquer this restraint as well by using data from humans – for analyzing pathological pathways in AD in a multidisciplinary setting.

It was a great honour to edit this book, though there were challenges, as it involved a lot of communication and networking between me and the editorial team. However, the end result was this all-inclusive book covering diverse themes in the field.

Finally, it is important to acknowledge the efforts of the contributors for their excellent chapters, through which a wide variety of issues have been addressed. I would also like to thank my colleagues for their valuable feedback during the making of this book.

Editor

Pathogenesis

Structure and Function of
the APP Intracellular Domain in Health and Disease

Ulrike Müller and Klemens Wild

Additional information is available at the end of the chapter

1. Introduction

Talking about Alzheimer's disease (AD) on a biochemical level needs to highlight the molecular „*corpus delicti*": the amyloid or senile plaques [1]. These plaques are extracellular fibrillar deposits in the cortex and hippocampus mainly composed of a single proteinaceous compound, the Aβ peptide comprising predominantly 40 or 42 amino acid residues (Aβ40, Aβ42) [2]. The Aβ peptides originate by sequential ectodomain shedding and regulated intramembrane proteolysis (RIP) of the amyloid precursor protein (APP), a type I integral membrane protein highly expressed in neurons including synaptic compartments. The responsible proteases, the famous β- and γ-secretase respectively, have been reviewed in detail and will not be part of this paper [3, 4]. Since the cloning of APP 25 years ago, more than 9,000 publications (about one per day!) are listed for this protein in the PubMed database indicating its pivotal position in the amyloid cascade hypothesis [5], which constitutes the widely accepted pathogenic cascade ultimately leading to AD. While some years ago the plaques themselves were thought to be the primary cause of disease, it is nowadays well recognized that soluble Aβ oligomers are responsible for many of the neurotoxic properties causing memory dysfunction and finally dementia.

Despite intense research efforts AD can so far only be insufficiently treated in a purely symptomatic way and disease-modifying drugs are most wanted but are still not available [6]. In order to get a glimpse of understanding AD pathology at a biochemical level, we therefore have to understand the molecular structure of the key-player APP and its connected protein network. The structure, however, needs to be correlated with the physiological functions and the deregulating mechanisms causing toxicity, cell death, and disease [7, 8]. Bearing this in mind, the simultaneously generated sister peptides of Aβ deserve a major focus, namely the amino-terminal fragment (N-APP286) derived from sAPPβ as a ligand for the death receptor

6 (DR6) [9], and the APP intracellular domain as created by the ε-cut of γ-secretase during the RIP process [3], which is the topic of this paper. We will start by getting the architecture of APP into place.

2. Architecture of the APP protein

APP can be divided into three domains (Figure 1). As a single pass type I membrane protein, the N-terminal ectodomain of APP (residues 18 to 624 neglecting the signal peptide, numbers refer to the neuronal splice form APP695, UniPROT entry: P05067-4) locates to the extracellular space. The single hydrophobic transmembrane domain (TMD, residues 625 to 648) is followed by the rather short APP intracellular domain (AICD, residues 649 to 695). More important than this topological classification is the distinction according to the fragments produced by secretase cleavage events [10]. The products produced by ectodomain shedding are sAPPα (residues 18 to 612; cleaved by α-secretases, members of the ADAM family of zinc metallo-proteases) and sAPPβ (residues 18 to 596; cleaved by β-secretase, an aspartic protease also known as BACE1 in the nervous system and BACE in peripheral tissue). The C-terminal fragments (CTFs) generated by ectodomain shedding are the still membrane embedded αCTF (CTF83) and βCTF (CTF99), respectively. The CTFs are subsequently cut in the RIP process by the intramembrane aspartate protease presenilin (1 or 2) as part of the γ-secretase complex, with αCTF being split into the p3 peptide and the AICD (residues 646 to 695) and βCTF into the Aβ peptide (Aβ40: residues 597 to 636; Aβ42: residues 597 to 638) and again the AICD.

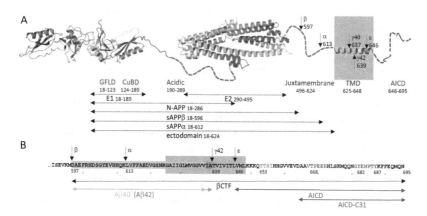

Figure 1. Architecture of APP and of its proteolytic fragments. A. Domain architecture of the neuronal splice variant APP695. Domains with known atomic structures (E1 and E2) and the TMD are shown as ribbon diagrams in a colour code from blue (N-terminus) to red (C-terminus). Dashed lines give structurally unknown regions. Proposed homodimeric interactions within E1 and E2 are shown in gray. Positions of secretase cleavage events and the respective breakdown products are labeled. B. Sequence and proteolytic fragments within βCTF. Aβ peptides, the TMD (gray), and sequence fingerprints within the AICD are colour coded.

In terms of three-dimensional structure, only substructures within the large APP ectodomain have been solved as independently folded subdomains. The N-terminal E1 domain is a two-lobe structure consisting of the growth factor like domain (GFLD, residues 18-123) and a copper-binding domain (CuBD, residues 124 to 189), both comprising mixed $\alpha\beta$ topologies rigidified by disulfide bridges [11-13]. The E1 domain is followed by a highly acidic, and probably unfolded, stretch of about 100 residues that passes on to the E2 domain (residues 290 to 495), consisting of two coiled-coils connected through a continuous central helix and resembling a spectrin family fold [14]. E1 and E2 domains have been implicated in APP dimerization [14-16], which is reported to be modified by the extracellular matrix [17], and to have significant impact on localization and cleavage events. In addition, dimerization might also involve the TMD region [16]. Besides dimerization, APP architecture (and likely function) is also influenced by a series of post-translational modifications, mainly by N- and O-glycosylation and phosphorylation [18], which will be discussed in detail below. The reminder of the ectodomain between E2 and the TMD, the so-called juxtamembrane region (residues 496 to 624), is again intrinsically disordered based on secondary structure prediction and contains the cleavage sites for the α- and β-secretases. The single TMD is clearly α helical, although with partial propensity in forming β structures. This propensity extends also to the juxtamembrane region with the fatal consequence, that after secretase cleavage the amyloid peptide folds into a β hairpin structure and aggregates to form the toxic oligomers and finally the amyloid fibrils. Finally, the AICD itself is again intrinsically disordered as shown by NMR and CD experiments [19, 20]. Importantly however, this small C-terminal stub has recently been shown to adopt different conformations reflecting its versatile functions. The structure-function relationship of the AICD shall be described in the following.

3. Biology of the AICD: Tales of a tail

When talking about the AICD, a clear distinction has to be made: the function (and probably also the structure) is different for AICD as part of APP at the membrane and for AICD as peptide generated by ϵ-cleavage of γ-secretase and first described by Passer et al. [21]. Within the AICD three sequence motifs have been identified to be of functional relevance. The first one is the [653]YTSI sequence, which has been implicated in the basolateral sorting of APP in polarized MDCK cells [22] and which is reminiscent to the YXXΦ (X: any residue; Φ: aromatic or large hydrophobic residue) consensus motif as tyrosine-based and clathrin-mediated endocytic sorting signal [23]. Indeed, when Tyr653 is mutated to alanine, APP is equally distributed on apical and basolateral membranes in MDCK cells [24]. Somewhat surprisingly, in neurons polarized sorting occurs independently of this signal [25]. Subcellular trafficking and neuronal APP sorting is still poorly understood [26] and remains a topic of intense investigation. This first motif contains three phosphorylatable residues (YTS), and it has been reported that at least Thr654 and Ser655 are phosphorylated in the adult rat brain under physiological conditions [27].

Much more attention has been drawn to the second fingerprint [667]VTPEER, as this site seems to be also critically involved in pathophysiological processes. While the function of the residues has remained elusive prior to the availability of structural data, Thr668 has since been established as the major phosphorylation site of APP and its physiological function has been investigated in the adult rat brain, post mitotic differentiating neurons and dividing cells [18]. Whereas pT668 in neurons is dominant in the fully-glycosylated mature APP, in differentiating cells the purely N-glycosylated immature protein as present in the endoplasmic reticulum and the early Golgi is of relevance. Accordingly, different kinases are responsible for Thr668 phosphorylation. In neurons, it is glycogen synthase kinase-3β (GSK3β) and cyclin-dependent kinase 5 (Cdk5), while Cdk1 and cdc2 kinase phosphorylate this residue in dividing cells. Moreover, when cells are exposed to stress, phosphorylation is taken over by c-Jun N-terminal kinase (JNK) [28].

Phosphorylation on Thr668 of APP depends on the presence of Pro669 and strongly affects Aβ production [29]. This is reminiscent of the Tau protein, where the phosphorylation of certain serine and threonine residues depends on adjacent proline residues and leads to tangle formation [29]. A first molecular explanation for the proline-dependency was revealed by studies showing that the prolyl isomerase Pin1, catalyzing the *cis-trans* isomerization of the Thr-Pro peptide bond, increases amyloidogenic APP processing and selectively elevates Aβ42 levels. Intriguingly, Pin1 is down regulated and/or inhibited by oxidation in neurons of Alzheimer's disease patients and *Pin1* knockout causes neurodegeneration (and tauopathy). Pin1 binds to Thr668-phosphorylated APP and accelerates Pro669 isomerization (by a factor of 10^3). Thus, the AICD swaps between two conformations, as visualized by NMR [29]. This conformational switch may in turn have crucial consequences with regard to the AICD protein interacting network, as shown for the neuronal adaptor protein Fe65 (Figure 2 and see below) [20, 30]. To evaluate in as much the phosphorylation state of Thr688 controls APP processing *in vivo*, knockin mice were generated in which Thr668 was changed to alanine (APP$_{TA/TA}$) [31, 32]. The APP$_{TA/TA}$ mutation, and thus absence of phosphorylation, did not significantly alter APP localization, processing, and Aβ generation, thus questioning the *in vivo* role of Thr668 phosphorylation. However, these studies cannot rule out the possibility that a pathological increase in Thr668 phosphorylation, as found in AD patients [33], will also modulate its function. In line with this notion, Thr668 phosphorylation has also been reported to influence APP cleavage by caspases between residues Asp664 and Ala665, producing the cytotoxic AICD-C31 fragment, a process that has been strongly implicated in AD pathogenesis [34].

The third and most intensely studied fingerprint within the AICD is the [681]GYENPTY sequence containing an NPXY motif, a well-established internalization signal for membrane proteins [35]. NPXY is a classical tyrosine-based sorting signal for transmembrane proteins to endosomes and lysosomes [23]. However, the signal has been shown to only mediate rapid internalization of a subset of type I membrane proteins, including APP as well as members of the low-density lipoprotein (LDL) receptor family and integrin β. These proteins are internalized via clathrin-coated pits. Nevertheless evidence for a direct interaction of NPXY motifs with the coat or the AP-2 adaptor is weak.

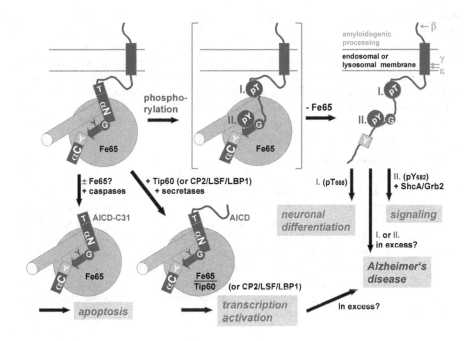

Figure 2. AICD in health and disease. Different fates of the AICD are exemplified for the main AICD interaction with Fe65-PTB2 (red T-box: TPEE, cyan Y-box: NPTY, G: glycine hinge, gray cylinder: C-terminal helix of Fe65-PTB2). In the non-phosphorylated state, AICD forms a stable complex with Fe65-PTB2 that assembles in ternary complexes with i.e. Tip60 or CP2/LSF/LBP1 via Fe65-PTB1. Upon cleavage by the secretases, the liberated complexes are involved in transcription activation. Alternatively, caspase cleavage within the AICD results in cytotoxic AICD-C31, which might compete with AICD for Fe65-PTB2 binding and induce apoptosis. Phosphorylation of either Thr668 (I.) or Tyr682 (II.) results in a destabilization of the Fe65-PTB2/AICD interaction (shown in brackets) and results in complex dissociation. Phosphorylation stimulates (I.) neuronal differentiation or (II.) initiates signaling cascades. Deregulation of the Fe65-PTB2/AICD interactions is strongly implicated in Alzheimer's disease progression.

Instead, the NPXY motif is well known to interact with adaptor proteins containing a domain known as phosphotyrosine-binding (PTB) or phosphotyrosine-interacting domain (PID) [36]. PTB domains reveal a fine tuned plasticity in ligand recognition, and besides recognizing phosphorylated NPXpY motifs, most PTB adaptor proteins can also bind to their ligand in a pY-independent manner. Accordingly, *in vitro* phosphorylation of Tyr687, which does not seem to occur in the brain [18], does i.e. not alter the binding affinity of AICD to its major PTB-containing adaptor protein Fe65.

In APP, the NPXY signal is extended by three residues at the N-terminal side (GYE), with especially Tyr682 being most critical for function [31, 37, 38]. The motif is present in many lysosomal glycoproteins that are endocytosed and targeted to the lysosomes [39]. In cell-culture studies, Tyr682 can be readily phosphorylated by the nerve growth factor receptor TrkA and the tyrosine kinases Abl and Src [40]. In brains of AD patients, it is known that at least βCTF is phosphorylated, whereas this is not the case for αCTF [41]. In addition, phosphorylation regulates both AICD peptide formation and AICD-dependent cellular responses (Figure 2). These data point to a sorting function regulated by Tyr682 phosphorylation, with non-phosphorylated APP kept at the plasma membrane and therefore processed by α-secretase, and a phosphorylation-dependent re-localization resulting in β-cleavage. Sorting implies docking to respective intracellular trafficking machineries and their adaptors, including PTB domain containing proteins. Consistently, an APP$_{YG/YG}$ mutation introduced into the endogenous APP locus by knock-in led to a marked shift toward the non-amyloidogenic pathway in brain with increased levels of full length APP, sAPPα, αCTF, unaltered βCTF and reduced sAPPβ and Aβ40 levels [31].

Sorting due to differentially phosphorylated residues is one side of the medal, signaling is the other [40]. Two signaling proteins are well known to require Tyr682 phosphorylation for binding to APP-CTFs, namely ShcA and Grb2. ShcA is a member of a family of cytoplasmic adaptor proteins (ShcA, ShcB, ShcC) that interacts with its PTB and Src homology2 (SH2) domains with receptor tyrosine kinases (RTKs) and activated growth factor receptors, which is the case also for SH2/SH3 domains containing Grb2 [42]. The initiated cascades are involved both in cell proliferation and gene transcription events, like i.e. the MAP kinase pathway. Again, binding occurs only to pTyr682 of βCTFs but not of αCTFs [41] (Figure 2). Whereas the reasons for the different binding preferences remain elusive, the underlying structural transitions within the AICD itself modulating sorting and signaling have been studied in some detail.

4. Structural transitions within the AICD

First structural insights on the AICD peptide came from NMR experiments, revealing most of the AICD to be unstructured. The transient structure (also termed intrinsic disorder: ID) of cytoplasmic domains of membrane proteins is well suited for the molecular recognition in intracellular signaling events for a number of reasons [43]: (i) modulation of the structural propensity provides ID proteins with the capability to combine high specificity with low affinity; (ii) binding diversity in which one region specifically recognizes differently shaped partners by structural accommodation at the binding interface, a phenomenon known as one-to-many signaling; (iii) binding commonality in which distinct sequences recognize a common binding site (with eventually different folds); (iv) the formation of large interaction surfaces as the ID region wraps up or surrounds its binding partner, making it possible to overcome steric restrictions; (v) faster rates of association by reducing dependence on orientation factors and by enlarging target sizes; (vi) faster rates of dissociation by unzipping mechanisms; (vii) the precise control and simple regulation of the binding thermodynamics; and (viii) the reduced life-time of ID proteins in the cell, possibly representing a mechanism of rapid turnover of important regulatory molecules. A prominent example of intrinsically disordered proteins is α-synuclein, a protein critically involved in Parkinson's disease, which binds to a multitude of partners differentially by alternative folding [44], a feature that equally applies to the intracellular domain of APP.

Although NMR experiments revealed the AICD to be intrinsically disordered, the TPEE and NPTY motifs where found to form type I β-turns and TPEE forms part of a helix-capping box [19] (Figure 3). Type I turns are the most frequent reverse turns in protein structures, which in total involve about $1/3^{rd}$ of all residues. Turns usually occur on the exposed protein surfaces and represent molecular recognition sites. In a capping box, the side chain of the first helical residue forms a hydrogen bond with the backbone of the fourth helical residue and, recipro-cally, the side chain of the fourth residue forms a hydrogen bond with the backbone of the first residue [45]. These boxes are known to stabilize the N-termini of α-helices, and preordering of the elements is thought to guide recognition of the intracellular protein network and to reduce the entropic costs for complex formation, a feature that applies as well for APP. In addition, the conformation of the TPEE motif and the propensity of forming the N-terminally capped α helix critically depend on the phosphorylation status of Thr668 [20, 46]. This structure-function relationship can be explored by the study of the AICD with its cytoplasmic interaction partners.

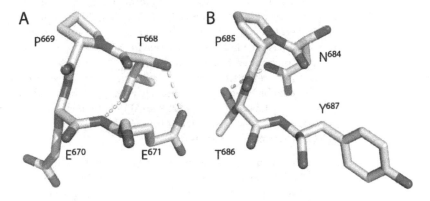

Figure 3. The TPEE and NPTY motifs. A. The TPEE motif forms a type I β-turn and a helix capping box with two char-acteristic hydrogen bonds (dashed yellow lines). B. The NPTY motif forms a similar type I β-turn.

5. Interaction partners of the AICD

More than 20 proteins have been reported to interact with the AICD [47] (Table 1). However, little is known whether these complexes occur also *in vivo* and what relevance they may have for cell physiology or AD pathogenesis. Basically, they can be classified in modifying, sorting, or signaling interactions. The modifying enzymes have been already mentioned and account for phosphorylation and prolyl *cis/trans* isomerization events. Basolateral sorting is guided by the protein PAT1, which is the only protein that has been shown to directly interact with the [653]YTSI motif and is associated with microtubules [48].

Knowledge about the interaction partners for the [667]VTPEER motif is similar scarce. Major binder for the motif, and as well for the complete AICD, are the multi-domain adaptor/ scaffolding proteins of the Fe65 family (Fe65, Fe65L1, and Fe65L2) [49]. The only additional binding partner to the [667]VTPEER motif is the dimeric adaptor protein 14-3-3γ, which seems to stabilize the AICD/Fe65 interaction [50]. Fe65 is enriched in brain, whereas Fe65L1 and Fe65L2 are more widely expressed. All three members contain a WW domain and two PTB domains (PTB1 and PTB2). Through the PTB2 domain, they interact with the AICD and can alter APP processing. After proteolytic processing of APP and release of the AICD to the cytoplasm, Fe65 can translocate to the nucleus to participate in gene transcription events (Figure 2), which is modulated by 14-3-3γ. This role is further mediated by interactions of Fe65-PTB1 with the transcription factors CP2/LSF/LBP1 [51] and Tip60 [52] and the WW domain with the nucleosome assembly factor SET [53]. Possible target genes identified by reporter assays include GSK3β, Neprilysin, KAI1, and the low-density lipoprotein receptor-related protein 1 (LRP1), but the physiological relevance for endogenous transcriptional regulation has been discussed controversially [54]. Fe65-PTB1 also interacts with two cell surface lipoproteins receptors, namely LRP1 [55] and ApoEr2 [56], forming trimeric complexes with APP. The Fe55 WW domain further binds to mammalian Ena (mEna) [57], through which it functions in regulation of the actin cytoskeleton, cell motility, and neuronal growth cone formation [49]. The interaction has been implicated in a role for AICD signaling, in synaptic plasticity and memory [58]. Moreover, Fe65 family proteins have attracted attention, as Fe65 or Fe65L1 double knockout mice revealed defects in cortical development with neuronal mispositioning and ectopia, resembling human lissencephaly type 2 [59]. Interestingly, very similar cortical defects were also found in APP-/-APLP1-/-APLP2-/- triple knockout mice lacking all APP family members, suggesting a lack of APP/Fe65 dependent signaling as the underlying cause of defects in both mouse mutants [60].

Fe65 binding to the AICD is unique, as its extended binding interface ranges from the [667]VTPEER up to the [681]GYENPTY motif and thus includes almost the entire AICD-C31 fragment (Figures 2 and 4A). Most other AICD interacting proteins recognize the [671]GYENPTY motif and neighbouring residues, with the interaction site spanning only about 10 residues. As [681]GYENPTY is essential for APP trafficking, the respective complexes can also alter APP processing. Like Fe65, the binders for this motif are PTB-containing proteins including members of the X11/Mint, JIP, Dab, and Shc families, as well as the Numb protein.

Mints consist of a divergent N-terminal region and conserved C-terminal sequences composed of one PTB domain and two tandem PDZ domains. Although their regulatory role for APP metabolism and transport is unresolved, it seems that they slow cellular APP processing and reduce Aβ40 and Aβ42 secretion [61] by suppressing translocation of APP into BACE- and γ-secretase-rich detergent-resistant membrane (DRM) domains, the so-called rafts [62, 66]. In addition, there is evidence for a functional role of the AICD interaction with X11/Mints for synapse formation [62, 67] and synaptic neurotransmitter release [68]. c-Jun N-terminal kinase (JNK) interacting protein-1 (JIP1), a scaffolding protein for the JNK kinase cascade, has been suggested to mediate anterograde transport of APP by the molecular motor kinesin-1. However, this initial view has been challenged recently, as in contrast to this model, APP constructs lacking the AICD are still transported to the nerve terminal by the fast axonal transport mechanism [63].

Protein	Interacting domain	Interacting region within AICD	Function	Processing*	Selected citations
PAT1	n.a.	YTSI	Basolateral sorting	α↑, β↓**	[48]
Fe65,	PTB2	AICD-C31:	Endocytosis, signaling and	β↓	[49]
Fe65L1, -L2	n.a.	VTPEER + GYENPTY	transcription activation, ...	n.a.	[50]
14-3-3-γ	PTB	VTPEER	AICD/Fe65 stabilization	β↓	[61] [62]
X11/Mint		GYENPTY	Exocytosis, synapse formation, ...		
JIP1	PTB	GYENPTY	Transport	β↓	[63]
Dab1	PTB	GYENPTY	Transport, signaling	α↑, β↓	[64]
ShcA/Grb2	PTB/SH2	G(pY)ENPTY	Signaling	-	[42]
Numb	PTB	GYENPTY	Notch crosstalk	***	[65]

Table 1. Selected interaction partners of the AICD. *Data depend on cell line studied and are sometimes conflicting. **Due to basolateral sorting and independent of PAT1 binding. Pat1 binding as such increases Aβ levels [48]. ***Numb isoform dependent. ↓ denotes changes of non-amyloidogenic (α) or amyloidogenic (β) APP processing.

The Dab family member Dab1 regulates neuronal migration in mammals as an essential component of the Reelin signaling pathway. Dab1 binds not only to APP family proteins [64] but is well known to also bind to ApoE receptors (ApoEr2, VLDLR, and LRP) [69]. Dab1 increases cell surface expression of APP and ApoEr2, increases α-cleavage of APP and ApoEr2, and decreases APP βCTF formation and Aβ production in transfected cells and in primary neurons. The Dab family represents a prototype of PTB domains that bind their ligands in a pY-independent manner [36]. In addition Dab proteins bind specifically to the phospho-inositide (PI) PI-4,5-P_2, which is predominantly located at the cellular membrane [70]. Binding of PTB domains to PIs is a common principle to locate and orientate the adaptors at the target membrane and to facilitate downstream events that accompany NPXY peptide binding. Since PTB domains structurally belong to the pleckstrin homology (PH) superfold family and PH domains are the prototypical PI binding domains, this function seems to be evolutionarily conserved within PTB domains [36]. The crystal structures of ternary complexes of Dabs bound to ApoEr2 [71] or APP [72] peptides and lipid revealed the lipid head group (IP_3) to be recognized by a large basic patch opposite the peptide-binding groove (Figure 4A). This patch, also termed as "phospholipid binding-crown", is conserved in many PTB domains [36].

Finally, binding of the AICD to the Numb PTB domain has been found to inhibit Notch signaling [65], thereby establishing a crosstalk between the APP family and Notch in the development of the peripheral nervous system (PNS) [73]. Like APP, the Notch receptor undergoes a series of proteolytic cleavages that release the Notch intracellular domain (NICD) that functions in transcriptional activation and subsequent signal transduction events, including proliferation, differentiation, or apoptotic cues [74]. Similar to the NICD, the AICD has been also found to regulate PI-mediated calcium signaling through a γ-secretase dependent pathway [75, 76]. Cells lacking APP were shown to exhibit deficits in calcium storage that could be reversed by transfection with APP constructs containing an intact AICD. Constructs lacking the AICD were not able to rescue the phenotype, strongly indicating that this domain is critically involved in endoplasmic reticulum (ER) calcium filling [76]. The multitude of interactions with the AICD raises the question of the spatial and temporal regulation of all these complexes, which needs a detailed structural analysis and a thorough biochemical characterization.

6. Structure-function relationship of AICD complexes

The structure-function relationship of AICD complexes is governed by the one-to-many principle with the intrinsically disordered AICD folding onto its manifold adaptor proteins, in particular the PTB domain containing proteins. The recurrent interaction pattern includes the recognition of the [681]GYENPTY sequence, which shall be described in the following. High resolution structures for this interaction are known for Dab1 and 2 [72], X11α [77], and the Fe65-PTB2 domains [30] (Figure 4A). All PTB domains comprise a pleckstrin homology (PH) fold consisting of a central β sandwich structure and a C-terminal α helix. Overall, complex formation can be described as an induced-fit docking of the AICD to a rigid PTB domain scaffold. Common to all the complexes is the binding of the [681]GYEN sequence to the β5 strand of the respective PTB domain by a mechanism called β completion, where a (antiparallel) β sheet is created between two polypeptide chains (*in trans*) (Figure 4D). This interaction occurs between the protein backbones and therefore strong sequence conservation is not present on the PTB domain side. The conservation of AICD Gly681 is explained as longer side chains would cause steric clashes with the PTB domains, as shown for the Fe65-PTB2/AICD interaction, where a G681A mutation abolishes the binding and Gal4-Tip60-dependent transactivation [78]. The importance of the flexible glycine becomes evident when comparing the solved PTB/AICD complexes (Figure 4B), revealing that Gly681 forms a hinge that allows for different AICD conformations in the N-terminal direction. The hinge function correlates with a peptide-flip of the glycine [30].

The side chain of Tyr682 is accommodated in the center of the interface and faces the C-terminal helix of PTB domains (Figures 3A and 3D). In all complexes it lays in a hydrophobic pocket, however, the conformations between the Fe65-PTB2 and Dab1 in respect to X11α and Dab2 complexes are different. The hydrophobic nature of the pocket explains the general conservation of a tyrosine or phenylalanine in this position in the context of NPXY sequences. All crystallized complexes are specific for non-phosphorylated Tyr682, which can be readily explained, as there is no space available to accommodate the extra phosphate moiety. This is in contrast to ShcA, where the binding site is more open [79], which apparently allows for binding of a phosphorylated Tyr682 (although no structure of this complex is available). The readout of the conserved glutamate is again different in the PTB complexes, although its function as selectivity filter seems to be minor. Whereas it forms i.e. a salt bridge with an arginine of X11α, in the Fe65-PTB2 complex it is fixed *in cis* to Lys688 following the NPTY motif.

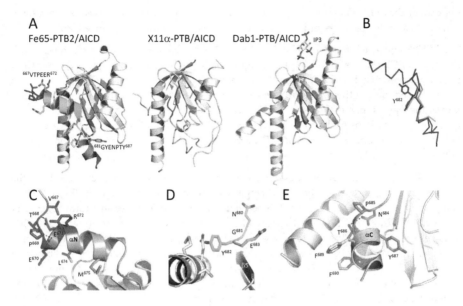

Figure 4. Structure of the AICD in PTB domain complexes. A. Crystal structures of AICD peptides in complex with PTB domains: Fe65-PTB2/AICD (PDB code 3DXC), X11α-PTB/AICD (1X11), and Dab1-PTB/AICD (1OQN). AICD peptides are colour coded from blue (N-terminus) to red (C-terminus) and PTB domains are given in gray. In Fe65-PTB2/AICD, the visible AICD structure corresponds to AICD-C31 and includes both the ^{667}VTPEER and the ^{681}GYENPTY sequences. Dab1 is also bound to the polar head group of the lipid PI-4,5-P$_2$ (IP3: inositol-1,4,5-triphosphate). B. Superposition of the three AICD fragments as shown in Figure 3A (complex with Fe65-PTB2: red; X11α: blue; Dab1: green). The alternative side chain conformations of Tyr682 are highlighted. C. Close-up view on the AICD helix αN in complex with Fe65-PTB2. The ^{667}VTPEER motif is highlighted in blue and hydrogen bonds within the capping box are given as dashed lines. D. Interaction of the ^{680}NGYE motif with Fe65-PTB2. The AICD stretch forms a β sheet *in trans* with strand β5 from the PTB domain. The side chain of Tyr682 is accommodated in a hydrophobic pocket created by the C-terminal helix of the PTB domain. E. Interaction of the ^{684}NPTY motif and helix αC of the AICD with Fe65-PTB2. Tyr687 is rather solvent exposed and helix αC is fixed to the PTB domain by hydrophobic interactions of two subsequent phenylalanines.

As already described, the ^{684}NPTY sequence is forming a type I β-turn structure, which is retained within the complexes and forms the N-terminal cap of an induced α-helix at the very C-terminus of AICD (helix αC) (Figure 4E). Asn684 has a conserved structural role, with the carboxamide of the side chain hydrogen bonding to the main chain of Thr686. As the carboxamide is also tightly bonded to the PTB domains, the preformed NPTY conformation is a major determinant and probably also a starting point for AICD folding and complex formation. The conserved proline initiates and stabilizes the subsequent helix as found in many α helices. The most prominent residue, however, is Tyr687, as the tyrosine at this position is the discriminator for the classification in pY-dependent and pY-independent PTB domains [36]. In all structurally solved AICD/PTB domain complexes the peptide is non-phosphorylated, which reflects the *in vivo* situation within neurons. The pY-independence is readily explained, as the binding pocket is rather solvent exposed, and besides some van-der-Waals interactions of the benzene ring the tyrosine is not coordinated further. The binding mode is quite different in pY-dependent Shc or IRS1 peptide complexes, where the phosphate moiety is read out by a set of conserved arginine residues and the binding pocket is much more pronounced [36].

The NPTY sequence is followed by the [688]KFFEQMQN[695] sequence, which forms the C-terminus of the AICD (Figures 4A and 4E). The conformation of this region is slightly different and not always present in the structures, as the complexes have mostly been formed with truncated synthetic peptides. In the Fe65-PTB2 (which contains the entire C-terminus) and X11α complexes, the region is part of the C-terminal helix αC. The helix is fixed to the PTB domains by hydrophobic interactions of the two phenylalanines (Phe689 and Phe690) with the C-terminal helices of the respective PTB domains. These helices are three turns longer than those of Shc [79] and IRS1 [80] PTBs, and therefore the total interaction surfaces are significantly larger.

In most PTB domain complexes bound to an NPXY motif the described surfaces comprise the entire interaction, however, there is a single exception to the rule: the Fe65-PTB2/AICD complex, where the interface is about three times as large and includes an additional α helix (helix αN, [669]PEERHLSKMQQ[679]) N-terminal to the [681]GYENPTY sequence (Figure 4C) [30]. This helix is N-terminally capped by the [667]VTPEER motif comprising the phosphorylatable Thr668 as already described. Like helix αC, helix αN is of amphipathic character and binds on a hydrophobic patch on the Fe65-PTB2 surface located in between strand β5 and the N-terminus of the C-terminal helix, which is almost perpendicularly crossed by helix αN. Whereas Leu674 and Met677 cover the hydrophobic patch, Glu670, His673, and Gln678 are involved in polar interactions with the PTB domain. With the exception of Glu670, the [667]VTPEER capping box is not touching the PTB domain, which is somewhat astonishing, as it was afore known that phosphorylation of Thr668 is detrimental to complex formation [20]. As described for free AICD, the side chain of Thr668 is hydrogen-bonded to the main chain of Glu671, and Pro668 is *in trans* configuration. Furthermore, the side chain of Glu671 is tied back to the main chain nitrogen of Thr668, and thus completing the rigid helix cap.

The most important question arising from structural data is how phosphorylation is able to regulate Fe65-PTB2/AICD complex formation in a process that is critically involved in Aβ generation and AD pathogenesis? Phosphorylation induces a *cis* configuration of Pro669 [46], which is incompatible with the formation of helix αN. As found by mutational studies [30], the destruction of the helix cap increases the entropy of the system and reduces the binding affinity, and once the helix is dissolved, the remaining interfaces are not sufficient for maintaining the complex. This molecular switch model is only valid for the Fe65-PTB2/AICD interaction, as all other PTB domains do not contact Thr668 and phosphorylation does therefore not alter their binding affinity [20]. Intriguingly, the Fe65-PTB2/AICD interface spans almost the entire AICD-C31 fragment, which has been implicated in apoptotic events. This raises the next question: what determines stability, lifetime, and eventually toxicity of the AICD?

7. AICD turnover

The turnover of APP is very fast (with a half life of cell surface APP of about 30-40 minutes only [81] and only about 10% of APP are estimated to reach the cellular membrane, whereas the majority of APP locates to the Golgi apparatus and trans-Golgi network [10]. APP not shed at the surface is internalized within minutes [82], delivered to endosomes, and if not degraded in lysosomes recycled to the cell surface [83]. AICD is even more difficult to study, as due to its small size it is rapidly degraded once it is released from the membrane by the insulin degrading enzyme (IDE) [84], that also degrades the Aβ peptide, by the proteasome [85], or by the endosomal/lysosomal system [86]. However, AICD found in the nucleus appears to be more stable, suggesting that AICD involved in signal transduction escapes rapid degradation [87]. Nuclear AICD is stabilized via interaction with Fe65 [88, 89], which accordingly has a dominant function in AICD mediated physiological and pathophysiological processes.

From a structural viewpoint it is evident that the enlarged and unique protein-protein interface coupled with high affinity binding prevents the AICD from degradation. Interestingly, AICD-C31 (starting at Ala665), which is believed to induce apoptosis and is enriched in AD brains [34], fits exactly in length with the AICD part interacting with Fe65-PTB2. Hence, two scenarios comprising a modulating role for Fe65 in AICD-C31 mediated neurotoxicity might be envisaged: (i), under physiological conditions Fe65 protects the AICD from caspase cleavage occurring at Asp664 and might therefore inhibit apoptosis as shown previously [90] and (ii), increased levels of AICD-C31 compete with AICD binding as part of full-length APP and therefore interfere with physiological Fe65 functions including nuclear signaling and trafficking of APP. In any case, modifying the protein-interacting network around the AICD seems to be a valid target for decreasing neurotoxicity and the treatment of AD.

8. Conclusion

Despite enormous efforts to develop an efficient treatment for AD, only symptomatic treatments with modest impact on the progress of the disease are available [6]. Drugs currently approved for the treatment of AD are either acetylcholine esterase inhibitors to increase the level of the neurotransmitter, which is depleted in AD brains, or antagonize the NMDA receptor to prevent abnormal neuronal stimulation [91]. None of them directly targets the amyloid cascade and would thereby allow for a disease-modifying treatment. Many current therapeutic approaches for AD focus on the reduction of the Aβ load either by inhibiting the involved secretases BACE and γ-secretase, or by augmenting the elimination of amyloid peptides, e.g. by active or passive immunotherapy [6]. Finally, a smaller number of trials have targeted ApoE4 levels or either tau phosphorylation or tau aggregation. None of the approaches was successful so far, which means that either there were not enough clinical trials or the ideas were too simplistic to be potent for a complex disease. Like for other complex diseases (i.e. hypertension or AIDS), a combination of drugs that have different modes of action could be the key to success.

In this sense, the AICD might be re-evaluated as a potential drug target. In contrast to Aβ, the AICD is a physiological highly relevant protein domain modulating a diverse set of important APP functions including trafficking and signal transduction. As both processes are also directly affecting Aβ production, upstream targeting of AICD might be beneficial as the Aβ pathology is prevented *a priori*. Moreover, the pathophysiology of the AICD and its breakdown product AICD-C31 has come into the focus of AD research and would be tackled directly. As the AICD by its nature is created intracellular, efficient compounds need to be able to pass the plasma membrane and to accumulate within neurons, as is i.e. the case for the NMDA receptor antagonist memantine [92]. However, the AICD is intrinsically disordered, and therefore the protein interaction network around the AICD might be the crucial target rather than the AICD itself. Major binding partners are the PTB domains, with their known ability to modulate Aβ production (like Fe65, ShcA, and X11α) and to specifically recognize and fold the AICD. Although protein-protein interactions are notoriously difficult to be targeted, the urgent need for a disease-modifying and efficient treatment for this devastating disease seems worth the trial.

Acknowledgements

UM and KW are supported by the Research Unit FOR1332 from the Deutsche Forschungsgemeinschaft (DFG). UM was further supported by NGFNplus and KW by DFG grant KW2649/1-4.

Author details

Ulrike Müller[1] and Klemens Wild[2*]

*Address all correspondence to: klemens.wild@bzh.uni-heidelberg.de

1 Institut für Pharmazie und Molekulare Biotechnologie, Universität Heidelberg, Germany

2 Biochemiezentrum der Universität Heidelberg (BZH), Universität Heidelberg, Germany

References

[1] Ballard, C, et al. *Alzheimer's disease.* Lancet, (2011). , 1019-1031.

[2] Masters, C. L, & Selkoe, D. J. *Biochemistry of Amyloid beta-Protein and Amyloid Deposits in Alzheimer Disease.* Cold Spring Harb Perspect Med, (2012). , a006262.

[3] Lichtenthaler, S. F, Haass, C, & Steiner, H. *Regulated intramembrane proteolysis--lessons from amyloid precursor protein processing.* J Neurochem, (2011). , 779-796.

[4] Dislich, B, & Lichtenthaler, S. F. *The Membrane-Bound Aspartyl Protease BACE1: Molecular and Functional Properties in Alzheimer's Disease and Beyond.* Front Physiol, (2012). , 8.

[5]   Tam, J. H, & Pasternak, S. H. *Amyloid and Alzheimer's disease: inside and out.* Can J Neurol Sci, (2012). , 286-298.

[6]   Huang, Y, & Mucke, L. *Alzheimer mechanisms and therapeutic strategies.* Cell, (2012). , 1204-1222.

[7]   Muller, U. C, & Zheng, H. *Physiological Functions of APP Family Proteins.* Cold Spring Harb Perspect Med, (2012). , a006288.

[8]   Pardossi-piquard, R, & Checler, F. *The physiology of the beta-amyloid precursor protein intracellular domain AICD.* J Neurochem, (2012). Suppl 1: , 109-124.

[9]   Nikolaev, A, et al. *APP binds DR6 to trigger axon pruning and neuron death via distinct caspases.* Nature, (2009). , 981-989.

[10] Haass, C, et al. *Trafficking and Proteolytic Processing of APP.* Cold Spring Harb Perspect Med, (2012). , a006270.

[11] Dahms, S. O, et al. *Structure and biochemical analysis of the heparin-induced E1 dimer of the amyloid precursor protein.* Proc Natl Acad Sci U S A, (2010). , 5381-5386.

[12] Barnham, K. J, et al. *Structure of the Alzheimer's disease amyloid precursor protein copper binding domain. A regulator of neuronal copper homeostasis.* J Biol Chem, (2003). , 17401-17407.

[13] Rossjohn, J, et al. *Crystal structure of the N-terminal, growth factor-like domain of Alzheimer amyloid precursor protein.* Nat Struct Biol, (1999). , 327-331.

[14] Wang, Y, & Ha, Y. *The X-ray structure of an antiparallel dimer of the human amyloid precursor protein E2 domain.* Mol Cell, (2004). , 343-353.

[15] Soba, P, et al. *Homo- and heterodimerization of APP family members promotes intercellular adhesion.* EMBO J, (2005). , 3624-3634.

[16] Kaden, D, et al. *The amyloid precursor protein and its homologues: structural and functional aspects of native and pathogenic oligomerization.* Eur J Cell Biol, (2012). , 234-239.

[17] Gralle, M, et al. *Solution conformation and heparin-induced dimerization of the full-length extracellular domain of the human amyloid precursor protein.* J Mol Biol, (2006). , 493-508.

[18] Suzuki, T, & Nakaya, T. *Regulation of amyloid beta-protein precursor by phosphorylation and protein interactions.* J Biol Chem, (2008). , 29633-29637.

[19] Ramelot, T. A, Gentile, L. N, & Nicholson, L. K. *Transient structure of the amyloid precursor protein cytoplasmic tail indicates preordering of structure for binding to cytosolic factors.* Biochemistry, (2000). , 2714-2725.

[20] Ando, K, et al. *Phosphorylation-dependent regulation of the interaction of amyloid precursor protein with Fe65 affects the production of beta-amyloid.* J Biol Chem, (2001). , 40353-40361.

[21] Passer, B, et al. *Generation of an apoptotic intracellular peptide by gamma-secretase cleavage of Alzheimer's amyloid beta protein precursor.* J Alzheimers Dis, (2000). , 289-301.

[22] Lai, A, et al. *Signal-dependent trafficking of beta-amyloid precursor protein-transferrin receptor chimeras in madin-darby canine kidney cells.* J Biol Chem, (1998). , 3732-3739.

[23] Bonifacino, J. S, & Traub, L. M. *Signals for sorting of transmembrane proteins to endosomes and lysosomes.* Annu Rev Biochem, (2003). , 395-447.

[24] Haass, C, et al. *Polarized sorting of beta-amyloid precursor protein and its proteolytic products in MDCK cells is regulated by two independent signals.* J Cell Biol, (1995). , 537-547.

[25] Back, S, et al. *beta-amyloid precursor protein can be transported independent of any sorting signal to the axonal and dendritic compartment.* J Neurosci Res, (2007). , 2580-2590.

[26] Brunholz, S, et al. *Axonal transport of APP and the spatial regulation of APP cleavage and function in neuronal cells.* Exp Brain Res, (2012). , 353-364.

[27] Oishi, M, et al. *The cytoplasmic domain of Alzheimer's amyloid precursor protein is phosphorylated at Thr654, Ser655, and Thr668 in adult rat brain and cultured cells.* Mol Med, (1997). , 111-123.

[28] Standen, C. L, et al. *Phosphorylation of thr(668) in the cytoplasmic domain of the Alzheimer's disease amyloid precursor protein by stress-activated protein kinase 1b (Jun N-terminal kinase-3).* J Neurochem, (2001). , 316-320.

[29] Pastorino, L, et al. *The prolyl isomerase Pin1 regulates amyloid precursor protein processing and amyloid-beta production.* Nature, (2006). , 528-534.

[30] Radzimanowski, J, et al. *Structure of the intracellular domain of the amyloid precursor protein in complex with Fe65-PTB2.* EMBO Rep, (2008). , 1134-1140.

[31] Barbagallo, A. P, et al. *Tyr(682) in the intracellular domain of APP regulates amyloidogenic APP processing in vivo.* PLoS One, (2010). , e15503.

[32] Sano, Y, et al. *Physiological mouse brain Abeta levels are not related to the phosphorylation state of threonine-668 of Alzheimer's APP.* PLoS One, (2006). , e51.

[33] Lee, M. S, et al. *APP processing is regulated by cytoplasmic phosphorylation.* J Cell Biol, (2003). , 83-95.

[34] Lu, D. C, et al. *Caspase cleavage of the amyloid precursor protein modulates amyloid beta-protein toxicity.* J Neurochem, (2003). , 733-741.

[35] Chen, W. J, Goldstein, J. L, & Brown, M. S. *NPXY, a sequence often found in cytoplasmic tails, is required for coated pit-mediated internalization of the low density lipoprotein receptor.* J Biol Chem, (1990). , 3116-3123.

[36] Uhlik, M. T, et al. *Structural and evolutionary division of phosphotyrosine binding (PTB) domains.* J Mol Biol, (2005). , 1-20.

[37] Perez, R. G, et al. *Mutagenesis identifies new signals for beta-amyloid precursor protein endocytosis, turnover, and the generation of secreted fragments, including Abeta42.* J Biol Chem, (1999). , 18851-18856.

[38] Barbagallo, A. P, et al. *The intracellular threonine of amyloid precursor protein that is essential for docking of Pin1 is dispensable for developmental function.* PLoS One, (2011). , e18006.

[39] Kornfeld, S, & Mellman, I. *The biogenesis of lysosomes.* Annu Rev Cell Biol, (1989). , 483-525.

[40] Schettini, G, et al. *Phosphorylation of APP-CTF-AICD domains and interaction with adaptor proteins: signal transduction and/or transcriptional role--relevance for Alzheimer pathology.* J Neurochem, (2010). , 1299-1308.

[41] Russo, C, et al. *Signal transduction through tyrosine-phosphorylated C-terminal fragments of amyloid precursor protein via an enhanced interaction with Shc/Grb2 adaptor proteins in reactive astrocytes of Alzheimer's disease brain.* J Biol Chem, (2002). , 35282-35288.

[42] Cattaneo, E, & Pelicci, P. G. *Emerging roles for SH2/PTB-containing Shc adaptor proteins in the developing mammalian brain.* Trends Neurosci, (1998). , 476-481.

[43] Uversky, V. N, Oldfield, C. J, & Dunker, A. K. *Showing your ID: intrinsic disorder as an ID for recognition, regulation and cell signaling.* J Mol Recognit, (2005). , 343-384.

[44] Uversky, V. N. *A Protein-chameleon conformational plasticity of alpha-synuclein, a disordered protein involved in neurodegenerative disorders.* J Biomol Struct Dyn, (2003). , 211-234.

[45] Seale, J. W, Srinivasan, R, & Rose, G. D. *Sequence determinants of the capping box, a stabilizing motif at the N-termini of alpha-helices.* Protein Sci, (1994). , 1741-1745.

[46] Ramelot, T. A, & Nicholson, L. K. *Phosphorylation-induced structural changes in the amyloid precursor protein cytoplasmic tail detected by NMR.* J Mol Biol, (2001). , 871-884.

[47] Muller, T, et al. *The amyloid precursor protein intracellular domain (AICD) as modulator of gene expression, apoptosis, and cytoskeletal dynamics-relevance for Alzheimer's disease.* Prog Neurobiol, (2008). , 393-406.

[48] Kuan, Y. H, et al. *PAT1a modulates intracellular transport and processing of amyloid precursor protein (APP), APLP1, and APLP2.* J Biol Chem, (2006). , 40114-40123.

[49] Mcloughlin, D. M, & Miller, C. C. *The FE65 proteins and Alzheimer's disease.* J Neurosci Res, (2008). , 744-754.

[50] Sumioka, A, et al. *Role of 14-3-3gamma in FE65-dependent gene transactivation mediated by the amyloid beta-protein precursor cytoplasmic fragment.* J Biol Chem, (2005). , 42364-42374.

[51] Minopoli, G, et al. *The beta-amyloid precursor protein functions as a cytosolic anchoring site that prevents Fe65 nuclear translocation.* J Biol Chem, (2001). , 6545-6550.

[52] Cao, X, & Sudhof, T. C. *A Transcriptionally correction of transcriptively] active complex of APP with Fe65 and histone acetyltransferase Tip60.* Science, (2001). , 115-120.

[53] Telese, F, et al. *Transcription regulation by the adaptor protein Fe65 and the nucleosome assembly factor SET.* EMBO Rep, (2005). , 77-82.

[54] Konietzko, U. *AICD nuclear signaling and its possible contribution to Alzheimer's disease.* Curr Alzheimer Res, (2012). , 200-216.

[55] Wagner, T, & Pietrzik, C. U. *The role of lipoprotein receptors on the physiological function of APP.* Exp Brain Res, (2012). , 377-387.

[56] Bu, G. *Apolipoprotein Ea nd its receptors in Alzheimer's disease: pathways, pathogenesis and therapy.* Nat Rev Neurosci, (2009). , 333-344.

[57] Sabo, S. L, et al. *The Alzheimer amyloid precursor protein (APP) and FE65, an APP-binding protein, regulate cell movement.* J Cell Biol, (2001). , 1403-1414.

[58] Ma, H, et al. *Involvement of beta-site APP cleaving enzyme 1 (BACE1) in amyloid precursor protein-mediated enhancement of memory and activity-dependent synaptic plasticity.* Proc Natl Acad Sci U S A, (2007). , 8167-8172.

[59] Guenette, S, et al. *Essential roles for the FE65 amyloid precursor protein-interacting proteins in brain development.* EMBO J, (2006). , 420-431.

[60] Herms, J, et al. *Cortical dysplasia resembling human type 2 lissencephaly in mice lacking all three APP family members.* EMBO J, (2004). , 4106-4115.

[61] Mueller, H. T, et al. *Modulation of amyloid precursor protein metabolism by X11alpha / Mint-1. A deletion analysis of protein-protein interaction domains.* J Biol Chem, (2000). , 39302-39306.

[62] Wang, Z, et al. *Presynaptic and postsynaptic interaction of the amyloid precursor protein promotes peripheral and central synaptogenesis.* J Neurosci, (2009). , 10788-10801.

[63] Szodorai, A, et al. *APP anterograde transport requires Rab3A GTPase activity for assembly of the transport vesicle.* J Neurosci, (2009). , 14534-14544.

[64] Howell, B. W, et al. *The disabled 1 phosphotyrosine-binding domain binds to the internalization signals of transmembrane glycoproteins and to phospholipids.* Mol Cell Biol, (1999). , 5179-5188.

[65] Roncarati, R, et al. *The gamma-secretase-generated intracellular domain of beta-amyloid precursor protein binds Numb and inhibits Notch signaling.* Proc Natl Acad Sci U S A, (2002). , 7102-7107.

[66] Saito, Y, et al. *X11 proteins regulate the translocation of amyloid beta-protein precursor (APP) into detergent-resistant membrane and suppress the amyloidogenic cleavage of APP by beta-site-cleaving enzyme in brain.* J Biol Chem, (2008). , 35763-35771.

[67] Ashley, J, et al. *Fasciclin II signals new synapse formation through amyloid precursor protein and the scaffolding protein dX11/Mint.* J Neurosci, (2005). , 5943-5955.

[68] Weyer, S. W, et al. *APP and APLP2 are essential at PNS and CNS synapses for transmission, spatial learning and LTP.* EMBO J, (2011). , 2266-2280.

[69] Hoe, H. S, & Rebeck, G. W. *Functional interactions of APP with the apoE receptor family.* J Neurochem, (2008). , 2263-2271.

[70] Mclaughlin, S, et al. *PIP(2) and proteins: interactions, organization, and information flow.* Annu Rev Biophys Biomol Struct, (2002). , 151-175.

[71] Stolt, P. C, et al. *Origins of peptide selectivity and phosphoinositide binding revealed by structures of disabled-1 PTB domain complexes.* Structure, (2003). , 569-579.

[72] Yun, M, et al. *Crystal structures of the Dab homology domains of mouse disabled 1 and 2.* J Biol Chem, (2003). , 36572-36581.

[73] Merdes, G, et al. *Interference of human and Drosophila APP and APP-like proteins with PNS development in Drosophila.* EMBO J, (2004). , 4082-4095.

[74] Artavanis-tsakonas, S, Rand, M. D, & Lake, R. J. *Notch signaling: cell fate control and signal integration in development.* Science, (1999). , 770-776.

[75] Hamid, R, et al. *Amyloid precursor protein intracellular domain modulates cellular calcium homeostasis and ATP content.* J Neurochem, (2007). , 1264-1275.

[76] Leissring, M. A, et al. *A physiologic signaling role for the gamma-secretase-derived intracellular fragment of APP.* Proc Natl Acad Sci U S A, (2002). , 4697-4702.

[77] Zhang, Z, et al. *Sequence-specific recognition of the internalization motif of the Alzheimer's amyloid precursor protein by the X11 PTB domain.* EMBO J, (1997). , 6141-6150.

[78] Cao, X, & Sudhof, T. C. *Dissection of amyloid-beta precursor protein-dependent transcriptional transactivation.* J Biol Chem, (2004). , 24601-24611.

[79] Zhou, M. M, et al. *Structure and ligand recognition of the phosphotyrosine binding domain of Shc.* Nature, (1995). , 584-592.

[80] Zhou, M. M, et al. *Structural basis for IL-4 receptor phosphopeptide recognition by the IRS-1 PTB domain.* Nat Struct Biol, (1996). , 388-393.

[81] Ring, S, et al. *The secreted beta-amyloid precursor protein ectodomain APPs alpha is sufficient to rescue the anatomical, behavioral, and electrophysiological abnormalities of APP-deficient mice.* J Neurosci, (2007). , 7817-7826.

[82] Lai, A, Sisodia, S. S, & Trowbridge, I. S. *Characterization of sorting signals in the beta-amyloid precursor protein cytoplasmic domain.* J Biol Chem, (1995). , 3565-3573.

[83] Haass, C, et al. *Targeting of cell-surface beta-amyloid precursor protein to lysosomes: alternative processing into amyloid-bearing fragments.* Nature, (1992). , 500-503.

[84] Edbauer, D, et al. *Insulin-degrading enzyme rapidly removes the beta-amyloid precursor protein intracellular domain (AICD).* J Biol Chem, (2002). , 13389-13393.

[85] Nunan, J, et al. *Proteasome-mediated degradation of the C-terminus of the Alzheimer's disease beta-amyloid protein precursor: effect of C-terminal truncation on production of beta-amyloid protein.* J Neurosci Res, (2003). , 378-385.

[86] Vingtdeux, V, et al. *Intracellular pH regulates amyloid precursor protein intracellular domain accumulation.* Neurobiol Dis, (2007). , 686-696.

[87] Cupers, P, et al. *The amyloid precursor protein (APP)-cytoplasmic fragment generated by gamma-secretase is rapidly degraded but distributes partially in a nuclear fraction of neurones in culture.* J Neurochem, (2001). , 1168-1178.

[88] Kimberly, W. T, et al. *The intracellular domain of the beta-amyloid precursor protein is stabilized by Fe65 and translocates to the nucleus in a notch-like manner.* J Biol Chem, (2001). , 40288-40292.

[89] Kinoshita, A, et al. *Direct visualization of the gamma secretase-generated carboxyl-terminal domain of the amyloid precursor protein: association with Fe65 and translocation to the nucleus.* J Neurochem, (2002). , 839-847.

[90] Cao, H, et al. *Characterization of an apoptosis inhibitory domain at the C-termini of FE65-like protein.* Biochem Biophys Res Commun, (2000). , 843-850.

[91] Cummings, J. L. *Alzheimer's disease.* N Engl J Med, (2004). , 56-67.

[92] Robinson, D. M, & Keating, G. M. *Memantine: a review of its use in Alzheimer's disease.* Drugs, (2006). , 1515-1534.

Chapter 2

The Amyloidogenic Pathway Meets the Reelin Signaling Cascade: A Cytoskeleton Bridge Between Neurodevelopment and Neurodegeneration

Daniel A. Bórquez, Ismael Palacios and
Christian González-Billault

Additional information is available at the end of the chapter

1. Introduction

Reelin is an extracellular matrix glycoprotein of ~400 kD, expressed in mammals during neurodevelopment by the Cajal-Retzius (CR) neurons, which are located in the marginal zone of the cortex and hippocampus [1], and by the cerebellar granule cells [2]. In adult stages, CR neurons degenerate in both structures [3], limiting Reelin production and secretion to GABAergic interneurons [4]. Meanwhile, the expression in the cerebellum remains being exclusive of granule cells [5]. During development, Reelin synthesis also occurs in structures like the hypothalamus, the olfactory bulb, the basal ganglia and the amygdale. In these last two brain regions, Reelin expression continues into adulthood but at low concentrations [1].

Reelin gene encompasses 450 kb of genomic DNA located on human chromosome 7q22 and in murine chromosome 5. Both genes contain 65 exons that encode a protein sharing a 94,2 (%) of identity [6-7]. The transcription initiation region and the exon 1 of the reelin gene is enriched in CG nucleotides, forming a large CpG island [8], which is associated with a methylation-dependent negative regulation of reelin transcription [9]. In fact, DNA methyltransferases and histone deacetylases inhibitors increase Reelin protein expression, most likely due to decreased reelin promoter methylation [10-11].

In addition to the epigenetic regulation, reelin gene show multiple *cis* elements, which contain binding sites for transcription factors involved in neurodevelopment such as Sp1, Tbr-1 and Pax6, and elements involved in cytoplasm-to-nucleus signal transduction as CREB and NF-κB [7,12]. Tbr-1 deficient mice show a clear disruption of cortical organization, accompanied by decreased Reelin levels [13]. On the other hand, retinoic acid, a known inducer of neuronal growth and differentiation, increase Pax6 and Sp1 levels leading to the activation of the reelin promoter and a subsequent increased Reelin protein synthesis [14].

The full length Reelin protein contains 3461 amino acids, organized from N- to C-terminal by the following domains and motifs: 1.- A signal peptide, 2.- F-spondin-like motif, 3.- 8 repeat domains, composed of a region A and region B spaced by EGF motif, and 4.- A region enriched in basic amino acids [2].

Reelin may undergo proteolytic cleavage at the beginning of the 3rd and 7th A-EGF-B repeat generating many fragments including the N-terminal, the intermediate segment and the C-terminal fragment. Cleavage may be precluded by zinc chelators, known inhibitors of metalloproteinases [15]. Recently a putative protease had been identified as p50 and p70 isoforms of a disintegrin and metalloproteinase with thrombospodin motif 4 (ADAMTS-4). The p50 isoform cleaves at N-terminal only, and p70 cleaves the N- and C-terminal sites [16]. The importance of the proteolytic processing remains unclear, however; several reports showed that the internalization of Reelin at target cells is independent of its cleavage. In turn, only the central region seems to be sufficient for Reelin functions. Reelin cleavage would be required to enable Reelin secretion, allowing the release of a central, active fragment from the extracellular matrix-attached full length protein [17-18]. In contrast to this notion, there are many studies showing that the N-terminal region is important for Reelin secretion (due to the presence of a signal peptide on this region) [19], and to promote the formation of homopolymers, which are essential for proper signal transduction [20]. There is still little evidence about the function of the C-terminal region. The *reeler* Orleans mutation characterized by a deletion of 220 nucleotides at the C-terminal, prevents the secretion of Reelin, suggesting a possible role for this region in normal Reelin functions [21].

2. Reelin in neurodevelopment

As outlined in the previous section, Reelin is a glycoprotein, which is expressed in CR neurons starting at embryonic day 11 (E11), mainly in the cortex, hippocampus and cerebellum. It expression remains high until day E18, when CR neurons begin to degenerate [1,3]. The importance of Reelin to neurodevelopment had been elucidated through numerous studies using a mice model exhibiting a spontaneous mutation (partial deletion) in the reelin gene, called the *reeler* mice [22]. These mice had pronounced defects in the correct neuronal positioning in the laminar structures of the brain. At day E11, postmitotic neurons located in the ventricular zone, migrate toward the pial surface to form the preplate. On E13, a new cohort of migrating neurons originated at the proliferative region separate the pre-plate. Pre-plate splitting originates two regions, the marginal zone and the sub-plate, which are positioned adjacent to the pial surface and near the ventricular zone, respectively. The marginal zone is rich in CR neurons, which are the primary source of Reelin during neurodevelopment. Several waves of postmitotic migrating neurons are positioned between the marginal zone and the sub plate, leading to the formation of the cortical plate. During the E14-E18 time lapse, four successive waves of postmitotic neurons migrate from the ventricular zone, through the sub-plate and neurons already positioned, to reach the marginal zone where the Reelin secreted by the CR neurons acts as a "stop signal" inducing the termination of the neuronal migration. This process is termed as "radial migration", and occurs through an inside-out mechanism, where early migrating neurons are placed at the inner aspects of the cortex [23]. Mechanistically, cortical neurons migrate using two different mechanisms, a glial-dependent process termed locomotion; and a glial-independent one termed nuclear translocation. During migration across the cortical plate, the neurons adopt morphology characterized by the presence of a cytoplasmic extension oriented toward the most outer aspect of the cortex, the leading process. A secondary cytoplasmic extension emerge orthogonally from the leading process and is termed the trailing process. While the leading process will be further developed as the dendritic arbor, the trailing process will become the axon [24].

The *reeler* mutant shows a clear disruption of the cortical layers, characterized by the absence of pre-plate splitting, generating a structure called the superplate [25]. Additionally, migrating neurons fail to establish an inside-out pattern of cortical layers [26]. Thus, in the *reeler* mutant, neurons that migrate earlier during development are placed in the outer aspect of the cortex, leading to an outside-in pattern of cortical layers [23,27-29].

Abnormal neuronal migration is not exclusively for the *reeler* mice cortex. Purkinje neurons in the cerebellum are also aberrantly organized. After birth, the Purkinje cell layer is absent, and a reduction of granule cells number is appreciated, these alterations result in a dramatic reduction of foliation pattern and diminished cerebellar size [30]. At the hippocampal region, the *reeler* mutant is characterized by the presence of non-compacted dentate gyrus and disorganized pyramidal layer [31].

Summarizing, Reeler brain shows smaller size and larger ventricles, the distribution of the dorsal, medial and ventral hippocampus is altered, the cortex display an inverted array of neurons in their layers and the cerebellum shows no foliation and alterations in the organization of its layers [32].

At the molecular level, the Reelin signaling pathway control several processes required for proper neuronal migration. For example, Reelin stabilize the leading process by inducing cofilin phosphorylation at Ser3, which regulates actin dynamics [33]. Furthermore, Reelin can also induce MAP1B phosphorylation through GSK-3β activation. MAP1B function is involved in formation of brain laminated areas, therefore, Reelin can modulate neuronal guidance through post-translational modifications of MAP1B [34]. These two examples show how Reelin can act coordinately to locally regulate the assembly of actin microfilaments and microtubules (Figure 1A).

In addition to its role in neurodevelopment, Reelin controls the formation of neural circuits, promoting the growth and branching of dendrites in hippocampal neurons [35]. Moreover, Reelin can enhance the formation of dendritic spines, supporting a role at the post-synaptic compartment [36].

Most of these cellular functions are dependent on a signaling pathway, triggered by the binding of Reelin to its two main receptors, the very-low density lipoprotein receptor

(VLDLR) and the ApolipoproteinE receptor 2 (ApoER2) [37]. The binding of Reelin to its receptor induce the phosphorylation of the adapter protein mDab1 on tyrosine residues [38].
mDab1 phosphorylation lead eventually to the modulation of cytoskeleton effectors molecules such as MAP1B and cofilin [23].

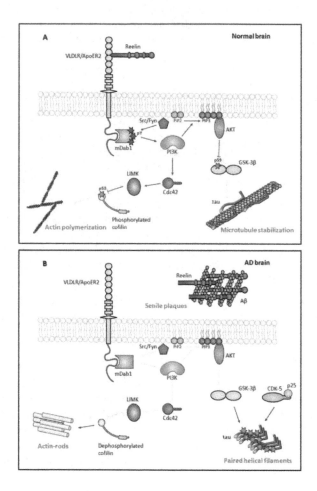

Figure 1. Reelin signaling pathway in normal brain and its impairment in AD brains. The panel A show the intracellular
events triggered by the binding of Reelin to its canonical membrane receptors, ApoER2 and VLDLR. mDab1 protein is specifically phosphorylated at tyrosine residues, which concomitantly with the activation of PI3K, regulate actin and microtubule dynamic behavior. LIMK-mediated phosphorylation of cofilin and the Akt inhibitory phosphorylation of GSK-3β are
essential to this regulation. On the other hand, in AD brains, diminished Reelin expression and its aggregation in amyloid-
like deposits, induce impairment in its signaling pathway (represented by gray lines). Decreased Reelin signaling triggers
the dephosphorylation of cofilin, promoting the formation of actin-rods. On the other hand, the activation of GSK-3β and
CDK-5, lead to hyperphosphorylation of tau protein inducing its aggregation into PHFs (panel B).

3. Reelin in the adult brain

Although Reelin function is mainly related to neurodevelopment, several recently studies assign roles in the adult brain, such as the development of dendrites and dendritic spines [36], modulation of synaptogenesis [39], modulation of synaptic plasticity [40-43] and neurotransmitter release [44]. The mechanism by which Reelin can modulate the synaptic transmission is not fully elucidated. Currently it is strongly suggested that Reelin acting through its canonical signaling pathway facilitates the phosphorylation of NR2A and NR2B subunits of the NMDA receptor, favoring the calcium influx into the postsynaptic neuron.

This intracellular calcium increase causes the insertion of the GluR1 subunit of AMPA receptors, allowing the phosphorylation and nuclear translocation of CREB [45]. CREB phosphorylation is required to elicit the formation of dendritic spines. In addition, Reelin reduces the number of silent synapses, facilitating the exchange of subunit NR2B by NR2A of NMDA receptor [46]. Therefore, Reelin modulates synaptic plasticity events involved in learning and memory processes in adults. Consistently with a role for Reelin in the control of neurotransmission, *reeler* mice show diminished expression of presynaptic (SNARE, SNAP-25) [44] and postsynaptic (PSD-95, PTEN) markers [43]. These defects cause failures in the release of neurotransmitters, impairing synaptic transmission.

4. Animals models for neuropsychiatric diseases

Owing to the importance that Reelin have in the correct structuration and lamination of the brain during development and in neuronal connectivity and synaptogenesis in the adult brain, its dysfunction has been directly related to the generation or susceptibility to acquire neuropsychiatric conditions such as depression and schizophrenia, or neurodegenerative diseases such as Alzheimer's disease (AD) [45].

The most tangible evidence supporting these putative relationships was obtained through studies of human brains derived from neuropsychiatric and neurodegenerative conditions. Decreased levels of Reelin are shown in postmortem samples from prefrontal cortex of patients with schizophrenia and bipolar disorders [47]. This decrease may be explained in schizophrenic patients by an abnormal hypermethylation of the *reelin* promoter, an epigenetic modification involved in gene silencing [48]. Furthermore, immunohistochemistry experiments in depressive and schizophrenic patients show decreased Reelin expression at the hippocampus [49]. On the other hand, diminished Reelin levels in the hippocampus of patients with AD had been reported, suggesting a direct correlation between the severity of the disease and the extent of decreased Reelin expression [50]. All of these antecedents provide evidence enough to feature a molecular link between decreased Reelin levels and neurodegenerative/psychiatric diseases.

In order to understand the etiology of neurodegenerative/psychiatric diseases, different animal models had been developed. A widely paradigm is the "two hit" model, which suggests that genetic and environmental factors may affect the development of central nervous system, acting as "the first hit". These early disorders are linked to long-term vulnerability, which after a "second hit" could cause the symptoms for a disease [51-52]. For diseases such as depression, autism and schizophrenia, the heterozygous *reeler* mice had been used as the genetic "first hit", while stress events after the birth or in adulthood are used as the environmental "second hit". The results indicate that heterozygous *reeler* mice, after a stressful event, such as maternal deprivation or corticosterone injection, exhibit significantly increased depressive or schizophrenic behaviors as compared with wild type littermates [53-54]. Indeed, *reeler* heterozygous animals in the absence of a stressful event, display a phenotype indistinguishable from control animals [55].

The "two hit" model has also been used to study the molecular mechanisms leading to the AD [56]. It is proposed that both oxidative stress and failures in mitotic signaling can independently triggers the onset of the disease; however both are necessary for their progression [57]. In addition, a correspondence had been established between the Reelin expression in the entorhinal cortex of aged rats with their cognitive abilities. A study revealed that aged "cognitively disabled" rats show a significant decreased of Reelin in neurons on layer II of the entorhinal cortex. Such a reduction in Reelin expression was not observed in juvenile or elderly "cognitively able" rats [58].

Since Reelin is expressed from development to adult stages, is conceivable that alterations in Reelin expression, induced by genetic or environmental factors generate a vulnerable stage, and a secondary factor, present in normal aging, may trigger the onset and progression of a pathological condition.

The Reelin-activated signaling pathways, which may be involved in the generation and development of AD are still unclear and will be discussed in next sections. In the last part of this section, we present some of the evidences that correlate altered levels of Reelin and AD. Pyramidal neurons placed in layer II of the entorhinal cortex and the hippocampus derived from AD patients brains exhibit decreased Reelin expression [50]. On the other hand, an increase in the full length and 180 kD proteolytic fragment of Reelin had been observed in the frontal cortex of AD derived samples [59]. The increase of this proteolytic fragment is attributed to problems with the proteolysis of Reelin, associated with decreased Rab11-endocytosis of full length Reelin [60]. In the other hand, an increase of Reelin is also observed in the frontal cortex of AD patients, which may involve a compensatory mechanism in response to the lower expression in disease-related most vulnerable areas like the entorhinal cortex and hippocampus [50].

The CR neurons participation in AD is a controversial issue. While electronic microscopy analysis suggested that CR neurons of the temporal cortex were dramatically reduced in AD patients [61], another study showed no difference between AD patients and normal, healthy subjects [62]. On the other hand, there are some polymorphisms in the Reelin gene which had been associated with AD. Seripa and colleagues reported significant differences in two analyzed polymorphisms in the Reelin gene, in a group of 223 Caucasians AD patients. These differences were exacerbated in female patients [63].

Finally, Reelin had been associated with the pathological hallmarks for AD, the senile plaques and the neurofibrillary tangles (NFT). Reelin can modulate tau phosphorylation, the
core protein of NFT [38]. It is also associated with senile plaques, large extracellular aggregates mainly formed for β-amyloid peptide (Aβ). Immunohistochemical studies revealed
that Reelin colocalizes with the amyloid precursor protein (APP) in the neuritic component
of typical AD plaques, at the hippocampus and cortex of mice expressing a mutant version
of APP [64]. Additionally, a reduction of Reelin-producing cells had been observed in older
mice and primates. This reduction is accompanied by the presence of Reelin aggregates and
memory deficits. Mice harboring APP with AD-associated mutations also showed Reelin aggregates, which co-localized with non-fibrillar amyloid plaques [65]. In addition, Reelin
forms oligomeric or protofibrillary deposits during aging, potentially creating a precursor
condition for Aβ plaque formation [66].

A direct relationship between decreased Reelin expression and increased levels of Aβ
peptide and plaque accumulation was provided by studies using transgenic mice carrying the APP Swedish and *reeler* mutation. The absence of Reelin expression resulted in an
age-dependent exacerbation of plaque pathology and increased NFTs in double mutants
as compared with the single APPsw mutant [67]. Finally, recent studies demonstrated a
feedforward mechanism by which Reelin would favor the formation of senile plaques;
and the subsequent Aβ peptide production would increase the Reelin levels by altering its
proteolytic processing in the cortex of mice and humans with AD [68].

5. Cytoskeletal abnormalities in Alzheimer´s disease

5.1. Tau protein and neurofibrillary tangles

Neurofibrillary tangles are amongst the standard characteristics of AD brains. These structures were firstly described by Alois Alzheimer more than a century ago and are composed of a densely packed array of fibers of 20 nm in diameter, called paired helical
filaments (PHF), which at the core are mainly composed by the microtubule-associated
protein, tau [69-70]. Tau protein stabilizes and enhances microtubule polymerization. It is
a heterogeneous protein giving rise to 6 isoforms derived from alternative splicing [71]. It
contains 3 or 4 imperfect repeats of 31 or 32 amino acids each in tandem which confers
the microtubule-binding properties of the protein. These repeats are enriched in basic
aminoacids that interact electrostatically with the mostly acidic C-terminal of β-tubulin
subunit [72]. Tau protein is highly phosphorylated in fetal brain [73], but minimally phosphorylated in normal adult brain [74]. The abnormal phosphorylation state of several residues in tau protein plays an important role modulating the affinity to microtubules and
promoting its aggregation [75] forming the core of PHFs [69,76-77]. Tau protein can be
phosphorylated by many protein kinases such as calcium-calmodulin dependent kinase
[78]; PKA [79-81] and PKC [82-83]. Interestingly, many of these residues are hyperphosphorylated in AD brains mainly due to an imbalance in the activity of kinases belongs to
the family of proline-directed Ser/Thr protein kinases (PDPKs), such as mitogen-activated

protein kinases (MAPK) [84], the glycogen synthase kinase (GSK)-3β [85], JNK [84], p38 [86] and Cyclin-dependent kinase (Cdk)-5 [87]. The abnormal phosphorylation state of tau protein is not only contributed by protein kinases, but also by deregulated protein phosphatases functions [88]. (Figure 1B)

5.2. Cofilin and actin-rods

NFTs are not the only intraneuronal cytoskeletal protein aggregates found in the brains of patients affected by AD. Hirano's bodies and actin-rods are two closely related aggregates primarily composed of actin and the actin binding protein, cofilin. Cofilin concertedly with the actin depolymerizing factor (ADF) constitutes the major modulators of actin dynamic assembly.

Hirano's bodies were originally described in 1965 and are defined as paracrystalline structures, eosinophilic intracellular arrangements resembling rod-shaped filaments of 7 nm. The actin-rods differ from Hirano's bodies by it smaller size, so it is hypothesized that these structures could be precursors of Hirano's bodies.

The formation of actin-rods in neurons seems to be the result of several neurodegenerative insults, such as ATP depletion, excitotoxic levels of glutamate, oxidative stress [89], and $A\beta_{1-42}$ oligomers [90]. A common event to all these stimuli triggers the formation of rods is the dephosphorylation (activation) of cofilin [89]. Cofilin/ADF is inactivated by phosphorylation of a highly conserved serine (Ser3), which precludes its binding to actin filaments and, therefore, its role as promoters of filament severing and actin subunits turnover at the minus end of filaments.

The Ser3 of ADF/cofilin is the only known substrate for the two isoforms of LIM domain kinases (LIM, an acronym for three *Caenorhabditis elegans* genes, *lin-11*, *isl-1* and *mec-3*). LIMKs is activated by phosphorylation at the Thr508, mediated by PAK or ROCK, two kinases that act as effectors for small GTPases Rac1 and RhoA respectively [91]. The regulation of signaling cascades, which target the functions of small GTPases, connect the dynamic control of the actin cytoskeleton with extracellular signals. In AD, different components of the signaling cascade involved in cofilin phosphorylation are altered, including decreased phosphorylation of PAK at Ser141, which is necessary for activation. Although a decrease in phosphorylation and activity of PAK is observed in large areas of cortex and hippocampus of AD brains, neurons located near to amyloid plaques exhibit strong staining for pSer141 PAK, suggesting that while the dephosphorylation is predominant in the brain of patients with AD, the amyloid fibrils present in amyloid plaques increases the activity of PAK [92].

Consistently, hippocampal neurons treated with fibrillar $A\beta_{1-42}$ show increased activity of PAK and its downstream substrate LIMK1 [93-94], most likely through a Rac1 and Cdc42 dependent mechanism [95]. Moreover, the treatment with oligomers of $A\beta_{1-40}$ has the opposite effect, decreasing the phosphorylation of PAK, indicating that oligomeric forms may be responsible for the overall reduction in PAK phosphorylation [92].

Similarly, cofilin dephosphorylation and the subsequent formation of actin-rods seem to be also a spatial-restricted phenomenon. In example, actin-rods occur in a subpopulation of neurons in organotypic slices treated with Aβ [96]. (Figure 1B)

The mechanisms involved in the Aβ-mediated cofilin dephosphorylation are dependent on changes in the activity of its upstream kinase, LIMK [90], and the activity of two known cofilin phosphatases, chronophin [97] and slingshot [94].

Interestingly, ATP depletion induces chronophin activation in a mechanism involving the dissociation of chronophin-HSP90 complex. This mechanism would be responsible for the formation of actin-rods under energy deprivation conditions [97].

6. Is the AD-associated Reelin reduction a major factor involved in the neuronal cytoskeleton pathology?

6.1. Reelin reduction in AD brains

There is an increasing body of evidence indicating that a deficiency in Reelin signaling may play a major role in the progression of AD. First, decreased Reelin expression is early observed in brains of AD transgenic mice model, even before Aβ deposition. Accordingly, Reelin expression is also decreased in brains of patients at the presymptomatic stages of AD. The progression of the disease causes in both cases, potentiate the Reelin deficiency from the hippocampus to the entorhinal cortex in mice and from the frontal cortex to the hippocampus and entorhinal cortex in humans [50,98]. The decrease in Reelin expression is linked to a reduction in CR cells at the cortical layer I in AD brains [61].

Reelin itself can form amyloid deposits in advanced stages of AD, which can or cannot be associated with Aβ senile plaques [64-66]. However, Aβ pathology seems to be a prerequisite for the formation of Reelin aggregates, as these only occur after formation of senile plaques [98].

On the other hand, the proteolytic fragments of Reelin showing aberrant glycosylation pattern are increased in the cerebrospinal fluid of patients with AD [59,99]. Altogether these antecedents support the hypothesis that the Reelin intracellular signaling is impaired at early stages of AD.

6.2. Cytoskeletal pathologies and Reelin signaling

Reelin signaling is triggered by the binding of Reelin to two members of the lipoprotein receptor family, the very low density lipoprotein receptor (VLDLR) and the ApoE receptor 2 (ApoER2)[100]. The signal is then transduced by a cytoplasmic adapter protein, the mammalian homologue for the *Drosophila* protein *disabled* (mDab)-1, which interacts with the NPXY motifs of the intracellular domain of several members of the LDL receptor family, including VLDLR and ApoER2.

As VLDLR/ApoER2 or mDab1 deficient mice exhibit a phenotype indistinguishable from *reeler* mice, it is suggested that both receptors and the adapter protein can be linearly placed on the same signal transduction pathway [37,101].

The binding of Reelin to its receptors induces mDab1 tyrosine phosphorylation, mediated by non-receptor tyrosine kinases from the Src family [102]. The mutation of these tyrosines residues by phenylalanines in a *knockin* mouse recapitulates several features of the *reeler* mouse, supporting that these phosphorylation events are required for proper Reelin signaling [103].

Several genetic models suggest that canonical Reelin signaling plays an essential role in controlling the phosphorylation state of tau and, therefore, modulating a critical event in the progression of AD (Table 1).

Mice deficient in various components of the Reelin signaling pathway, including Reelin itself, VLDLR, ApoER2 and Dab1 show increased tau phosphorylation in several AD-associated epitopes, such as those recognized by the antibodies AT8 (pSer202/205) and PHF1 (pSer396/404) [38,104-106].

The increase in tau phosphorylation is caused by increased activity of two main kinases, Cdk5 and GSK-3β [105], suggesting that Reelin is playing a negative control over the activities of these kinases.

GSK-3β is normally inhibited by phosphorylation at its N-terminal region by the protein kinase Akt, mainly at the Ser9. Reelin signaling in turn, activates Akt through its recruitment to membrane domains rich in phosphatidylinositol 3-phosphate (PIP3), whose formation is involved the activity of the phosphatidilinositol 3-kinase (PI3K). Reelin activates PI3K by potentiating the interaction between tyrosine phosphorylated-mDab1 and the p85α subunit of PI3K [107-108].

Moreover, it has been proposed that the increased activity of Cdk5 in Dab1 or Reelin deficient mice may be due to a remarkable increase of the proteolyzed form of a Cdk5 activator, called p25 [105]. This fragment induces a non-physiological activation of Cdk5, which is present mainly in pathological conditions, including brains of patients with AD [109]. Since the proteolysis of the Cdk5 activator is due to the activity of calpain, it may be hypothesized that the Reelin signaling pathway could regulate calpain-dependent proteolysis of p35.

It has been proposed that Cdk5 could not be directly regulated by the Reelin signaling cascade, because cortical neurons treated with Reelin do not exhibit any significant change in the Cdk5 activity [107] or a diminished phosphorylation state of Cdk5-dependent substrates [110]. However, it may not be ruled out that a subset of substrates still not analyzed can be phosphorylated by Cdk5 due to impairment in Reelin signaling.

Protein	Functions in Reelin signaling	Association with Alzheimer´s disease	References
Reelin	Extracellular matrix glycoprotein	Diminished levels in restricted areas of AD brain. Reelin-deficient mice show increased tau phosphorylation	[50, 98]
ApoER2	Reelin receptor	VLDLR and ApoER2 dKO mice present elevated levels of phosphorylated tau	[38]
VLDLR	Reelin receptor	VLDLR and ApoER2 dKO mice present elevated levels of phosphorylated tau	[38]
mDab1	Intracellular adapter for Reelin receptors	mDab1-deficient mice show increased tau phosphorylation and early death.	[106]
PI3K	Lipid kinase essential for membrane recruiting of Akt	Impairment in PI3K-Akt pathway was observed in aged APP-PS1 transgenic mice.	[112]
Akt	Phosphorylates and inhibits GSK-3β	Impairment in PI3K-Akt pathway was observed in aged APP-PS1 transgenic mice.	[112]
GSK-3β	Major tau kinase	Phosphorylates tau at AD-associated epitopes	[85]
tau	Microtubule-associated protein. Promotes microtubule assembly and stabilization	Hyperphosphorylated tau constitutes the core of NFTs	[77]
Cdc42	Small GTPase associated with actin dynamics	A lesser Aβ-induced actin-rod formation is observed in cdc42 null neurons	[96]
LIMK1	Major effector of Rho-family GTPases. Phosphorylates and inactivates cofilin	The expression of constitutively active LIMK1 reduces Aβ-induced actin-rods in hippocampal slices	[90]
Cofilin	Actin binding protein with F-actin depolymerizing activity	Ser3 dephosphorylation triggers its aggregation into actin-rods	[89]

Table 1. Association of Reelin signaling pathway with Alzheimer´s disease

The Reelin signaling pathway can target not only microtubule cytoskeleton, but also the actin microfilament formation. Acting through its canonical signaling pathway that involve receptors VLDLR and ApoER2, the adapter protein Dab1 and activation of PI3K, Reelin is able to activate the small GTPases Rac1 and Cdc42, increasing actin polymerization. These changes in small Rho GTPases are responsible of increased mobility of growth cones and promote the appearance of filopodia in the axon of cortical neurons in culture [111]. The stabilization of actin filaments is mediated directly by an increase in activation of LIMK and phosphorylation of cofilin Ser3 [33]. LIMK and cofilin phosphorylation are two key events that regulate actin microfilament turnover in a Rac-dependent manner. Currently, there are no studies showing a causal relationship between impaired Reelin signaling and molecular changes affecting cofilin phosphorylation that could regulate the formation of actin-rods. However, it is tempting to speculate that further studies may solve a linkage between the decreased Reelin signaling observed in AD brains and abnormal actin dynamics.

Acknowledgements

Supported by Fondecyt 1095089 to CG-B.

Author details

Daniel A. Bórquez, Ismael Palacios and Christian González-Billault

*Address all correspondence to: chrgonza@uchile.cl

Cell and Neuronal Dynamics Laboratory, Faculty of Sciences, Universidad de Chile, Santiago, Chile

References

[1] Alcantara S, Ruiz M, D'Arcangelo G, Ezan F, de Lecea L, Curran T, Sotelo C, Soriano E. Regional and cellular patterns of reelin mRNA expression in the forebrain of the developing and adult mouse. Journal of Neuroscience 1998;18(19) 7779-7799.

[2] Tissir F, Goffinet AM. Reelin and brain development. Nature Reviews Neuroscience 2003;4(6) 496-505.

[3] Ringstedt T, Linnarsson S, Wagner J, Lendahl U, Kokaia Z, Arenas E, Ernfors P, Ibanez CF. BDNF regulates reelin expression and Cajal-Retzius cell development in the cerebral cortex. Neuron 1998;21(2) 305-315.

[4] Pesold C, Impagnatiello F, Pisu MG, Uzunov DP, Costa E, Guidotti A, Caruncho HJ. Reelin is preferentially expressed in neurons synthesizing gamma-aminobutyric acid in cortex and hippocampus of adult rats. Proceedings of the National Academy of Sciences of the United States of America 1998;95(6) 3221-3226.

[5] Lacor PN, Grayson DR, Auta J, Sugaya I, Costa E, Guidotti A. Reelin secretion from glutamatergic neurons in culture is independent from neurotransmitter regulation.

Proceedings of the National Academy of Sciences of the United States of America 2000;97(7) 3556-3561.

[6] DeSilva U, D'Arcangelo G, Braden VV, Chen J, Miao GG, Curran T, Green ED. The human reelin gene: isolation, sequencing, and mapping on chromosome 7. Genome Research 1997;7(2) 157-164.

[7] Royaux I, Lambert de Rouvroit C, D'Arcangelo G, Demirov D, Goffinet AM. Genomic organization of the mouse reelin gene. Genomics 1997;46(2) 240-250.

[8] Chen Y, Sharma RP, Costa RH, Costa E, Grayson DR. On the epigenetic regulation of the human reelin promoter. Nucleic Acids Research 2002;30(13) 2930-2939.

[9] Matrisciano F, Tueting P, Dalal I, Kadriu B, Grayson DR, Davis JM, Nicoletti F, Guidotti A. Epigenetic modifications of GABAergic interneurons are associated with the schizophrenia-like phenotype induced by prenatal stress in mice. Neuropharmacology 2012.

[10] Mitchell CP, Chen Y, Kundakovic M, Costa E, Grayson DR. Histone deacetylase inhibitors decrease reelin promoter methylation in vitro. Journal of Neurochemistry 2005;93(2) 483-492.

[11] Kundakovic M, Chen Y, Costa E, Grayson DR. DNA methyltransferase inhibitors coordinately induce expression of the human reelin and glutamic acid decarboxylase 67 genes. Molecular Pharmacology 2007;71(3) 644-653.

[12] Grayson DR, Chen Y, Costa E, Dong E, Guidotti A, Kundakovic M, Sharma RP. The human reelin gene: transcription factors (+), repressors (-) and the methylation switch (+/-) in schizophrenia. Pharmacology & Therapeutics 2006;111(1) 272-286.

[13] Hevner RF, Shi L, Justice N, Hsueh Y, Sheng M, Smiga S, Bulfone A, Goffinet AM, Campagnoni AT, Rubenstein JL. Tbr1 regulates differentiation of the preplate and layer 6. Neuron 2001;29(2) 353-366.

[14] Chen Y, Kundakovic M, Agis-Balboa RC, Pinna G, Grayson DR. Induction of the reelin promoter by retinoic acid is mediated by Sp1. Journal of Neurochemistry 2007;103(2) 650-665.

[15] Lambert de Rouvroit C, de Bergeyck V, Cortvrindt C, Bar I, Eeckhout Y, Goffinet AM. Reelin, the extracellular matrix protein deficient in reeler mutant mice, is processed by a metalloproteinase. Experimental Neurology 1999;156(1) 214-217.

[16] Hisanaga A, Morishita S, Suzuki K, Sasaki K, Koie M, Kohno T, Hattori M. A disintegrin and metalloproteinase with thrombospondin motifs 4 (ADAMTS-4) cleaves Reelin in an isoform-dependent manner. FEBS Letters 2012.

[17] Jossin Y, Gui L, Goffinet AM. Processing of Reelin by embryonic neurons is important for function in tissue but not in dissociated cultured neurons. Journal of Neuroscience 2007;27(16) 4243-4252.

[18] Jossin Y, Ignatova N, Hiesberger T, Herz J, Lambert de Rouvroit C, Goffinet AM. The central fragment of Reelin, generated by proteolytic processing in vivo, is critical to its function during cortical plate development. Journal of Neuroscience 2004;24(2) 514-521.

[19] D'Arcangelo G, Nakajima K, Miyata T, Ogawa M, Mikoshiba K, Curran T. Reelin is a secreted glycoprotein recognized by the CR-50 monoclonal antibody. Journal of Neuroscience 1997;17(1) 23-31.

[20] Utsunomiya-Tate N, Kubo K, Tate S, Kainosho M, Katayama E, Nakajima K, Mikoshiba K. Reelin molecules assemble together to form a large protein complex, which is inhibited by the function-blocking CR-50 antibody. Proceedings of the National Academy of Sciences of the United States of America 2000;97(17) 9729-9734.

[21] de Bergeyck V, Nakajima K, Lambert de Rouvroit C, Naerhuyzen B, Goffinet AM, Miyata T, Ogawa M, Mikoshiba K. A truncated Reelin protein is produced but not secreted in the 'Orleans' reeler mutation (Reln[rl-Orl]). Brain Research: Molecular Brain Research 1997;50(1-2) 85-90.

[22] D'Arcangelo G, Miao GG, Curran T. Detection of the reelin breakpoint in reeler mice. Brain Research: Molecular Brain Research 1996;39(1-2) 234-236.

[23] Gupta A, Tsai LH, Wynshaw-Boris A. Life is a journey: a genetic look at neocortical development. Nature Reviews Genetics 2002;3(5) 342-355.

[24] O'Rourke NA, Dailey ME, Smith SJ, McConnell SK. Diverse migratory pathways in the developing cerebral cortex. Science 1992;258(5080) 299-302.

[25] Caviness VS, Jr. Neocortical histogenesis in normal and reeler mice: a developmental study based upon [3H]thymidine autoradiography. Brain Research 1982;256(3) 293-302.

[26] Ogawa M, Miyata T, Nakajima K, Yagyu K, Seike M, Ikenaka K, Yamamoto H, Mikoshiba K. The reeler gene-associated antigen on Cajal-Retzius neurons is a crucial molecule for laminar organization of cortical neurons. Neuron 1995;14(5) 899-912.

[27] Frotscher M. Dual role of Cajal-Retzius cells and reelin in cortical development. Cell and Tissue Research 1997;290(2) 315-322.

[28] Curran T, D'Arcangelo G. Role of reelin in the control of brain development. Brain Research: Brain Research Reviews 1998;26(2-3) 285-294.

[29] Tissir F, Lambert de Rouvroit C, Goffinet AM. The role of reelin in the development and evolution of the cerebral cortex. Brazilian Journal of Medical and Biological Research 2002;35(12) 1473-1484.

[30] Goffinet AM, So KF, Yamamoto M, Edwards M, Caviness VS, Jr. Architectonic and hodological organization of the cerebellum in reeler mutant mice. Brain Research 1984;318(2) 263-276.

[31] Stanfield BB, Cowan WM. The development of the hippocampus and dentate gyrus in normal and reeler mice. Journal of Comparative Neurology 1979;185(3) 423-459.

[32] Badea A, Nicholls PJ, Johnson GA, Wetsel WC. Neuroanatomical phenotypes in the reeler mouse. NeuroImage 2007;34(4) 1363-1374.

[33] Chai X, Forster E, Zhao S, Bock HH, Frotscher M. Reelin stabilizes the actin cytoskeleton of neuronal processes by inducing n-cofilin phosphorylation at serine3. Journal of Neuroscience 2009;29(1) 288-299.

[34] Gonzalez-Billault C, Del Rio JA, Urena JM, Jimenez-Mateos EM, Barallobre MJ, Pascual M, Pujadas L, Simo S, Torre AL, Gavin R, Wandosell F, Soriano E, Avila J. A role of MAP1B in Reelin-dependent neuronal migration. Cerebral Cortex 2005;15(8) 1134-1145.

[35] Niu S, Renfro A, Quattrocchi CC, Sheldon M, D'Arcangelo G. Reelin promotes hippocampal dendrite development through the VLDLR/ApoER2-Dab1 pathway. Neuron 2004;41(1) 71-84.

[36] Niu S, Yabut O, D'Arcangelo G. The Reelin signaling pathway promotes dendritic spine development in hippocampal neurons. Journal of Neuroscience 2008;28(41) 10339-10348.

[37] Trommsdorff M, Gotthardt M, Hiesberger T, Shelton J, Stockinger W, Nimpf J, Hammer R, Richardson J, Herz J. Reeler/Disabled-like disruption of neuronal migration in knockout mice lacking the VLDL receptor and ApoE receptor 2. Cell 1999;97(6) 689-1390.

[38] Hiesberger T, Trommsdorff M, Howell BW, Goffinet A, Mumby MC, Cooper JA, Herz J. Direct binding of Reelin to VLDL receptor and ApoE receptor 2 induces tyrosine phosphorylation of disabled-1 and modulates tau phosphorylation. Neuron 1999;24(2) 481-489.

[39] Borrell V, Del Rio JA, Alcantara S, Derer M, Martinez A, D'Arcangelo G, Nakajima K, Mikoshiba K, Derer P, Curran T, Soriano E. Reelin regulates the development and synaptogenesis of the layer-specific entorhino-hippocampal connections. Journal of Neuroscience 1999;19(4) 1345-1358.

[40] Chen Y, Beffert U, Ertunc M, Tang TS, Kavalali ET, Bezprozvanny I, Herz J. Reelin modulates NMDA receptor activity in cortical neurons. Journal of Neuroscience 2005;25(36) 8209-8216.

[41] Herz J, Chen Y. Reelin, lipoprotein receptors and synaptic plasticity. Nature Reviews Neuroscience 2006;7(11) 850-859.

[42] Qiu S, Zhao LF, Korwek KM, Weeber EJ. Differential reelin-induced enhancement of NMDA and AMPA receptor activity in the adult hippocampus. Journal of Neuroscience 2006;26(50) 12943-12955.

[43] Ventruti A, Kazdoba TM, Niu S, D'Arcangelo G. Reelin deficiency causes specific defects in the molecular composition of the synapses in the adult brain. Neuroscience 2011;189 32-42.

[44] Hellwig S, Hack I, Kowalski J, Brunne B, Jarowyj J, Unger A, Bock HH, Junghans D, Frotscher M. Role for Reelin in neurotransmitter release. Journal of Neuroscience 2011;31(7) 2352-2360.

[45] Knuesel I. Reelin-mediated signaling in neuropsychiatric and neurodegenerative diseases. Progress in Neurobiology 2010;91(4) 257-274.

[46] Qiu S, Weeber EJ. Reelin signaling facilitates maturation of CA1 glutamatergic synapses. Journal of Neurophysiology 2007;97(3) 2312-2321.

[47] Guidotti A, Auta J, Davis JM, Di-Giorgi-Gerevini V, Dwivedi Y, Grayson DR, Impagnatiello F, Pandey G, Pesold C, Sharma R, Uzunov D, Costa E. Decrease in reelin and glutamic acid decarboxylase67 (GAD67) expression in schizophrenia and bipolar disorder: a postmortem brain study. Archives of General Psychiatry 2000;57(11) 1061-1069.

[48] Abdolmaleky HM, Cheng KH, Russo A, Smith CL, Faraone SV, Wilcox M, Shafa R, Glatt SJ, Nguyen G, Ponte JF, Thiagalingam S, Tsuang MT. Hypermethylation of the reelin (RELN) promoter in the brain of schizophrenic patients: a preliminary report. American Journal of Medical Genetics Part B, Neuropsychiatric Genetics 2005;134B(1) 60-66.

[49] Fatemi SH, Earle JA, McMenomy T. Reduction in Reelin immunoreactivity in hippocampus of subjects with schizophrenia, bipolar disorder and major depression. Molecular Psychiatry 2000;5(6) 654-663, 571.

[50] Chin J, Massaro CM, Palop JJ, Thwin MT, Yu GQ, Bien-Ly N, Bender A, Mucke L. Reelin depletion in the entorhinal cortex of human amyloid precursor protein transgenic mice and humans with Alzheimer's disease. Journal of Neuroscience 2007;27(11) 2727-2733.

[51] Maynard TM, Sikich L, Lieberman JA, LaMantia AS. Neural development, cell-cell signaling, and the "two-hit" hypothesis of schizophrenia. Schizophrenia Bulletin 2001;27(3) 457-476.

[52] Girirajan S, Rosenfeld JA, Cooper GM, Antonacci F, Siswara P, Itsara A, Vives L, Walsh T, McCarthy SE, Baker C, Mefford HC, Kidd JM, Browning SR, Browning BL, Dickel DE, Levy DL, Ballif BC, Platky K, Farber DM, Gowans GC, Wetherbee JJ, Asamoah A, Weaver DD, Mark PR, Dickerson J, Garg BP, Ellingwood SA, Smith R, Banks VC, Smith W, McDonald MT, Hoo JJ, French BN, Hudson C, Johnson JP, Ozmore JR, Moeschler JB, Surti U, Escobar LF, El-Khechen D, Gorski JL, Kussmann J, Salbert B, Lacassie Y, Biser A, McDonald-McGinn DM, Zackai EH, Deardorff MA, Shaikh TH, Haan E, Friend KL, Fichera M, Romano C, Gecz J, DeLisi LE, Sebat J, King MC, Shaffer LG, Eichler EE. A recurrent 16p12.1 microdeletion supports a two-hit model for severe developmental delay. Nature Genetics 2010;42(3) 203-209.

[53] Laviola G, Ognibene E, Romano E, Adriani W, Keller F. Gene-environment interaction during early development in the heterozygous reeler mouse: clues for modelling of major neurobehavioral syndromes. Neuroscience and Biobehavioral Reviews 2009;33(4) 560-572.

[54] Lussier AL, Romay-Tallon R, Kalynchuk LE, Caruncho HJ. Reelin as a putative vulnerability factor for depression: examining the depressogenic effects of repeated corticosterone in heterozygous reeler mice. Neuropharmacology 2011;60(7-8) 1064-1074.

[55] Teixeira CM, Martin ED, Sahun I, Masachs N, Pujadas L, Corvelo A, Bosch C, Rossi D, Martinez A, Maldonado R, Dierssen M, Soriano E. Overexpression of Reelin prevents the manifestation of behavioral phenotypes related to schizophrenia and bipolar disorder. Neuropsychopharmacology 2011;36(12) 2395-2405.

[56] Zhu X, Lee HG, Perry G, Smith MA. Alzheimer disease, the two-hit hypothesis: an update. Biochimica et Biophysica Acta 2007;1772(4) 494-502.

[57] Zhu X, Castellani RJ, Takeda A, Nunomura A, Atwood CS, Perry G, Smith MA. Differential activation of neuronal ERK, JNK/SAPK and p38 in Alzheimer disease: the 'two hit' hypothesis. Mechanisms of Ageing and Development 2001;123(1) 39-46.

[58] Stranahan AM, Haberman RP, Gallagher M. Cognitive decline is associated with reduced reelin expression in the entorhinal cortex of aged rats. Cerebral Cortex 2011;21(2) 392-400.

[59] Botella-Lopez A, Burgaya F, Gavin R, Garcia-Ayllon MS, Gomez-Tortosa E, Pena-Casanova J, Urena JM, Del Rio JA, Blesa R, Soriano E, Saez-Valero J. Reelin expression and glycosylation patterns are altered in Alzheimer's disease. Proceedings of the National Academy of Sciences of the United States of America 2006;103(14) 5573-5578.

[60] Hibi T, Hattori M. The N-terminal fragment of Reelin is generated after endocytosis and released through the pathway regulated by Rab11. FEBS Letters 2009;583(8) 1299-1303.

[61] Baloyannis SJ. Morphological and morphometric alterations of Cajal-Retzius cells in early cases of Alzheimer's disease: a Golgi and electron microscope study. International Journal of Neuroscience 2005;115(7) 965-980.

[62] Riedel A, Miettinen R, Stieler J, Mikkonen M, Alafuzoff I, Soininen H, Arendt T. Reelin-immunoreactive Cajal-Retzius cells: the entorhinal cortex in normal aging and Alzheimer's disease. Acta Neuropathologica 2003;106(4) 291-302.

[63] Seripa D, Matera MG, Franceschi M, Daniele A, Bizzarro A, Rinaldi M, Panza F, Fazio VM, Gravina C, D'Onofrio G, Solfrizzi V, Masullo C, Pilotto A. The RELN locus in Alzheimer's disease. Journal of Alzheimer's Disease 2008;14(3) 335-344.

[64] Wirths O, Multhaup G, Czech C, Blanchard V, Tremp G, Pradier L, Beyreuther K, Bayer TA Reelin in plaques of beta-amyloid precursor protein and presenilin-1 double-transgenic mice. Neuroscience Letters 2001;316(3) 145-148.

[65] Knuesel I, Nyffeler M, Mormede C, Muhia M, Meyer U, Pietropaolo S, Yee BK, Pryce CR, LaFerla FM, Marighetto A, Feldon J. Age-related accumulation of Reelin in amyloid-like deposits. Neurobiology of Aging 2009;30(5) 697-716.

[66] Doehner J, Madhusudan A, Konietzko U, Fritschy JM, Knuesel I. Co-localization of Reelin and proteolytic AbetaPP fragments in hippocampal plaques in aged wild-type mice. Journal of Alzheimer's Disease 2010;19(4) 1339-1357.

[67] Kocherhans S, Madhusudan A, Doehner J, Breu KS, Nitsch RM, Fritschy JM, Knuesel I. Reduced Reelin expression accelerates amyloid-beta plaque formation and tau pathology in transgenic Alzheimer's disease mice. Journal of Neuroscience 2010;30(27) 9228-9240.

[68] Botella-Lopez A, Cuchillo-Ibanez I, Cotrufo T, Mok SS, Li QX, Barquero MS, Dierssen M, Soriano E, Saez-Valero J. Beta-amyloid controls altered Reelin expression and processing in Alzheimer's disease. Neurobiology of Disease 2010;37(3) 682-691.

[69] Kosik KS, Joachim CL, Selkoe DJ. Microtubule-associated protein tau (tau) is a major antigenic component of paired helical filaments in Alzheimer disease. Proceedings of the National Academy of Sciences of the United States of America 1986;83(11) 4044-4048.

[70] Weingarten MD, Lockwood AH, Hwo SY, Kirschner MW. A protein factor essential for microtubule assembly. Proceedings of the National Academy of Sciences of the United States of America 1975;72(5) 1858-1862.

[71] Lee G, Cowan N, Kirschner M. The primary structure and heterogeneity of tau protein from mouse brain. Science 1988;239(4837) 285-288.

[72] Lee G, Neve RL, Kosik KS. The microtubule binding domain of tau protein. Neuron 1989;2(6) 1615-1624.

[73] Lindwall G, Cole RD. The purification of tau protein and the occurrence of two phosphorylation states of tau in brain. Journal of Biological Chemistry 1984;259(19) 12241-12245.

[74] Seubert P, Mawal-Dewan M, Barbour R, Jakes R, Goedert M, Johnson GV, Litersky JM, Schenk D, Lieberburg I, Trojanowski JQ, Lee VM. Detection of phosphorylated Ser262 in fetal tau, adult tau, and paired helical filament tau. Journal of Biological Chemistry 1995;270(32) 18917-18922.

[75] Iqbal K, Alonso Adel C, Grundke-Iqbal I. Cytosolic abnormally hyperphosphorylated tau but not paired helical filaments sequester normal MAPs and inhibit microtubule assembly. Journal of Alzheimer's Disease 2008;14(4) 365-370.

[76] Grundke-Iqbal I, Iqbal K, Tung YC, Quinlan M, Wisniewski HM, Binder LI. Abnormal phosphorylation of the microtubule-associated protein tau (tau) in Alzheimer cytoskeletal pathology. Proceedings of the National Academy of Sciences of the United States of America 1986;83(13) 4913-4917.

[77] Ihara Y, Nukina N, Miura R, Ogawara M. Phosphorylated tau protein is integrated into paired helical filaments in Alzheimer's disease. Journal of Biochemistry 1986;99(6) 1807-1810.

[78] Steiner B, Mandelkow EM, Biernat J, Gustke N, Meyer HE, Schmidt B, Mieskes G, Soling HD, Drechsel D, Kirschner MW, Goedert M, Mandelkow E. Phosphorylation of microtubule-associated protein tau: identification of the site for Ca2(+)-calmodulin dependent kinase and relationship with tau phosphorylation in Alzheimer tangles. EMBO Journal 1990;9(11) 3539-3544.

[79] Andorfer CA, Davies P. PKA phosphorylations on tau: developmental studies in the mouse. Developmental Neuroscience 2000;22(4) 303-309.

[80] Liu SJ, Zhang JY, Li HL, Fang ZY, Wang Q, Deng HM, Gong CX, Grundke-Iqbal I, Iqbal K, Wang JZ. Tau becomes a more favorable substrate for GSK-3 when it is pre-phosphorylated by PKA in rat brain. Journal of Biological Chemistry 2004;279(48) 50078-50088.

[81] Jensen PH, Hager H, Nielsen MS, Hojrup P, Gliemann J, Jakes R. alpha-synuclein binds to Tau and stimulates the protein kinase A-catalyzed tau phosphorylation of serine residues 262 and 356. Journal of Biological Chemistry 1999;274(36) 25481-25489.

[82] Hoshi M, Nishida E, Miyata Y, Sakai H, Miyoshi T, Ogawara H, Akiyama T. Protein kinase C phosphorylates tau and induces its functional alterations. FEBS Letters 1987;217(2) 237-241.

[83] Correas I, Diaz-Nido J, Avila J. Microtubule-associated protein tau is phosphorylated by protein kinase C on its tubulin binding domain. Journal of Biological Chemistry 1992;267(22) 15721-15728.

[84] Reynolds CH, Utton MA, Gibb GM, Yates A, Anderton BH. Stress-activated protein kinase/c-jun N-terminal kinase phosphorylates tau protein. Journal of Neurochemistry 1997;68(4) 1736-1744.

[85] Hanger DP, Hughes K, Woodgett JR, Brion JP, Anderton BH. Glycogen synthase kinase-3 induces Alzheimer's disease-like phosphorylation of tau: generation of paired helical filament epitopes and neuronal localisation of the kinase. Neuroscience Letters 1992;147(1) 58-62.

[86] Reynolds CH, Betts JC, Blackstock WP, Nebreda AR, Anderton BH. Phosphorylation sites on tau identified by nanoelectrospray mass spectrometry: differences in vitro between the mitogen-activated protein kinases ERK2, c-Jun N-terminal kinase and P38, and glycogen synthase kinase-3beta. Journal of Neurochemistry 2000;74(4) 1587-1595.

[87] Baumann K, Mandelkow EM, Biernat J, Piwnica-Worms H, Mandelkow E. Abnormal Alzheimer-like phosphorylation of tau-protein by cyclin-dependent kinases cdk2 and cdk5. FEBS Letters 1993;336(3) 417-424.

[88] Trojanowski JQ, Lee VM. Phosphorylation of paired helical filament tau in Alzheimer's disease neurofibrillary lesions: focusing on phosphatases. FASEB Journal 1995;9(15) 1570-1576.

[89] Minamide LS, Striegl AM, Boyle JA, Meberg PJ, Bamburg JR. Neurodegenerative stimuli induce persistent ADF/cofilin-actin rods that disrupt distal neurite function. Nature Cell Biology 2000;2(9) 628-636.

[90] Davis RC, Marsden IT, Maloney MT, Minamide LS, Podlisny M, Selkoe DJ, Bamburg JR. Amyloid beta dimers/trimers potently induce cofilin-actin rods that are inhibited by maintaining cofilin-phosphorylation. Molecular Neurodegeneration 2011;6(10).

[91] Bernard O Lim kinases, regulators of actin dynamics. International Journal of Biochemistry & Cell Biology 2007;39(6) 1071-1076.

[92] Zhao L, Ma QL, Calon F, Harris-White ME, Yang F, Lim GP, Morihara T, Ubeda OJ, Ambegaokar S, Hansen JE, Weisbart RH, Teter B, Frautschy SA, Cole GM. Role of p21-activated kinase pathway defects in the cognitive deficits of Alzheimer disease. Nature Neuroscience 2006;9(2) 234-242.

[93] Heredia L, Helguera P, de Olmos S, Kedikian G, Sola Vigo F, LaFerla F, Staufenbiel M, de Olmos J, Busciglio J, Caceres A, Lorenzo A. Phosphorylation of actin-depolymerizing factor/cofilin by LIM-kinase mediates amyloid beta-induced degeneration: a potential mechanism of neuronal dystrophy in Alzheimer's disease. Journal of Neuroscience 2006;26(24) 6533-6542.

[94] Mendoza-Naranjo A, Contreras-Vallejos E, Henriquez DR, Otth C, Bamburg JR, Maccioni RB, Gonzalez-Billault C. Fibrillar amyloid-beta1-42 modifies actin organization affecting the cofilin phosphorylation state: a role for Rac1/cdc42 effector proteins and the slingshot phosphatase. Journal of Alzheimer's Disease 2012;29(1) 63-77.

[95] Mendoza-Naranjo A, Gonzalez-Billault C, Maccioni RB. Abeta1-42 stimulates actin polymerization in hippocampal neurons through Rac1 and Cdc42 Rho GTPases. Journal of Cell Science 2007;120(Pt 2) 279-288.

[96] Davis RC, Maloney MT, Minamide LS, Flynn KC, Stonebraker MA, Bamburg JR. Mapping cofilin-actin rods in stressed hippocampal slices and the role of cdc42 in amyloid-beta-induced rods. Journal of Alzheimer's Disease 2009;18(1) 35-50.

[97] Huang TY, Minamide LS, Bamburg JR, Bokoch GM. Chronophin mediates an ATP-sensing mechanism for cofilin dephosphorylation and neuronal cofilin-actin rod formation. Developmental Cell 2008;15(5) 691-703.

[98] Herring A, Donath A, Steiner KM, Widera MP, Hamzehian S, Kanakis D, Kolble K, Elali A, Hermann DM, Paulus W, Keyvani K. Reelin Depletion is an Early Phenomenon of Alzheimer's Pathology. Journal of Alzheimer's Disease 2012;30(4) 963-979.

[99] Saez-Valero J, Costell M, Sjogren M, Andreasen N, Blennow K, Luque JM. Altered levels of cerebrospinal fluid reelin in frontotemporal dementia and Alzheimer's disease. Journal of Neuroscience Research 2003;72(1) 132-136.

[100] D'Arcangelo G, Homayouni R, Keshvara L, Rice DS, Sheldon M, Curran T. Reelin is a ligand for lipoprotein receptors. Neuron 1999;24(2) 471-479.

[101] Howell B, Hawkes R, Soriano P, Cooper J. Neuronal position in the developing brain is regulated by mouse disabled-1. Nature 1997;389(4c369df1-0b52-a4f8-d881-0c77f39fea11) 733-740.

[102] Howell B, Herrick T, Cooper J. Reelin-induced tyrosine [corrected] phosphorylation of disabled 1 during neuronal positioning. Genes & Development 1999;13(6) 643-651.

[103] Howell B, Herrick T, Hildebrand J, Zhang Y, Cooper J. Dab1 tyrosine phosphorylation sites relay positional signals during mouse brain development. Current Biology 2000;10(10) 877-962.

[104] Matsuki T, Zaka M, Guerreiro R, van der Brug MP, Cooper JA, Cookson MR, Hardy JA, Howell BW. Identification of Stk25 as a genetic modifier of Tau phosphorylation in Dab1-mutant mice. PLoS One 2012;7(2) e31152.

[105] Ohkubo N, Lee YD, Morishima A, Terashima T, Kikkawa S, Tohyama M, Sakanaka M, Tanaka J, Maeda N, Vitek MP, Mitsuda N. Apolipoprotein E and Reelin ligands modulate tau phosphorylation through an apolipoprotein E receptor/disabled-1/glycogen synthase kinase-3beta cascade. FASEB Journal 2003;17(2) 295-297.

[106] Brich J, Shie FS, Howell BW, Li R, Tus K, Wakeland EK, Jin LW, Mumby M, Churchill G, Herz J, Cooper JA. Genetic modulation of tau phosphorylation in the mouse. Journal of Neuroscience 2003;23(1) 187-192.

[107] Beffert U, Morfini G, Bock HH, Reyna H, Brady ST, Herz J. Reelin-mediated signaling locally regulates protein kinase B/Akt and glycogen synthase kinase 3beta. Journal of Biological Chemistry 2002;277(51) 49958-49964.

[108] Bock HH, Jossin Y, Liu P, Forster E, May P, Goffinet AM, Herz J. Phosphatidylinositol 3-kinase interacts with the adaptor protein Dab1 in response to Reelin signaling and is required for normal cortical lamination. Journal of Biological Chemistry 2003;278(40) 38772-38779.

[109] Patrick GN, Zukerberg L, Nikolic M, de la Monte S, Dikkes P, Tsai LH. Conversion of p35 to p25 deregulates Cdk5 activity and promotes neurodegeneration. Nature 1999;402(6762) 615-622.

[110] Beffert U, Weeber EJ, Morfini G, Ko J, Brady ST, Tsai LH, Sweatt JD, Herz J. Reelin and cyclin-dependent kinase 5-dependent signals cooperate in regulating neuronal migration and synaptic transmission. Journal of Neuroscience 2004;24(8) 1897-1906.

[111] Leemhuis J, Bouche E, Frotscher M, Henle F, Hein L, Herz J, Meyer DK, Pichler M, Roth G, Schwan C, Bock HH. Reelin signals through apolipoprotein E receptor 2 and Cdc42 to increase growth cone motility and filopodia formation. Journal of Neuroscience 2010;30(44) 14759-14772.

[112] Jimenez S, Torres M, Vizuete M, Sanchez-Varo R, Sanchez-Mejias E, Trujillo-Estrada L, Carmona-Cuenca I, Caballero C, Ruano D, Gutierrez A, Vitorica J. Age-dependent

accumulation of soluble amyloid beta (Abeta) oligomers reverses the neuroprotective effect of soluble amyloid precursor protein-alpha (sAPP(alpha)) by modulating phosphatidylinositol 3-kinase (PI3K)/Akt-GSK-3beta pathway in Alzheimer mouse model. Journal of Biological Chemistry 2011;286(21) 18414-18425.

Chapter 3

Mechanism of Alzheimer Amyloid β-Protein Precursor Localization to Membrane Lipid Rafts

Yuhki Saito, Takahide Matsushima and
Toshiharu Suzuki

Additional information is available at the end of the chapter

1. Introduction

Alzheimer's disease (AD) is a group of common neurodegenerative diseases associated with progressive dementia with aging. The principal pathological hallmarks of AD are senile plaques and neurofibrillary tangles in the brain, which are found at significantly higher frequencies in AD patients than age-matched healthy (non-AD) subjects [1]. Senile plaques consist mainly of 39–43 amino-acid amyloid-β (Aβ) peptide, which is generated by sequential proteolytic processing of amyloid β-protein precursor (APP) (Figure 1) [2]. Common Aβ species generated in the human and murine brain are Aβ40 and Aβ42. Mutations in *APP* and *Presenilin*, which have been identified as familial AD-causative genes, result in increased Aβ production and/or an increased ratio of neurotoxic Aβ42.

Aβ is generated by sequential processing of APP with β- and γ-secretase, the catalytic unit of which is presenilin. Findings reported during the late 1980s and early 1990s led to the proposal of the "Aβ cascade hypothesis" of AD onset, which states that Aβ generation is a primary cause of AD [3]. Several lines of evidence indicate that the amyloidogenic processing of APP, including Aβ generation, occurs in membrane microdomains termed lipid rafts [4]. However, the molecular mechanisms underlying APP translocation to lipid rafts remain unclear. In this chapter, regulatory mechanisms for lipid raft translocation of APP and APP C-terminal fragments (APP CTFs) generated primarily by the cleavage of APP are described.

Membrane lipid rafts are known as sites of amyloidogenic processing of APP and enriched with active β-secretase, while non-amyloidogenic cleavage of APP by α-secretase is performed outside lipid rafts. Neural adaptor protein X11-like (X11L) regulates the translocation of mature APP (mAPP), which is the *N*- and *O*-glycosylated form and real substrate of secretases in the late protein secretory pathway, to lipid rafts. APP bound to X11L preferentially localizes to sites outside of lipid rafts and escapes from active β-secretase [5]. Dissociation of the APP-X11L complex leads to APP entry into lipid rafts, suggesting that dysfunction of X11L in its interaction with APP may recruit more APP to lipid rafts and increase the generation of Aβ [5].

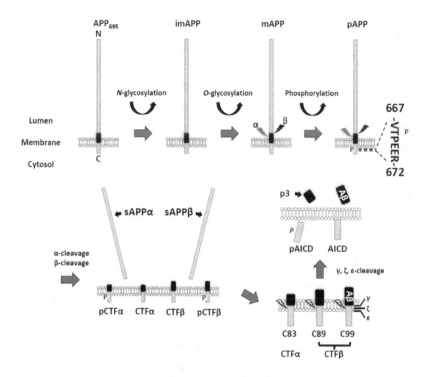

Figure 1. The schema of APP metabolism and post-translational modification of APP. APP is subjected to *N*-glycosylation at ER to form imAPP followed by *O*-glycosylation at the *medial-/trans*-Golgi apparatus to form mAPP. Residue Thr668 of mAPP is specifically phosphorylated in brain. mAPP is cleaved in sequential proteolytic events mediated by β-secretase or α-site APP cleaving enzyme, and the γ-secretase complex. β-secretase primarily cleaves APP in the luminal domain to generate sAPPβ and CTFβ (C99 and C89). C99 contains an intact Aβ sequence. γ-secretase complex mediates the cleavage of CTFβ at ε, ζ, and γ-sites to generate Aβ and AICD peptides. α-site APP cleaving enzyme generates sAPPα and CTFα (C83). CTFα cleavage by γ-secretase complex then generates p3 peptide and AICD.

In contrast to APP, APP CTF translocation to lipid rafts seems to involve another regulatory system that also includes active γ-secretase to cleave APP CTFs. The translocation of CTFs to lipid rafts is regulated by APP phosphorylation. The cytoplasmic region of APP is well known to demonstrate neuron-specific phosphorylation at Thr668 (numbering for the APP695 isoform). However, the maximum phosphorylation level of APP is 10–20% in the brain, and its physiological function is not clear [6].

A recent study found that the phosphorylation level of APP CTFs was much higher than that of full-length APP, and phosphorylated CTFs (pCTFs), but not nonphosphorylated CTFs (nCTFs), were preferentially located outside of detergent-resistant, lipid raft-like membrane microdomains, indicating that Thr668 phosphorylation appears to function on the APP CTF rather than full-length APP [7]. Recent analysis revealed that pCTFs are relatively movable within the membrane as integral membrane proteins, while nCTFs are susceptible to being anchored to a lipid raft by direct binding of the C-terminal tail to membrane lipids. Once in lipid rafts, nCTFs can be preferentially captured and cleaved by γ-secretase. Interestingly, phosphorylation levels of amyloidogenic CTFβ were significantly decreased in aged brain [7]. Two molecular mechanisms of APP and APP CTF translocation to ripid rafts are described in the following section.

2. Metabolism and post-translational modification of APP

APP, which is a type I membrane protein, is subjected to N-glycosylation at the endo plasmic reticulum (ER) to form immature APP (imAPP) followed by O-glycosylation at the *medial-/trans*-Golgi apparatus to form mature APP (mAPP) (Figure 1). mAPP is then transported through the *trans*-Golgi network to the plasma membrane, where it enters the late secretory pathway and is metabolized by either amyloidogenic or amyloidolytic (non-amyloiodgenic) processing [6, 8]. In the amyloidogenic pathway, APP is cleaved in sequential proteolytic events mediated by β-secretase (β-site APP cleaving enzyme 1 or BACE1) and the γ-secretase complex comprised of four core subunits, presenilins (PS1 or PS2), anterior pharynx defective 1 (APH-1), presenilin enhancer 2 (PEN2), and nicastrin. β-secretase primarily cleaves APP in the luminal domain to generate soluble APPβ (sAPPβ) and membrane-associated APP carboxyl terminal fragments (CTFβ/C99 and CTFβ'/C89). C99 contains an intact Aβ sequence (Figure 1). γ-secretase complex mediates the cleavage of CTFβ at ε, ζ, and γ-sites to generate Aβ and APP intracellular domain (AICD) peptides. Non-amyloidogenic cleavage of APP is mediated by α-site APP cleaving enzyme (α-secretase, including ADAM9, ADAM10, and ADAM17) to generate sAPPα and CTFα (C83), which contains only the carboxyl half of Aβ peptide. CTFα cleavage by γ-secretase complex then generates p3 peptide and AICD.

Residue Thr668 of the APP cytoplasmic region is located within the 667-VTPEER-672 motif and is phosphorylated (number corresponding to the APP695 isoform) in the late secretory pathway in neurons. Protein kinases such as GSK3β (glycogen synthase kinase-3β), CDK5 (cyclin-dependent kinase-5), CDK1/CDC2, and JNK (c-Jun N-terminal kinase) are thought to mediate this phosphorylation of APP [6]. APP CTFs are also phosphorylated at Thr668 and detected as phosphopeptide pC99, pC89, and pC83 by western blot analysis using a phosphorylation-state-specific anti-APP Thr668 antibody or pAPP antibody (Figure 2A). Typical APP CTF species in the brain appear as five bands: pC99, nC99, pC89, a mixture of nC89 plus pC83, and nC83. Treatment of CTFs with phosphatase is effective for the identification of the respective species. Levels of the phosphorylated CTFβ species pC99 and pC89 were significantly higher than those of their nonphosphorylated forms, nC99 and nC89, while phosphorylated CTFα, pC83, demonstrated a trend toward decreased levels in comparison to nonphosphorylated CTFα, nC83 (Figure 2B). The relative ratio of total phosphorylated CTFs was equivalent to that of nonphosphorylated CTFs (Figure 2C), although phosphorylated CTFβ and CTFβ' were predominant compared to their nonphosphorylated forms. These observations indicate that pCTFs and nCTFs are present at equal levels in the brain as potential substrates for γ-secretase.

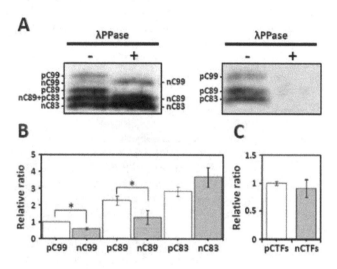

Figure 2. Level of CTF species in brain membrane fractions. (A) CTF species in brain membrane preparations. (B) and (C) Levels of CTF species in brain membrane preparations. Levels of the phosphorylated CTFβ species (pC99 and pC89) were significantly higher than those of their nonphosphorylated forms, nC99 and nC89.

The 667-VTPEER-672 motif, including the phosphorable amino acid Thr668, forms a type I β-turn and N-terminal helix-capping box structure to stabilize its C-terminal helix structure [9]. Therefore, phosphorylation of Thr668 induces significant conformational changes in the cytoplasmic region of APP (Figure 3) that affect its interaction with FE65, a neuronal adaptor protein [10]. The usual procedure to explore the function of a protein phosphorylation site is to mimic the phosphorylation state by amino acid substitutions of Asp or Glu for the appropriate Thr and Ser residues. However, this strategy may not be suitable in the case of APP phosphorylation, as the substitution of Asp for Thr668 did not alter the carboxyl terminal helix state as remarkably as phosphorylation of Thr668 (Figure 3A). By contrast, substitution of Thr668 with Ala668 in APP has been found to mimic effectively the nonphosphorylated state in the helix structure of the APP cytoplasmic domain. Figure 3B presents a schematic illustration of the Thr668-dependent conformational changes. Thr668Ala mutation mimics the nonphosphorylated state of APP, but Thr668Asp mutation did not completely mimic the phosphorylation structure of APP. Therefore, to reveal the role of APP phosphorylation at Thr668, careful analysis for the phosphorylation state of both APP and the APP metabolic fragments in the brain are described here.

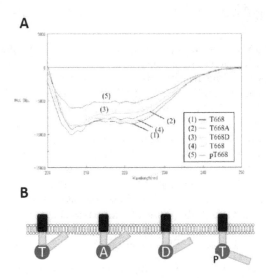

Figure 3. Circular dichroism (CD) spectra of APP cytoplasmic peptides (A) and schematic of changes to the APP cytoplasmic domain dependent on Thr668 residue modification (B). The substitution of Asp for Thr668 did not alter the carboxyl terminal helix state as remarkably as phosphorylation of Thr668. By contrast, substitution of Thr668 with Ala668 in APP has been found to mimic effectively the nonphosphorylated state in the helix structure of the APP cytoplasmic domain.

3. Lipid rafts and Alzheimer's disease

Dynamic and highly ordered membrane microdomains, termed lipid rafts, are rich in cholesterol and sphingolipids such as seramide, gangliosides, glycerophospholipids, and sterols. The average diameter of lipid rafts has been estimated at 50 nm. However, several classes of lipid rafts that vary in size and duration can exist in a cell [11]. Lipid rafts are formed in the Golgi and transported to the plasma membrane [12], where they serve as platforms for cell signaling, pathogen entry, cell adhesion, and protein sorting. Lipid rafts are biochemically defined as the detergent-resistant membrane (DRM) fraction [12]. Aβ generation and aggregation occur in lipid rafts, suggesting that lipid rafts play an important role in APP processing and subsequent AD pathogenesis. A growing body of evidence indicates that active β- and γ-secretases are located in membrane microdomains [13-15]. S-Palmitoylation of BACE1 at residues Cys474/478/482/485 is essential for the localization of BACE1 to lipid rafts [13,14]. S-Palmitoylation of nicastrin at Cys689 and of APH1 at Cys182 and Cys245 contributed to their stability and the lipid raft association of these nascent subunits, but did not affect the lipid raft localization of PS1 and PEN2 or the assembly of γ-secretase complex [15]. Taken together, lipid raft localization of secretases involved in amyloidogenic APP cleavage is regulated by their post-translational modification. However, the factors that determine lipid raft localization of APP remain unclear.

4. X11 protein regulation of APP localization to lipid rafts

X11 family proteins (X11s), consisting of X11/X11α/Mint1, X11L/X11β/Mint2, and X11L2/X11γ/Mint3, are encoded by separate genes on human chromosomes 9, 15, and 19 and mouse chromosomes 19, 7, and 10, respectively. X11s contain an evolutionarily conserved central phosphotyrosine binding/interaction (PTB/PI) domain and two C-terminal PDZ domains [16]. The PTB/PI and PDZ domains are well-characterized protein-protein interaction domains, and X11 proteins interact with various types of proteins, including APP, alcadein, apoER2, munc18, KIF17, kalirin, hyperpolarization-activated cyclic nucleotide-gated (HCN) channel, and Arfs, through their PTB/PI and PDZ domains. Interaction of X11L with APP can stabilize APP metabolism and intracellular trafficking, which induce the suppression of Aβ generation [16-18]. Metabolic analysis of APP in X11 and/or X11L knockout mice confirmed that X11s modulated APP metabolism and suppressed Aβ generation as an endophenotype *in vivo* [5, 19, 20]. X11 or X11L transgenic mice crossed to commonly used AD model mice (APPswe transgenic mice) demonstrated reduced amyloid deposition along with decreased levels of Aβ40 and Aβ42 in the brain compared to APPswe transgenic mice [21, 22].

The molecular mechanisms underlying the suppression of APP amyloidogenic metabolism by X11 and X11L have been addressed in a recent analysis. In the brains of mice lacking X11 and/or X11L, levels of CTFβ and Aβ were increased relative to wild-type animals (Figure 4) [5].

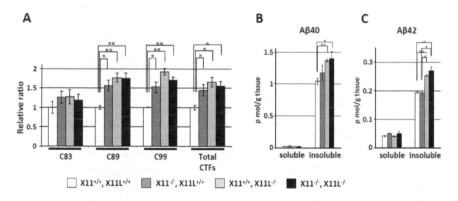

Figure 4. Quantification of APP CTFs in the hippocampus of wild-type, X11-deficient, X11L-deficient, and X11/X11L doubly deficient mice. Levels of CTFβ and Aβ were increased in X11s deficient mice, indicating that amyloidogenic metabolism of APP was enhanced in X11s deficient mice.

The absence of X11s resulted in more APP and APP CTF translocation to DRMs and enhanced colocalization of APP or APP CTFs with BACE1 in DRMs but not in non-DRMs (Figure 5A and B) [5]. Interestingly, X11s were recovered in membrane fractions, and they largely localized to non-DRMs but not DRMs (Figure 5C), indicating that APP can associate exclusively with X11s outside of DRMs to prevent APP translocation to lipid rafts, where amyloidogenic metabolism of APP occurs (Figure 6).

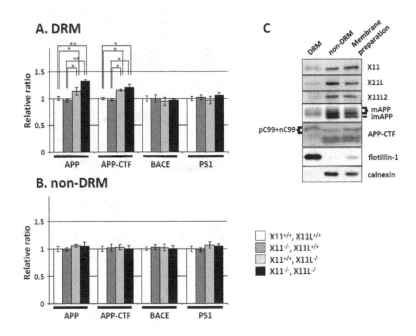

Figure 5. Quantification of APP, APP CTFs, BACE, and PS1 in (A) DRM and (B) non-DRM fractions from wild-type, X11-deficient, X11L-deficient, and X11/X11L doubly deficient mouse cortex. Higher levels of mAPP and CTFβ were recovered in DRM of the X11L-deficient and the X11/X11L doubly deficient mouse brain. (C) Localization of membrane-attached X11 proteins to DRM and non-DRM fractions. X11s were recovered in membrane fractions, and they largely localized to non-DRMs but not DRMs.

The Dysfunction of X11s in aged neurons may thus contribute to sporadic AD etiology. The dysfunction of X11s could lead to a weakening of the association between X11s and APP, resulting in greater translocation of APP to DRMs. Alteration in the lipid composition of membranes may enlarge lipid raft areas or increase the number of lipid rafts, which could also enhance APP translocation to DRMs. These qualitative alterations in X11s and/or lipid metabolism could result in increased β-cleavage of APP even if β-secretase itself is not enzymopathic.

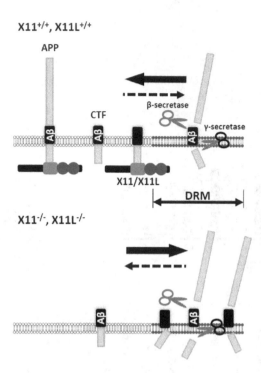

Figure 6. Possible role of X11 proteins in regulating the DRM association and β-site cleavage of APP. X11s associate with APP outside of DRMs and prevent translocation of APP into DRM. When X11L dissociates from APP, the APP translocates into DRMs, and that fraction of APP molecules is cleaved by BACE which is active in DRM (upper panel). In the absence of X11s, APP molecules are not anchored outside of DRMs, and more APP translocates into DRMs, resulting in increased β-site cleavage of APP (lower panel). The arrows indicate translocation direction of APP.

5. Regulation of APP CTF translocation to lipid rafts by Thr668 phosphorylation

Because similar amounts of nCTFs and pCTFs were found in mouse brain (Figure 2C), generation of similar levels of the APP intracellular cytoplasmic domain fragments, nonphosphorylated AICD (nAICD) and phosphorylated AICD (pAICD), is expected if γ-secretase cleaves nCTFs and pCTFs equivalently. However, membrane prepared from mouse brain generated higher levels of nAICD than pAICD in an *in vitro* γ-secretase assay (Figure 7A). Incubation of membrane preparations demonstrated a time-dependent, nearly linear increase in the generation of nAICD and pAICD during the 0–2 h time period, and the reaction essentially reached a plateau in the 2–4 h period (Figure 7B and C). Dephosphorylation and degradation of pAICD did not occur in this assay. Importantly, the ratio of pAICD to AICD generation was constant throughout the incubation time (1–4 h) with the relative ratio (amount of pAICD/amount of nAICD) measuring 0.35 ± 0.10 at the 2 h point (Figure 7D). Taken together, these *in vitro* analyses indicate that both phosphorylated and nonphosphorylated CTFs are kinetically equivalent as a substrate for γ-secretase, but the results also show that the generation of pAICD was significantly lower when compared to that of nAICD. These observations suggest that pCTFs are located at a distance from active γ-secretase in the membrane, while nCTFs are positioned nearer to the active enzyme.

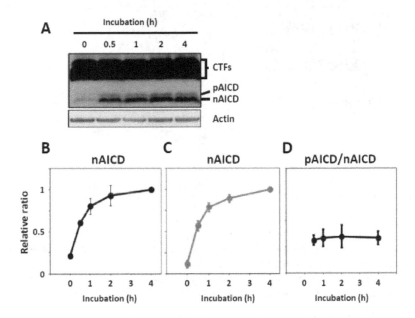

Figure 7. *In vitro* kinetic analysis of phosphorylated and nonphosphorylated CTF cleavage by γ secretase. (A) *In vitro* γ-secretase assay with membrane preparations from wild-type mouse brain. (B) and (C) kinetic analysis of AICD generated by incubation of membrane preparations. (D) the production ratio of pAICD to nAICD (pAICD/nAICD) at the indicated times are shown. Both phosphorylated and nonphosphorylated CTFs are kinetically equivalent as a substrate for γ-secretase, but the results also show that the generation of pAICD was significantly lower when compared to that of nAICD.

Thr668 phosphorylation could regulate APP CTF translocation to the lipid raft microdomain. To examine this hypothesis, γ-secretase-enriched lipid raft-like membrane microdomains were prepared as DRMs using CHAPSO. Application of CHAPSO is preferable for the isolation of DRMs, including active γ-secretase complexes, compared to procedures using other detergents such as Triton X-100 [23, 24]. Components of the active γ-secretase complex, both PS1 N- and C-terminal fragments and PEN2, were predominantly recovered in the DRM fraction along with a small amount of APP CTFs (~20% measured) [7]. Phosphorylation levels of APP CTFs in the DRM and non-DRM fractions were examined, and the respective nCTFs and pCTFs were compared as a relative ratio in which pC99 in the DRM was set to 1.0 (Figure 8).

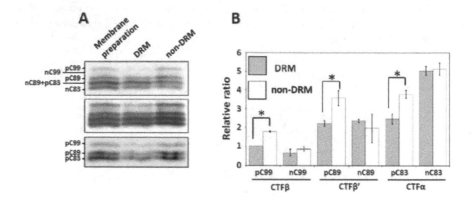

Figure 8. Quantification of pCTFs and nCTFs in DRM and non-DRM fractions. (A) Identification of APP CTFs in DRM and non-DRM fractions. (B) CTFs levels in DRM and non-DRM fractions. Significantly higher levels of the phosphorylated species pC99, pC89, and pC83 were found in the non-DRM fractions.

Significantly higher levels of the phosphorylated species pC99, pC89, and pC83 were found in the non-DRM fractions compared to the DRM fractions. Additionally, the phosphorylation level of total APP CTFs in DRM was significantly lower than that in non-DRM. These results indicate that phosphorylated CTFs are preferentially localized outside of the DRM/lipid raft-like membrane microdomain and thus prevented from cleavage by γ-secretase.

How does phosphorylation of Thr668 regulate the localization of APP CTFs between DRM and non-DRM? A recent structural analysis revealed that the cytoplasmic domain tail of APP can interact with membrane lipids [25]. Since phosphorylation of APP at Thr668 induces a significant change in its cytoplasmic domain conformation (Figure 2) [9, 10, 26], phosphorylation of the APP cytoplasmic domain at Thr668 can influence the association of the APP cytoplasmic tail with membrane lipids.

Liposomes prepared with endogenous lipids from the membrane fractions of mouse brain have been used as a model for neural membranes [27]. Synthetic cytoplasmic APP 648–695 peptide with (pC47) or without (nC47) a phosphate group at residue Thr668 was incubated with the liposomes, and the liposome-bound peptides were recovered and analyzed by immunoblotting. Notably, nonphosphorylated APP cytoplasmic peptide (nC47) bound strongly to the liposomes, while phosphorylated peptide (pC47) demonstrated no detectable association (Figure 9A) [7]. This trend was also confirmed by examining the AICD, which lacks the transmembrane domain due to ε-cleavage by γ-secretase [28, 29]. Most nAICD was recovered in the brain membrane fraction (~75%) rather than in the soluble cytoplasmic fraction (~25%), while comparatively more pAICD was found in the cytoplasmic fraction (~45%) (Figure 9B).

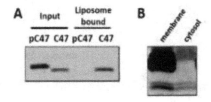

Figure 9. Liposome-binding ability of APP cytoplasmic domain and ist localization in mouse brain. (A) The binding ability of the phosphorylated APP cytoplasmic domain peptide with liposomes composed of lipids from mouse brain membranes. (B) distribution of AICD endogenously generated in mouse brain. Nonphosphorylated nC47 and AICD bound strongly to the liposome and membrane fraction.

Therefore, the nonphosphorylated forms of APP CTFs and AICD tend to bind membrane lipids, mediated by their C-termini, and phosphorylation of APP CTFs and AICD at Thr668 functions to prevent direct membrane association, apparently by changing the conformation of their cytoplasmic regions. In addition to these observations, pCTFβ levels were significantly decreased with age in cynomolgus monkey brains [7], indicating that the preservation of APP CTF phosphorylation levels correlates with the suppression of γ-cleavage.

To conclude this section, first, almost equal amounts of pCTFs and nCTFs are present in mouse brain, while lower amounts of pAICD are generated compared to nAICD. Second, both pAICD and nAICD are kinetically equivalent substrates for γ-secretase. These observations suggest that pCTFs are sequestered away from the membrane region where γ-secretase is active (DRM/lipid raft-like membrane microdomain) [15], and that pCTFs are located outside of the DRM/lipid raft-like membrane microdomain due to a change in the conformation of their cytoplasmic tail, to which the membrane lipids bind. Thus, the pCTFs can quickly disperse from the DRM/lipid raft-like membrane microdomain with their increased mobility in the membrane (Figure 10).

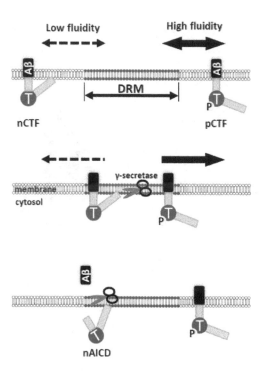

Figure 10. Possible role of APP CTF phosphorylation at Thr668 in regulating its fluidity within the membrane and its cleavage by γ-secretase.

6. Conclusions

X11L abundantly present in non-DRM traps APP outside of the DRM and prevents contact between APP and the β-secretases located within the DRM. Phosphorylation of APP at Thr668 induces conformational changes to the APP cytoplasmic domain and reduces the affinity of the APP C terminal to lipids. This change alters APP CTF fluidity and decreases the probability of APP CTF presence in lipid rafts, in which contact between APP CTFs and γ-secretase occurs. In conclusion, translocation of APP and APP CTFs to lipid rafts is regulated by neuronal adaptor protein X11L and Thr668 phosphorylation of APP CTFs.

Abbrevations

ADAM: a disintegrin and metalloprotease domain, APH-1: anterior pharynx defective 1, AICD: APP intracellular domain, APP: amyloid precursor protein, APP CTFs: APP C-terminal fragments, BACE1: β-site APP cleaving enzyme 1/β-secretase, CDK5: cyclin-dependent kinase-5, CD spectra: Circular dichroism spectra, DRM: detergent-resistant membrane, GSK3:βglycogen synthase kinase-3β, JNK: c-Jun N-terminal kinase, imAPP: immature APP, mAPP: mature APP, pAICD; nAICD; nonphosphorylated AICD, nCTFs; nonphosphorylated CTFs, phosphorylated AICD, pCTFs; phosphorylated CTFs, PS: presenilins, PEN2; presenilin enhancer 2, PTB/PI domain; phosphotyrosine binding/interaction domain; sAPP; soluble APP, X11L; X11-like.

Author details

Yuhki Saito, Takahide Matsushima and Toshiharu Suzuki

Laboratory of Neuroscience, Graduate School of Pharmaceutical Sciences, Hokkaido University, Sapporo, Japan

References

[1] Braak H, Braak E. Neuropathological stageing of Alzheimer-related changes. Acta. Neuropathol. 1991;82(4): 239-259.

[2] Selkoe DJ. Alzheimer's disease: genes, proteins, and therapy. Physiol Rev 2001;81(2): 741-766.

[3] Hardy JA and Higgins GA. Alzheimer's disease: the amyloid cascade hypothesis. Science 1992; 256: 184-185.

[4] Vetrivel KS and Thinakaran G. Membrane rafys in Alzheimer's disease beta-amyloid production. Biochem. Biophys. Acta. 2010; 1801: 860-867.

[5] Saito Y, Sano Y, Vassar R, Gandy S, Nakaya T, Yamamoto T. and Suzuki T. X11 proteins regulate the translocation of amyloid beta-protein precursor (APP) into detergent-resistant membrane and suppress the amyloidogenic cleavage of APP by beta-site-cleaving enzyme in brain. J. Biol. Chem. 2008;283(51): 35763-71.

[6] Suzuki T and Nakaya T. Regulation of amyloid beta-protein precursor by phosphorylation and protein interactions. J Biol Chem 2008;31(44): 29633-37.

[7] Matsushima T, Saito Y, Elliott JI, Iijima-Ando K, Nishimura M, Kimura N, Hata S, Yamamoto T, Nakaya T, Suzuki T. Membrane-microdomain Localization of Amyloid

β-Precursor Protein (APP) C-terminal Fragments is Regulated by Phosphorylation of the Cytoplasmic Thr668 Residue. J Biol Chem 2012; 287(23): 19715-24.

[8]   Thinakaran G and Koo EM. Amyloid precursor protein trafficking, processing and function. J. Biol. Chem. 2008; 283 (44): 29615-29619.

[9]   Ramelot TA, Gentile LN, Nicholson LK. Transient structure of the amyloid precursor protein cytoplasmic tail indicates preordering of structure for binding to cytosolic factors. Biochemistry 2000;39(10): 2714-25.

[10] Ando K, Oishi M, Takeda S, Iijima K, Isohara T, Nairn AC, Kirino Y, Greengard P, Suzuki T. Role of phosphorylation of Alzheimer's amyloid precursor protein during neuronal differentiation. J Neurosci 1999;19(11): 4421-7.

[11] Hancock JF. Lipid rafts: contentious only from simplistic standpoints. Nat Rev Mol Cell Biol 2006;7(6): 456-62.

[12] Brown DA, London E. Functions of lipid rafts in biological membranes. Annu Rev Cell Dev Biol 1998;14: 111-36.

[13] Benjannet S, Elagoz A, Wickham L, Mamarbachi M, Munzer JS, Basak A, Lazure C, Cromlish JA, Sisodia S, Checler F, Chretien M, Seidah NG. Posttranslational processing of beta-secretase (beta-amyloid-converting enzyme) and its ectodomain shedding. The pro- and transmembrane/cytosolic domains affect its cellular activity and amyloid-beta production, J Biol Chem 2001;276(14): 10879–87.

[14] Vetrivel KS, Meckler X, Chen Y, Nguyen PD, Seidah NG, Vassar R, Wong PC, Fukata M, Kounnas MZ, Thinakaran G. Alzheimer disease Abeta production in the absence of S-palmitoylation-dependent targeting of BACE1 to lipid rafts, J Biol Chem 2009;284 (6): 3793–803.

[15] Cheng H, Vetrivel KS, Drisdel RC, Meckler X, Gong P, Leem JY, Li T, Carter M, Chen Y, Nguyen P, Iwatsubo T, Tomita T, Wong PC, Green WN, Kounnas MZ, Thinakaran G. S-palmitoylation of gamma-secretase subunits nicastrin and APH-1, J Biol Chem 2009;284(3): 1373–84.

[16] Tomita S, Ozaki T, Taru H, Oguchi S, Takeda S, Yagi Y, Sakiyama S, Kirino Y, Suzuki T. Interaction of a neuron-specific protein containing PDZ domains with Alzheimer's amyloid precursor protein. J Biol Chem 1999; 274(4): 2243-54.

[17] Araki Y, Tomita S, Yamaguchi H, Miyagi N, Sumioka A, Kirino Y, Suzuki T. Novel cadherin-related membrane proteins, Alcadeins, enhance the X11-like protein-mediated stabilization of amyloid beta-protein precursor metabolism. J Biol Chem 2003; 278(49): 49448-49458.

[18] Taru H, Suzuki T. Regulation of the physiological function and metabolism of AβPP by AβPP binding proteins. J Alzheimers Dis 2009;18(2): 253-265.

[19] Sano Y, Syuzo Takabatake A, Nakaya T, Saito Y, Tomita S, Itohara S, Suzuki T. Enhanced amyloidogenic metabolism of the amyloid beta-protein precursor in the X11L-deficient mouse brain. J Biol Chem 2006;281(49): 37853-37860.

[20] Kondo M, Shiono M, Itoh G, Takei N, Matsushima T, Maeda M, Taru H, Hata S, Yamamoto T, Saito Y, Suzuki T. Increased amyloidogenic processing of transgenic human APP in X11-like deficient mouse brain. Mol Neurodegener 2010; 15;5:35.

[21] Lee JH, Lau KF, Perkinton MS, Standen CL, Shemilt SJ, Mercken L, Cooper JD, McLoughlin DM, Miller CC. The neuronal adaptor protein X11alpha reduces Abeta levels in the brains of Alzheimer's APPswe Tg2576 transgenic mice. J Biol Chem 2003; 278(47): 47025-29.

[22] Lee JH, Lau KF, Perkinton MS, Standen CL, Rogelj B, Falinska A, McLoughlin DM, Miller CC. The neuronal adaptor protein X11beta reduces amyloid beta-protein levels and amyloid plaque formation in the brains of transgenic mice. J Biol Chem 2004;279(47): 49099-104.

[23] Wahrle S, Das P, Nyborg AC, McLendon C, Shoji M, Kawarabayashi T, Younkin LH, Younkin SG,. Golde TE. Cholesterol-dependent gamma-secretase activity in buoyant cholesterol-rich membrane microdomains. Neurobiol Dis 2002;9(1). 11-23.

[24] Vetrivel KS, Cheng H, Lin W, Sakurai T, Li T, Nukina N, Wong PC, Xu H, Thinakaran G. Association of gamma-secretase with lipid rafts in post-Golgi and endosome membranes. J Biol Chem 2004;279(43): 44945-54.

[25] Beel AJ, Mobley CK, Kim HJ, Tian F, Hadziselimovic A, Jap B, Prestegard JH, Sanders CR. Structural studies of the transmembrane C-terminal domain of the amyloid precursor protein (APP): does APP function as a cholesterol sensor? Biochemistry 2008; 47(36): 9428-46.

[26] Ramelot TA, Nicholson LK. Phosphorylation-induced structural changes in the amyloid precursor protein cytoplasmic tail detected by NMR. J Mol Biol 2001; 307(3): 871-884.

[27] Sumioka A, Yan D, Tomita S. TARP phosphorylation regulates synaptic AMPA receptors through lipid bilayers. Neuron 2010; 66(5): 755-67.

[28] Gu Y, Misonou H, Sato T, Dohmae N, Takio K, Ihara Y. Distinct intramembrane cleavage of the beta-amyloid precursor protein family resembling gamma-secretase-like cleavage of Notch. J Biol Chem 2001;276(38): 35235-38.

[29] Qi-Takahara Y, Morishima-Kawashima M, Tanimura Y, Dolios G, Hirotani N, Horikoshi Y, Kametani F, Maeda M, Saido TC, Wang R, Ihara Y. Longer forms of amyloid beta protein: implications for the mechanism of intramembrane cleavage by gamma-secretase. J Neurosci 2005; 25(2): 436-45.

γ-Secretase — Regulated Signaling and Alzheimer's Disease

Kohzo Nakayama, Hisashi Nagase,
Chang-Sung Koh and Takeshi Ohkawara

Additional information is available at the end of the chapter

1. Introduction

Alzheimer's disease (AD) is an incurable and progressive neurodegenerative disorder and the most common form of dementia that occurs with aging. The main hallmarks of this disease are the extracellular deposition of amyloid plaques and the intracellular aggregation of tangles in the brain [1, 2]. Although the causes of both the onset and progression of AD are still uncertain, much evidence, including results of genetic analysis, indicates that amyloid precursor protein (APP) itself and its proteolytic processing are responsible for AD. Indeed, familial forms of AD (FAD) have mutations [3] or a duplication of the *APP* gene [4] or mutations in the presenilin1 or 2 (*PS1* or *PS2*) genes [5-7] that code for a catalytic component of the γ-secretase complex [8].

Although APP plays a central role in AD [1, 2], the physiological function of this membrane protein is not clear [9]. On the other hand, γ-secretase was first identified as a protease that cleaves APP within the transmembrane domain and produces amyloid-β (Aβ) peptides [10], which are the main constituent of amyloid plaques and are thought to be involved in AD pathogenesis. However, similar to the physiological functions of APP, those of γ-secretase are also still unclear [11, 12].

The signaling hypothesis suggests that the primary function of γ-secretase is to regulate signaling of type 1 membrane proteins (the amino terminus is extracellular, and the carboxy terminus is cytoplasmic); this was proposed by analogy of Notch signaling [13-15]. Notch is a family of evolutionarily conserved type 1 membrane proteins that mediate the fates of numerous cells in both invertebrates and vertebrates [16-18]. The molecular mechanism of the Notch signaling pathway is unique because it is controlled by proteolytic cleavage reactions [19, 20]. In the canonical Notch signaling pathway, ligands bind to the extracellular domain of Notch expressed on neighboring cells and trigger sequential proteolytic cleavage. Finally, the intracellular domain (ICD) of Notch (NICD) is released from the cell membrane by γ-secretase; NICD then translocates into the nucleus where it modulates gene expression through binding to transcription factors. Therefore, γ-secretase plays a central regulatory role in Notch signaling.

Recently, more than five dozen type 1 transmembrane proteins, including Notch and APP, have been reported as substrates for γ-secretase [21]. The ICDs of these proteins are also released from the cell membrane [13-15, 22]. Furthermore, it has been shown that some of these ICDs exist in the nucleus. These processes are very similar to those involved in Notch signaling. Thus, the common enzyme γ-secretase modulates the proteolysis and turnover of putative signaling molecules; this suggests that mechanisms similar to the Notch signaling pathway may widely contribute to γ-secretase–regulated signaling [13-15, 23]. Indeed, it has been shown that the ICD of APP (AICD), which is released from the cell membrane by γ-secretase, also translocates to the nucleus [24-26] and may function as a transcriptional regulator [27, 28]. These observations suggest the existence of APP signaling.

To test the hypothesis that APP has a signaling mechanism similar to that of Notch, we established embryonic carcinoma P19 cell lines that overexpressed AICD [29], which may mimic signaling mechanisms. Although neurons differentiated from these cell lines, AICD expression induced dynamic changes in gene expression profile and neuron-specific apoptosis [30]. These results suggest that APP also has a signaling mechanism, which may be closely related to AD.

In this chapter, we first summarize current research progress regarding Notch, APP, and γ-secretase. We also focus on the signaling hypothesis; γ-secretase–regulated mechanisms similar to Notch signaling may widely play roles in signaling events involving type 1 transmembrane proteins, including APP. Next, we review recent evidence supporting the existence of APP signaling. Furthermore, we discuss the possibility that APP signaling is involved in the onset and progression of AD.

2. γ-Secretase controls Notch signaling

Notch is a family of evolutionarily conserved type 1 membrane proteins with a mass of about 300 kDa [31] that mediates fates of numerous cells in both invertebrates and vertebrates [16, 17]. For example, cells expressing the major ligand Delta inhibit the neural differentiation of neighboring Notch-expressing cells during neurogenesis. Disruption of or disorder in Notch signaling leads to developmental defects or cancer in mammals [18].

While *Drosophila* has only one Notch gene, four Notch isoforms (Notch1 to 4) have been identified in mammals. The typical Notch protein contains 36 tandem epidermal growth factor (EGF)-like repeats in its extracellular domain, and six tandem ankyrin-like (CDC10) repeats, a nuclear localization signal, and a PEST sequence in its intracellular domain [31]. The 11th and 12th EGF-like repeats are essential for binding to its ligands [32]. Notch is cleaved in the trans-Golgi network, apparently by furin-like covertase, and is expressed on the cell surface as a heterodimer [33].

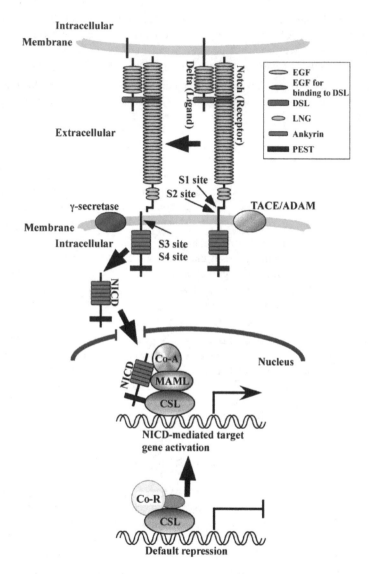

Figure 1. Notch signaling pathway. Notch proteins are expressed on the cell surface as heterodimers after cleavage at the S1 site by furin. The binding of Notch to the ligand triggers sequential proteolytic cleavage of the regulated intramembrane proteolysis (RIP). When Notch binds to the ligand, Notch is cleaved at the S2 site in the juxtamembrane region by TACE or ADAM protease. Next, the remaining protein stub is further cleaved by γ-secretase at the S3 and S4 sites within the transmembrane domain and NICD is released from the membrane. Then, NICD translocates into the nucleus and binds to the CSL together with MAML. The resultant CSL–NICD–MAML complex removes co-repressors (Co-R) from CSL transcription factor and recruits a co-activator (Co-A), resulting in conversion from repressor to activator. Finally, the complexes of CSL-NICD-MAML-Co-activators promote transcription of the target genes.

Drosophila has two different Notch ligands, Delta [34] and Serrate [35]. In mammals, two families of Notch ligands, Delta-like protein family (Dll1, 3, and 4) [36-38] and Jagged family (Jagged 1 and 2) [39, 40], have been identified. The extracellular domains of all these ligands also contain variable number of EGF-like repeats, e.g., *Drosophila* Delta has nine, while most vertebrate Deltas have eight, and *Caenorhabditis elegans* Lag-2 has two repeats. All these ligands share a single copy of a 2nd cysteine-rich conservative motif called the DSL (Delta: Serrate: Lag-2) domain [41], which is essential for binding to Notch [42].

As shown in Fig.1, in the canonical Notch signaling pathway, ligands bind to the extracellular domain of Notch proteins on neighboring cells and trigger sequential proteolytic cleavage reactions; this is called the regulated intramembrane proteolysis (RIP) mechanism [43]. Precise steps of Notch processing are mentioned in section 4.2 of this chapter. In brief, first, Notch is cleaved within the juxtamembrane (JM) domain by metalloproteases to remove most of the extracellular region [44, 45]. Next, the remaining protein stub is further cleaved by γ-secretase within the transmembrane (TM) domain and NICD is released from the membrane [46-48]. The released NICD translocates to the nucleus and controls the expression of certain genes through binding to transcription factors. Thus, γ-secretase plays a central regulatory role in Notch signaling.

Members of the CSL transcription factor family (CBF1/RBP-jκ in mammals, Su(H) in *Drosophila*, and Lag-1 in *C. elegans*) are major downstream targets of Notch signaling [19]. NICD binds to CSL transcription factors, and six tandem ankyrin-like repeats in NICD are essential for binding to CSL transcription factors [49]. NICD also binds to Mastermind-like proteins (MAML family in mammals) [50], thus forming the CSL-NICD-MAML complex. The formation of these complexes results in removal of co-repressors from CSL and recruitment of co-activators, such as P/CAF and P300 [50, 51]. Through this process, the CSL complex is converted from a transcriptional repressor to an activator. Finally, these complexes bind to the *cis*-acting DNA sequences of target genes, such as Hes (Hairy/Enhancer of split in *Drosophila*), which encode the basic helix-loop-helix (bHLH) transcription factors, and promote their transcription [52].

3. Amyloid Precursor Protein (APP)

3.1. Overview of APP

APP was identified as a cDNA cloned using a partial amino acid sequence of the Aβ fragment isolated from the amyloid plaque of AD brains [53]. This cDNA coded for an evolutionarily conserved type 1 transmembrane protein. Fig. 2 shows schematic diagram of APP protein. Although APP is expressed in many tissues, this protein especially accumulates in the synapses of neurons. The human *APP* gene is about 240 kb in length containing at least 18 exons [54] and is localized on the long arm of chromosome 21 [53], an extra copy of which is present in patients with Down's syndrome (trisomy 21). Several alternative splicing isoforms of APP have been found, which differ mainly in the absence (APP-695, predominantly expressed in neurons) or presence (APP-751 and APP-770) of the Kunitz protease inhibitor (KPI) domain toward the N-terminus of the protein [55].

As described below, APP undergoes sequential proteolytic cleavage reactions to generate the extracellular fragment, intracellular fragment (AICD), and Aβ fragment that is located in the membrane-spanning region. Note that both the extracellular fragment and AICD are generated at the same time as Aβ. Extensive post-translational modifications of APP, such as glycosylation, phosphorylation, and tyrosine sulfation, have been observed.

Mammals have two other members of APP family called APP-like protein 1 (APLP1) and 2 (APLP2) [56]. APLP1 expression is restricted to neurons. On the other hand, expression of APLP2 is detected in many tissues, although it is highly enriched in the brain. These APP family proteins share conserved domains, such as the E1 and E2, in the extracellular region. The E1 domain contains several subdomains, such as a growth factor-like domain and a metal-binding motif [57]. The E2 domain has a coiled coil dimerization motif and may bind proteoglycans in the extracellular matrix [58].

Interestingly, the amino acid sequence of the Aβ fragment is not highly conserved and is unique to APP; on the other hand, the highest degree of sequence conservation is found in the ICD not only within the APP homologues [29] but also within the APP family [9]. This strong sequence conservation most likely reflects functional importance of the ICDs in the APP family proteins.

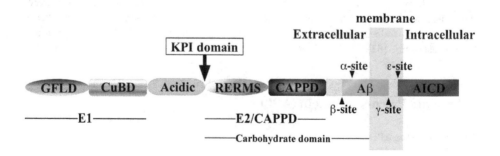

Figure 2. Schematic domain structure of APP. APP protein family shares the conserved E1 and E2 domains in their extracellular region. The E1 domain contains N-terminal growth factor-like domain (GFLD) and copper-binding domain (CuBD). The E1 domain is linked via acidic domain to the carbohydrate domain including E2 domain, which consists of RERMS sequence and central APP domain (CAPPD). E2 domain is followed by the Aβ region, and the intracellular domain (AICD) which is the most conserved region. Although the Kunitz protease inhibitor (KPI) domain is present at the indicated site in APP-751 and APP-770, APP-695 lacks this domain.

3.2. Proposed APP functions

Although the physiological functions of APP are not clear, several possibilities have been proposed. The most considerable functions are synapse formation and repair [59, 60]. Indeed, APP expression is upregulated after neural injury as well as during neuronal differentiation [59, 60]. After translation in the soma, APP is transported in an anterograde manner to the synaptic region, where the amount of APP is correlated with synaptogenesis. APP knockout mice show impaired long-term potentiation and declined memory without remarkable neuronal loss [61]. This evidence also supports this idea.

It has also been suggested that APP acts as a cell adhesion molecule and plays a role in cell–cell interaction. Indeed, the E1 and E2 domains can interact with extracellular matrix proteins and heparan sulfate proteoglycans [57, 58]. In addition, it has also been shown that extracellular domains of APP family proteins can interact with each other *in trans*. Therefore, APP family proteins may bind to each other in a homophilic or heterophilic manner to enhance cell–cell adhesion [62].

As APP may have a signaling mechanism, as described in detail below, the idea that APP is a cell-surface receptor is interesting. Indeed, several candidates of ligand for APP have been proposed. For example, F-spondin [63] and Nogo-66 [64] receptor bind to the extracellular domain of APP and regulate the production of Aβ. In addition, Aβ itself can also bind to the extracellular domain of APP [65].

3.3. Aβ amyloid

Aβ is the main constituent of an amyloid plaque, which is thought to be the hallmark and a major cause of AD pathogenesis in the brain. Thus, the amyloid hypothesis is generally accepted as the mechanism of the onset and progression of AD. The traditional amyloid hypothesis is that overproduced Aβ forms insoluble amyloid plaques, which are commonly observed in the AD brain and are believed to be the toxic form of APP and responsible for neurodegeneration [66].

As detailed in section 4.2., Aβ is generated after sequential cleavage of APP by β- and γ-secretases. Although these fragments range from 36 to 43 amino acid residues in length, Aβ40 and Aβ42 are the most common isoforms. Aβ40 is predominant over Aβ42, but Aβ42 is more amyloidogenic [67] and is, therefore, thought to be closely associated with AD. Furthermore, similar amyloid plaques are found in particular variants of Lewy body dementia [68] and in the muscle disease inclusion body myositis [69]. Aβ also forms aggregates that coat cerebral blood vessels in cerebral amyloid angiopathy (CAA), which is observed in over 90% of AD patients [70].

Deposition of Aβ in the AD brain is thought to be formed due to imbalances between the production of Aβ and its removal from the brain through various clearance mechanisms, including enzyme-mediated degradation [71]. Therefore, mechanisms of not only production but also degradation of Aβ have been studied extensively. As a result, several candidates for Aβ degradation enzymes are proposed. Neprilysin (NEP) and insulin-degrading enzyme (IDE) are expressed in neurons as well as within the vasculature and the levels of both these enzymes are reduced in AD [71]; therefore, these enzymes have been well studied in relation to AD. Interestingly, it has been reported that *APOE* e4, which is the most-established genetic risk factor for the onset of AD and CAA, is associated with reduced levels of both enzymes [72, 73]. Furthermore, other candidates for Aβ degradation enzymes have been proposed, including endothelin-converting enzymes 1 and 2 (ECE-1 and ECE-2) [74] and angiotensin-converting enzyme (ACE) [75]. The levels of plasmin and plasminogen activators (uPA and tPA) and ECE-2 have also been shown to be reduced in the AD brain [71].

4. γ-Secretase

4.1. Overview of γ-secretase

γ-Secretase was first identified as a protease that cleaves APP within the TM domain and produces Aβ peptides [10], which is thought to be a major cause of the pathogenesis in the AD brain.

γ-Secretase is a complicated complex composed of PS, nicastrin (NCT), anterior pharynx defective-1 (Aph-1), and PS enhancer-2 protein (Pen-2) [8, 11, 12]. Two PS genes, *PS1* located on chromosome 14 [5] and *PS2* located on chromosome 1 [6, 7], have been identified by genetic linkage analyses as the genes responsible for early-onset FAD. The *PS1* and *PS2* genes encode proteins with eight or nine transmembrane domains of 467 and 448 amino acids, respectively, with about 65% sequence identity between the two proteins. Both proteins are the catalytic components of the γ-secretase complex. Although both PS1 and PS2 are expressed ubiquitously in the brain and peripheral tissues of adult mammals, PS1 expression level is significantly higher than that of PS2 [76]. NCT is a single-pass membrane protein and may recognize the substrate proteins of γ-secretase [77]. Indeed, the extracellular domain of NCT resembles an aminopeptidase, but lacks catalytic residues. Thus, this domain can interact with the free N-terminal of stubs of γ-secretase substrates generated by ectodomain shedding [78]; hence, shedding of γ-secretase substrates may be essential for the production of free N-termini of these proteins retained in the membrane to be recognized by NCT. Aph-1 may act as a scaffold during the process of γ-secretase complex assembly, and Pen-2 may act as a trigger for the proteolytic cleavage of PS in order to activate it [11, 12].

The physiological functions of γ-secretase have not been clarified. However, this protease can cleave a surprisingly large number of transmembrane proteins [79]. Indeed, more than five dozen proteins, most of which are type 1 membrane proteins, have been reported as γ-secretase substrates [21]. Interestingly, these substrates have a wide range of biological functions. Representative γ-secretase substrates are shown in Table 1.

Substrate	Function	PS or ICD function
ApoER2	Lipoprotein receptor, neuronal migration	Activates nuclear reporter
APP	Precursor to Aβ, adhesion, trophic properties, axonal transport?	Ab generation, release of ICD, Complex with Fe65/Tip60, Cell death?
APLP1/2	Cell adhesion?	Forms complex with Fe65 and Tip60
β-Catenin	Transduce Wnt signals stabilize adherens junctions	Facilitates phosphorylation
CD43	Signal transduction	Signaling molecule?
CD44	Cell adhesion	Activates TRE-mediated nuclear transcription
CSF1-R	Protein tyrosine kinase	Unknown
CXCL16 & CX3CL1	Membrane chemokine ligands	Unknown
DCC	Axon guidance, tumor suppressor	Activates nuclear reporter
Delta	Notch ligand	Transcriptional regulation
E-cadherin	Cell adhesion	Promotes disassembly of adhesion complex
ERBB4	Receptor tyrosine kinase	Regulates heregulin-induced growth inhibition
HLA-A2	MHC class I molecule	Unknown
IFN-αR2	Subunit of type I IFN-α receptor	Transcriptional regulation
Insulin receptor	Receptor tyrosine kinase	Accumulates in nucleus
IGIF-R	Receptor tyrosine kinase	Unknown
IL-1RI	Cytokine receptor	Unknown
IL-1RII	Cytokine receptor	Unknown
Jagged	Notch ligand	Modulates AP-1-mediated transcription
LAR	Receptor tyrosine phosphatase	Accumulates in nucleus
LDLR	Lipoprotein receptor	Unknown
LRP	Scavenger and signaling receptor	Activates nuclear reporter
Na channel β-subunit	Cell adhesion, an auxiliary subunit of voltage-gated Na channel	Alters cell adhesion and migration
N-cadherin	Cell adhesion	Promotes CBP degradation
Nectin-1α	Adherens junction, synapse receptor	Remodeling of cell junctions?
Notch1-4	Signaling receptor	Transcriptional regulation
NRADD	Apoptosis in neuronal cells	Modulates glycosylation/maturation of NRADD
P75NTR	Neurotrophin co-receptor, dependence receptor	Modulates p75-TrkA complex? Nuclear signaling?
γ-Protocadherin	Cell adhesion, neuronal differentiation	Regulation of gene transcription?
Syndecan-3	Cell surface proteoglycan co-receptor	Regulation of membrane-targeting of CASK
Telencephalin	Cell adhesion	Turnover of telencephalin
Tyrosinase,Tyrosinase-related protein 1/2	Pigment synthesis	Intracellular transport of Post-Golgi Tyr-containing vesicles
Vasorin	TGF-β inhibitor	Unknown

Table 1. Substrates for γ-secretase

4.2. Some γ-secretase substrates share a common proteolytic process

Fig.3 shows the proteolytic processes of Notch, APP, and CD44. There are surprising simi-larities between these processes and all of these processes follow the RIP mechanism. For ex-ample, in the canonical Notch signaling pathway, ligands bind to the extracellular domain of Notch on neighboring cells and trigger sequential proteolytic cleavage reactions (the RIP mechanism) and shedding at the S2 site by TACE or ADAM protease making the truncated Notch [44, 45]. Truncated Notch is further cleaved by γ-secretase in at least two sites within the TM domain [46-48], i.e., at the S3 site to release NICD and at the S4 site to release the remaining small peptide (Nβ). As mentioned above, NICD, which is released from the cell membrane to the cytoplasm by γ-secretase, translocates to the nucleus where its activity is expressed through binding to transcription factors.

The proteolytic process of APP is very similar to that of Notch and also follows the RIP mechanism. Cleavage of APP by α- secretase [80] or β-secretase [81] at the α- or β-site, re-spectively, within the JM region results in shedding of almost the entire extracellular do-main and generates membrane-tethered α- or β-carboxy terminal fragments (CTFs). Several zinc metalloproteinases, such as TACE and ADAM [82, 83], and the aspartyl protease BACE2 [84] can cleave APP at the α-site, while BACE1 (β-site APP cleaving enzyme) cleaves APP at the β-site [81]. Once the extracellular domain has been shed, the remaining stub is further cleaved at least twice by γ-secretase within the TM domain at γ- and ε-sites resulting in production of either non-amyloidogenic p3 peptide (in combination with α-secretase) or amyloidogenic Aβ (in combination with BACE1), respectively, and AICD [11, 12]. As dis-cussed in the next paragraph, although a large proportion of AICD is rapidly degraded in the cytoplasm, a small amount of the remaining AICD may translocate to the nucleus.

It has been reported that several other type 1 membrane proteins also follow the RIP mecha-nism and their ICDs are released from the cell membrane [13, 14, 22]. For example, as shown in Fig.3, the process of sequential proteolytic cleavage of CD44, which is important for im-mune system function, is very similar to those of Notch and APP [22]. In addition, the ICD of this protein (CD44ICD) also translocates to the nucleus (Fig.3).

As discussed here, several γ-secretase substrates follow the RIP mechanism. The ICDs of these substrates are released from the cell membrane by γ-secretase, and these ICDs translo-cate to the nucleus. These processes are very similar to those involved in Notch signaling. Therefore, the observations that the common enzyme, γ-secretase, modulates proteolysis and the turnover of possible signaling molecules led to the attractive idea, the signaling hy-pothesis, which suggests that mechanisms similar to those occurring in the Notch signaling pathway may contribute widely to γ-secretase–regulated signaling mechanisms.

Actually, Dll1, a major ligand of Notch, is cleaved sequentially by metalloproteases and γ-secretase, and ICD of Dll1 (Dll1IC) is released from the cell membrane and then translocates to the nucleus [85, 86]. Furthermore, we have shown that Dll1IC then binds to Smad 2 and 3, which are transcription factors involved in the TGF-β/activin signaling pathway, and may alter transcription of specific genes that are involved in neuronal differentiation [87]. These results suggest that Dll1 also has a signaling mechanism similar to that of Notch.

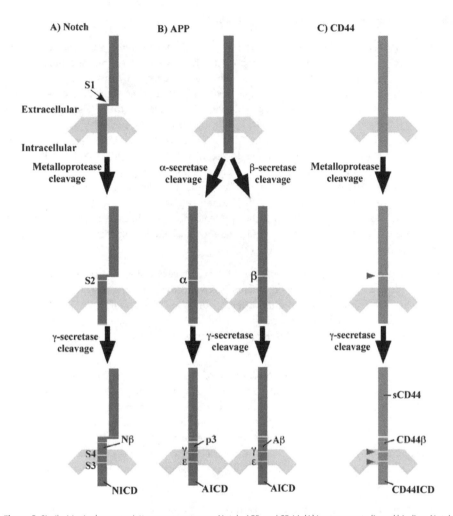

Figure 3. Similarities in the proteolytic processes among Notch, APP, and CD44. (A) In response to ligand binding, Notch undergoes shedding due to metalloprotease cleavage at the S2 site within the juxtamembrane domain. After shedding the extracellular domain, the remaining Notch stub is further cleaved by γ-secretase at S3 and S4 sites within the transmembrane domain. This sequential proteolysis produces NICD and Nβ fragment. (B) Cleavage of APP by α-secretase or β-secretase at the α-site or β-site, respectively, within the juxtamembrane domain results in shedding of almost the entire extracellular domain and generates membrane-tethered α- or β-carboxy terminal fragments (CTFs). Several zinc metalloproteinases and BACE2 can cleave APP at the α-site, while BACE1 cleaves APP at the β-site. After shedding the extracellular domain, the remaining stub is further cleaved at least twice within the transmembrane domain at γ- and ε-sites by γ-secretase, producing either p3 peptide (in combination with α-secretase) or Aβ (in combination with BACE1), respectively, and AICD. (C) Several stimuli, such as PKC activation and Ca²⁺ influx, trigger ectodomain cleavage of CD44 by a metalloprotease at the site within the juxtamembrane domain, resulting in the secretion of soluble CD44 (sCD44). After shedding the extracellular domain, the remaining CD44 stub is further cleaved by γ-secretase at two sites within the transmembrane domain. This sequential proteolysis produces the CD44ICD and CD44β, an Aβ-like peptide.

4.3. Is γ-secretase a proteasome of the membrane?

As mentioned above, more than five dozen γ-secretase substrates, most of which are type 1 membrane proteins, have been reported. This raises the simple question against the signaling hypothesis, why so many membrane proteins can transmit signals to the nucleus. In reply to this question, another possibility that γ-secretase acts as a proteasome of the membrane has been proposed [11, 12]. Indeed, as the ICDs of these substrates including AICD, which are released by γ-secretase, are rapidly degraded [24, 88], it is usually difficult to detect their ICDs by western blotting. Furthermore, ectodomain shedding seems to be constitutive for some substrates, and ligand binding has been reported to enhance only cleavage of Notch [47], Delta [87], Syndecan-3 [89], and ERBB4 [90]. In addition, much evidence supporting the signaling hypothesis was obtained in overexpression assays that differ somewhat from normal physiological conditions. Based on these observations, the proteasome hypothesis suggesting that the primary function of γ-secretase is to facilitate the selective disposal of type 1 membrane proteins has been proposed [11, 12].

Although the proteasome hypothesis for γ-secretase is reasonable and potent, there is no doubt that the certain signaling mechanisms regulated by γ-secretase, such as Notch signaling, exist. Therefore, it is likely that different functions of γ-secretases reflect their variant complexes in different combinations with multiple components, such as Aph-1, Pen2, and/or PS isoforms, with different cellular functions, such as roles in signaling or degradation.

In addition, it seems that a small proportion of ICDs of these substrates that are released by γ-secretase are sufficient for signaling mechanisms. Generally, γ-secretase substrates like APP are considerably more abundant than transcription factors, which are usually rare molecules. Although a large proportion of ICDs of these substrates are rapidly degraded, a small amount of the remaining ICDs may be sufficient for their signaling functions with small quantities of transcription factors. Thus, the majority of ICDs of these substrates may be degraded, and only a small proportion may play roles in signaling.

In relation to this issue, an attractive idea has been proposed in which a certain stimulus controls APP signaling through phosphorylation and dephosphorylation of AICD. Since AICD is stabilized [91] and translocated into the nucleus by Fe65 [26], it is thought that Fe65 is essential for the signaling function of AICD. Non-phosphorylated AICD can bind to Fe65 and form a complex; thus, this complex is stabilized and immediately translocates to the nucleus, where it mediates the expression of target genes in association with Tip60. On the other hand, phosphorylated AICD cannot bind to Fe65. Therefore, phosphorylated AICD without Fe65 cannot translocate to the nucleus. Phosphorylated AICD that remains in the cytosol is rapidly degraded by degradation enzymes such as the proteasome and/or IDE. Indeed, it has been reported that phosphorylation at Thr^{668} in the APP-695 isoform strongly inhibited binding to Fe65 [92, 93].

5. The role of AICD

5.1. Signaling functions of AICD

As mentioned above, the observations that the common enzyme, γ-secretase, modulates proteolysis and the turnover of possible signaling molecules led to the signaling hypothesis. This suggests that mechanisms similar to the Notch signaling pathway may contribute widely to γ-secretase–regulated signaling mechanisms, including APP signaling. If APP signaling exists, it may be closely related to AD.

Actually, there is accumulating evidence for the existence of APP signaling and its contribution to the onset and progression of AD. As mentioned above, the highest degree of sequence conservation within the APP homologues is found in the ICD [9, 29]. This sequence conservation suggests the functional importance of AICD, which may reflect the existence of APP signaling. In addition, several AICD-interacting proteins, which may regulate AICD stability, cellular localization, and transcriptional activity, have been identified. Based on this, several models of APP signaling have also been proposed. As mentioned above, it has been suggested that AICD recruits Fe65 proteins and translocates into the nucleus where the AICD-Fe65-Tip60 ternary complex may control transcription of target genes [27]. Furthermore, *NEP* gene expression requires binding of the AICD to its promoter [94].

Transgenic mice overexpressing both AICD and Fe65 showed abnormal activity of glycogen synthase kinase 3 beta (Gsk3b protein) [95], leading to hyperphosphorylation and aggregation of tau. This results in microtubule destabilization and the reduction of nuclear β-catenin levels causing a loss of cell-cell contact that may contribute to neurotoxicity in AD. Subsequent neurodegeneration and working memory deficits were also observed in these transgenic mice [96]. In other experiments, similar transgenic mice exhibited abnormal spiking events in their electroencephalograms and susceptibility to kainic acid-induced seizures independent of Aβ [97]. Furthermore, the function of c-Abl kinase in the transcriptional regulation of AICD was reported and c-Abl was shown to modulate AICD-dependent cellular responses, transcriptional induction, as well as apoptotic responses [98]. Interestingly, elevated AICD levels have also been reported in AD brains [96]. In addition, AICD was detected in the nucleus in injured brains [99]. Taken together, it is likely that APP signaling changes the expression of certain genes, which may cause AD pathology.

To explore APP signaling, we established several AICD-overexpressing embryonic carcinoma P19 cell lines [29]. Undifferentiated AICD-overexpressing cells retained epithelial cell-like morphology and healthy as well as control cells. Although neurons were differentiated from these cell lines after aggregation culture with all-*trans*-retinoic acid (RA) treatment, AICD expression induced neuron-specific cell death. Indeed, as shown in Fig.4, while neurons from control cells that carried the vector alone were healthy, almost all neurons differentiated from AICD-overexpressing P19 cells showed severe degeneration, becoming spherical with numerous vacuoles and detaching from the culture dishes 4 days after the induction of differentiation.

Since DNA fragmentation was detected, these cells died by apoptosis. In addition, all terminal deoxynucleotidyl transferase (TdT)-mediated deoxyuridine triphosphate (dUTP)-biotin nick end-labeling (TUNEL)-positive cells were also Tuj1-positive neurons. Taken together, we concluded that AICD could induce neuron-specific apoptosis [29]. The effects of AICD were restricted to neurons, with no effects observed in non-neural cells.

Thus, although further studies are required, these results strongly suggest that AICD plays a role in APP signaling and induces neuronal cell death, which may closely relate to the onset and progression of AD.

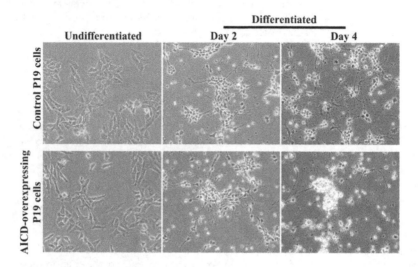

Figure 4. Expression of AICD in P19 cells induced neuronal cell death. After aggregation culture with RA, AICD-expressing P19 and control P19 cells carrying vector alone were replated and cultured for the indicated periods on dishes and allowed to differentiate. Undifferentiated AICD-expressing P19 cells retained epithelial cell-like morphology similar to control cells, while the differentiated cells became round and showed a bipolar morphology with neurite extension. Two days after replating (Day 2), all cell lines grew well and neurons with long neurites appeared. Four days after replating (Day 4), control cells still grew well as clusters and many neurons had differentiated from these cells. However, many AICD-expressing P19 cells showed severe degeneration, becoming spherical with numerous vacuoles and detached from the culture dishes.

5.2. AICD changes the gene expression profile

If APP signaling exists, AICD should change the expression of certain genes. To examine this possibility and identify the genes involved in this neuron-specific apoptosis, we performed DNA microarray analyses to evaluate the changes in the expression of more than 20,000 independent genes induced by AICD through the process of neuron-specific apoptosis [30]. Gene expression levels were deduced by hybridization signal intensity on the DNA microarrays, and the data from AICD-overexpressing cells were compared to data from control cells at the same 3 points during culture: 1) the undifferentiated state; 2) after 4 days of aggregation with RA (aggregated state); and 3) 2 days after replating (differentiated state). According to our expectations, AICD was shown to alter the expression of a great many genes; in the presence of AICD, the expression levels of 277 genes were upregulated by more than 10-fold, while those of 341 genes were downregulated to less than 10% of the original level [30].

Gene Symbol	Gene Name	Function	Relative Expression Levels (fold)		
			Undifferentiated	Aggregated	Differentiated
Non-regulated genes (housekeeping genes)					
Actb	β-actin	cytoskeleton protein	-1.2	1.2	1
Sdha	succinate dehydrogenase subunit A	electron transporter in the TCA cycle and respiratory chain	-1.1	-1.6	-1.2
Eef1a1	eukaryotic translation elongation factor-1 alpha 1	essential component for the elongation phase during protein translation	1	-1.1	1.2
Upregulated genes					
Ptprt	protein tyrosine phosphatase receptor T	protein tyrosine phosphatase that regulates STAT3 activity	906	204	116
Cpb1	carboxypeptidase B1	hydrolysis of C-terminal end of basic amino acid peptide bond	16	296	222
Nr2e1	tailless homolog	transcription factor that is essential for neural stem cell proliferation and self renewal	5.8	244	54
Myh1	myosin heavy chain 1	one of the components of the motor protein myosin	-4.2	259	-1.1
Dnahc7c	axonemal dynein heavy chain	essential for motility of cilia and flagellae	133	41	43
Alkbh3	alkylation repair homolog 3	AlkB enzyme that repairs methylation damage in DNA and RNA	69	80	43
Ctgf	connective tissue growth factor	skeletogenesis/vasculogenesis by modulating BMP, Wnt, and IGF-I signals	90	54	40
Downregulated genes					
Hes5	hairy and enhancer of split 5	transcription factor that inhibits neurogenesis	-8.7	-3039	-2515
Slc10a6	sodium-dependent organic anion transporter	transport of sulfoconjugated steroid hormones and bile acids	-145	-785	-1212
Nid1	nidogen-1	extracellular matrix linker protein	-304	-165	-507
LOC213332	analog of Na+-dependent glucose transporter 1	putative glucose transporter	-232	-325	-306
Dtx1	Deltex1	regulator of Notch signaling pathway	-30	-85	-691
Rbp4	retinol-binding protein 4	retinol transporter from the liver to extrahepatic tissues	-525	-100	-24
Col3a1	collagen type III alpha 1	extracellular matrix protein	4.1	-29	-234

Relative expression levels (fold) were estimated from the intensities of hybridization signals. Housekeeping gene expression was unaltered in AICD-overexpressing P19 and control P19 cells in all states, suggesting that these genes are not affected by AICD. These results also indicated that the observed differences in expression were not due to technical problems, such as uneven hybridization or poor RNA quality.

Table 2. Expression levels of 7 upregulated and 7 downregulated genes, as well as 3 housekeeping genes

AICD strongly induced expression of several genes, representative examples of which are listed in Table 2. For example, AICD-overexpressing P19 cells showed strong expression of the protein tyrosine phosphatase receptor T (*Ptprt*) gene at all sampling points: 906-fold, 204-fold, and 116-fold upregulation, in undifferentiated, aggregated, and differentiated states, respectively, compared with control cells. In contrast to these upregulated genes, the expression of several genes was strongly inhibited by AICD. Although *Hes5* expression was markedly increased through the process of neural differentiation, with an increase of almost 300-fold in control cells, AICD inhibited this induction. As shown in Fig.5, these results were confirmed by RT-PCR. Thus, AICD may induce both upregulation and downregulation of certain genes, suggesting that AICD plays an important role in APP signaling.

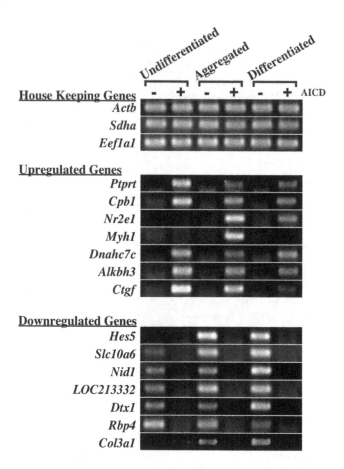

Figure 5. RT-PCR analysis of representative 7 upregulated genes and 7 downregulated genes, as well as 3 housekeeping genes, in P19 cells overexpressing AICD. The RNA samples same as applied to DNA microarray analysis was used in this RT-PCR analysis.

We performed Gene Ontology (GO) analysis and classified these upregulated and downregulated genes according to the GO terms [30]; however, we did not find genes that were significantly related to cell death among those with altered expression. Furthermore, we evaluated AICD-induced changes in the expression of genes thought to be involved in cell death in AD [30]; however, we found no significant changes in expression of these genes. Thus, it is likely that AICD does not directly induce the expression of genes involved in cell death, but the extreme dynamic changes in gene expression disrupt the homeostasis of certain neurons and thus give rise to neuron-specific cell death. Taken together, these results strongly suggest the existence of APP signaling.

6. Can Aβ clarify all aspects of the onset and progression of AD?

Autosomal dominant mutations in and around the Aβ region of the *APP* gene, which accelerate proteolytic processing, are responsible for hereditary early-onset AD [3]. The human *APP* gene is located on the long arm of chromosome 21 [53], an extra copy of which is present in individuals with Down's syndrome (trisomy 21). Patients with Down's syndrome develop AD by 40 years of age, most likely due to this gene dosage effect [4]. In addition, both PS1 and PS2, which are catalytic components of the γ-secretase complex, were identified by genetic linkage analyses as the genes responsible for FAD [5-7]. In many cases, familial diseases can provide an understanding of the sporadic ones. Therefore, both APP itself and its proteolytic processing may be responsible for the onset and progression of not only FAD but also sporadic AD.

As mentioned above, Aβ is the main constituent of amyloid plaque, which is thought to play a major role in the pathogenesis of AD; its presence is a hallmark of the AD brain. Thus, the amyloid hypothesis is generally accepted as the mechanism of the onset and progression of AD. Although an alternative hypothesis has also been proposed, which suggests that soluble Aβ oligomers rather than insoluble amyloid plaques are responsible for the onset and progression of AD because the soluble form of the Aβ oligomer is toxic for neurons [100, 101], Aβ still plays a central role in this idea.

However, several doubts have recently been raised regarding the amyloid hypothesis that Aβ plays a central role in the onset and progression of AD. One of the most critical arguments against this hypothesis is the presence of high levels of Aβ deposition in many nondemented elderly people [102], suggesting that Aβ amyloid plaques are not toxic. Indeed, transgenic mice overproducing Aβ show amyloid deposition mimicking that seen in the AD brain but do not show neurodegeneration [61]. Furthermore, several anti-Aβ drugs and vaccines have failed to show efficacy in phase III clinical trials [103]. Surprisingly, long-term follow-up studies showed unexpected problems [104]. Immunization of AD patients with the anti-Aβ vaccine, AN-1792, cleared Aβ amyloid plaques. Actually, patients with high titers of antibody against Aβ showed virtually complete plaque removal. However, there was no evidence of improvement in survival and/or cognitive function, even in patients with high titers of anti-Aβ antibody [104]. Although several interpretation for this lack of improvement have been proposed, these results lead to the idea that both soluble and insoluble forms of Aβ may not be involved in the onset and progression of AD.

Based on these observations, it has been suggested that AD may be caused by an APP-derived fragment, just not necessarily Aβ [105]. As both extracellular fragments and AICD are generated at the same time as Aβ, acceleration of proteolytic processing leads to overproduction of not only Aβ but also of both the extracellular fragments and AICD. Therefore, it is likely that the extracellular fragments and/or AICD are responsible for the onset and progression of AD. Indeed, AICD has been shown to induce neuron-specific apoptosis, which leads to AD pathology, as mentioned above.

In addition, it has also been proposed that APP is a ligand of Death receptor 6 (DR6) [106], which mediates cell death and is expressed at high levels in the human brain regions most affected by AD. APP is cleaved by β-secretase, releasing the extracellular domain (sAPPβ), which is further cleaved by an as yet unknown mechanism to release a 35 kDa N-terminal fragment (N-APP). This N-APP fragment binds DR6 to trigger neurodegeneration through caspase 6 in axons and caspase 3 in cell bodies [106]. These results suggest that N-APP may also be involved in the onset and progression of AD.

7. The model of APP signaling

Through this chapter, we discussed the possibility of the existence of APP signaling. It is likely that disorders of this signaling mechanism are involved in the onset and progression of AD. As AICD is generated at the same time as Aβ, acceleration of proteolytic processing leads to overproduction of not only Aβ but also AICD in AD brain as discussed above. Furthermore, we showed that AICD alters the expression of certain genes and induces neuron-specific apoptosis [29, 30].

If the APP signaling hypothesis is correct, certain molecules involved in APP signaling may be attractive candidates for the targets of drug discovery for treating AD. Fig.6 is a schematic model of APP signaling. As mentioned above, after cleavage within the JM domain by α- or β-secretase, AICD is released from the membrane by γ-secretase. Inhibiters for these proteases are being studied extensively.

As mentioned in section 4.3, non-phosphorylated AICD can bind to the nuclear adaptor protein Fe65 [92, 93], which is essential for translocation of AICD to the nucleus. However, phosphorylated AICD cannot bind to Fe65. These results suggest the possibility that a certain stimulus controls APP signaling through phosphorylation and dephosphorylation of AICD. It has also been shown that the majority of cell membrane-associated APP is phosphorylated specifically at Thr^{668} in neurons [107]. Therefore, phosphorylated AICD, which is released from the cell membrane to the cytoplasm by γ-secretase, cannot bind to Fe65 and thus cannot translocate to the nucleus. Phosphorylated AICD left in the cytosol is rapidly degraded, probably by the proteasome and/or IDE [88]. However, if AICD is dephosphorylated by certain phosphatase, AICD can binds to Fe65. Thus, AICD/Fe65 complexes may immediately translocate to the nucleus, where they mediate expressions of certain target genes in association with histone acetyltransferase Tip60 [27]. Besides dephosphorylation of AICD, if phosphorylation of membrane-associated APP is inhibited, non-phosphorylated AICD may also increase. Therefore, it is likely that non-phosphorylated AICD is involved in the onset and progression of AD.

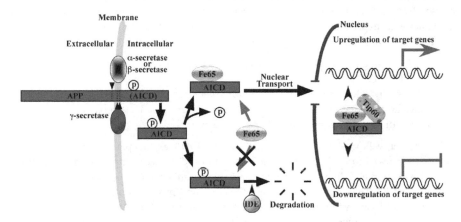

Figure 6. Model of APP signaling pathway. The majority of cell membrane-associated APP is phosphorylated within its ICD in neurons. After cleavage of JM domain by α- or β-secretase, AICD is released from the membrane by γ-secretase. Phosphorylated AICD cannot bind to the nuclear adaptor protein Fe65, which is thought to be essential for transloca-tion of AICD to the nucleus, and thus cannot translocate to the nucleus. Phosphorylated AICD left in the cytosol is rap-idly degraded, probably by the proteasome and/or insulin-degrading enzyme (IDE). On the other hand, dephosphorylated AICD binds to Fe65. Therefore, dephosphorylated AICD/Fe65 complexes immediately translocate to the nucleus, where they meidate up- and downregulation of certain target genes in association with Tip60.

In addition to these possibilities, it is also likely that AICD is ineffective in the normal brain, because almost all AICD is degraded rapidly, and APP signaling cannot be transmitted. However, both AICD and Aβ are overproduced in the AD brain compared to normal brain. Thus, although the majority of AICD is degraded, a small amount of the remaining AICD may play a role in signaling and cause neuron-specific cell death in the AD brain. In addi-tion, if the degrading activity of AICD is reduced or lost in the AD brain, APP signaling, which leads to neuron-specific cell death, may be enhanced. Thus, compounds that inhibit translocation of AICD to the nucleus will be good candidates for AD therapy. From this point of view, protein phosphatase inhibitors and chemicals that impair the interaction be-tween AICD and Fe65 may be potential ones.

8. Conclusion

γ-Secretase was first identified as a protease that cleaves APP within the transmembrane do-main and produces Aβ peptides, which are the main hallmark of AD and are thought to be involved in the pathogenesis in the AD brains. However, the physiological functions of this protease remain to be clarified.

The signaling hypothesis for γ-secretase suggesting that its primary function is to regulate the signaling of type 1 membrane proteins was proposed by analogy of Notch signaling. In the canonical Notch signaling pathway, ligands bind to the extracellular domain of Notch expressed on neighboring cells, and trigger sequential proteolytic cleavage. Finally, NICD is released from the cell membrane by γ-secretase and translocates into the nucleus where it modulates gene expression through binding to transcription factors. Thus, γ-secretase plays a central regulatory role in Notch signaling.

While APP is thought to play central roles in the onset and progression of AD, the physiological functions of this protein also have not yet been fully elucidated. However, it has been shown that AICD, which is released from the cell membrane by γ-secretase, also translocates to the nucleus and may function as a transcriptional regulator. These observations suggest the existence of a signaling mechanism similar to that of Notch.

In this chapter, we focused on the signaling aspects of APP and its pathological roles in AD. Indeed, we showed that AICD alters gene expression and induces neuron-specific apoptosis. Thus, it is likely that APP has a signaling mechanism similar to that of Notch and that APP signaling is at least partially responsible for the onset and progression of AD. If the APP signaling hypothesis is correct, several molecules involved in APP signaling may be attractive candidates for the targets of drug discovery for treating AD. Thus, extensive studies about this issue are expected.

Abbreviations

AD, Alzheimer's disease;

Aβ, amyloid-β;

APP, amyloid precursor protein;

AICD, the intracellular domain of APP;

Aph-1, anterior pharynx defective-1;

CAA, cerebral amyloid angiopathy;

Dll, Delta-like protein

Dll1IC, the intracellular domain of Dll1;

EGF, epidermal growth factor;

FAD, familial AD;

Hes, Hairy/Enhancer of split;

ICD, intracellular domain;

IDE, insulin-degrading enzyme;

JM, juxtamembrane;

KPI, Kunitz inhibitor domain;

NICD, the intracellular domain of Notch;

NCT, nicastrin;

NEP, neprilysin;

PS, presenilin;

Pen-2, PS enhancer-2 protein;

RIP, regulated intramembrane proteolysis;

RA, all-trans-retinoic acid;

TM, transmembrane;

Acknowledgments

Our works described here were supported by the grants-in-aid from the Ministry of Education, Culture, Sports, Science, and Technology of Japan. Some parts of this manuscript have been taken from our publications in Cellular and Molecular Neurobiology Volume 31, Number 6, 887-900 (2011) and in Current Psychopharmacology, Volume 1, Number 2, 155-166 (2012).

Author details

Kohzo Nakayama[1,4*], Hisashi Nagase[2], Chang-Sung Koh[3] and Takeshi Ohkawara[1]

*Address all correspondence to: kohzona@shinshu-u.ac.jp

1 Department of Anatomy, Shinshu University, School of Medicine, Matsumoto, Nagano, Japan

2 Department of Immunology and Infectious Diseases, Shinshu University, School of Medicine, Japan

3 Department of Biomedical Sciences, Shinshu University, School of Health Sciences, Matsumoto, Nagano, Japan

4 Department of Developmental and Regenerative Medicine, Mie University, Graduate School of Medicine, Tsu, Mie, Japan

References

[1] Hardy J. Amyloid, the presenilins and Alzheimer's disease. Trends Neurosci. 1997;20:154-9.

[2] Selkoe DJ. Alzheimer's disease: genes, proteins, and therapy. Physiol Rev. 2001;81:741-66.

[3] Goate A, Chartier-Harlin MC, Mullan M, Brown J, Crawford F, Fidani L, et al. Segregation of a missense mutation in the amyloid precursor protein gene with familial Alzheimer's disease. Nature. 1991;349:704-6.

[4] Lott IT, Head E. Alzheimer disease and Down syndrome: factors in pathogenesis. Neurobiol Aging. 2005;26:383-9.

[5] Sherrington R, Rogaev EI, Liang Y, Rogaeva EA, Levesque G, Ikeda M, et al. Cloning of a gene bearing missense mutations in early-onset familial Alzheimer's disease. Nature. 1995;375:754-60.

[6] Levy-Lahad E, Wasco W, Poorkaj P, Romano DM, Oshima J, Pettingell WH, et al. Candidate gene for the chromosome 1 familial Alzheimer's disease locus. Science. 1995;269:973-7.

[7] Rogaev EI, Sherrington R, Rogaeva EA, Levesque G, Ikeda M, Liang Y, et al. Familial Alzheimer's disease in kindreds with missense mutations in a gene on chromosome 1 related to the Alzheimer's disease type 3 gene. Nature. 1995;376:775-8.

[8] Iwatsubo T. The gamma-secretase complex: machinery for intramembrane proteolysis. Curr Opin Neurobiol. 2004;14:379-83.

[9] Zheng H, Koo EH. The amyloid precursor protein: beyond amyloid. Mol Neurodegener. 2006;1:5.

[10] Haass C, Selkoe DJ. Cellular processing of beta-amyloid precursor protein and the genesis of amyloid beta-peptide. Cell. 1993;75:1039-42.

[11] Kopan R, Ilagan MX. Gamma-secretase: proteasome of the membrane? Nat Rev Mol Cell Biol. 2004;5:499-504.

[12] Selkoe DJ, Wolfe MS. Presenilin: running with scissors in the membrane. Cell. 2007;131:215-21.

[13] Nakayama K, Nagase H, Hiratochi M, Koh CS, Ohkawara T. Similar mechanisms regulated by gamma-secretase are involved in both directions of the bi-directional Notch-Delta signaling pathway as well as play a potential role in signaling events involving type 1 transmembrane proteins. Curr Stem Cell Res Ther. 2008;3:288-302.

[14] Nakayama K, Nagase H, Koh CS, Ohkawara T. gamma-Secretase-Regulated Mechanisms Similar to Notch Signaling May Play a Role in Signaling Events, Including

APP Signaling, Which Leads to Alzheimer's Disease. Cell Mol Neurobiol. 2011;31:887-900.

[15] Nakayama K, Nagase H, Koh C-S, Ohkawara T. Gamma-Secretase-Regulated Signaling: Notch, APP, and Alzheimer's Disease. Current Psychopharmacology. 2012;1:155-66.

[16] Artavanis-Tsakonas S, Matsuno K, Fortini ME. Notch signaling. Science. 1995;268:225-32.

[17] Lewis J. Notch signalling and the control of cell fate choices in vertebrates. Semin Cell Dev Biol. 1998;9:583-9.

[18] Bolos V, Grego-Bessa J, de la Pompa JL. Notch signaling in development and cancer. Endocr Rev. 2007;28:339-63.

[19] Artavanis-Tsakonas S, Rand MD, Lake RJ. Notch signaling: cell fate control and signal integration in development. Science. 1999;284:770-6.

[20] Justice NJ, Jan YN. Variations on the Notch pathway in neural development. Curr Opin Neurobiol. 2002;12:64-70.

[21] McCarthy JV, Twomey C, Wujek P. Presenilin-dependent regulated intramembrane proteolysis and gamma-secretase activity. Cell Mol Life Sci. 2009;66:1534-55.

[22] Nagase H, Koh CS, Nakayama K. gamma-Secretase-regulated signaling pathways, such as notch signaling, mediate the differentiation of hematopoietic stem cells, development of the immune system, and peripheral immune responses. Curr Stem Cell Res Ther. 2011;6:131-41.

[23] Koo EH, Kopan R. Potential role of presenilin-regulated signaling pathways in sporadic neurodegeneration. Nat Med. 2004;10 Suppl:S26-33.

[24] Cupers P, Orlans I, Craessaerts K, Annaert W, De Strooper B. The amyloid precursor protein (APP)-cytoplasmic fragment generated by gamma-secretase is rapidly degraded but distributes partially in a nuclear fraction of neurones in culture. Journal of neurochemistry. 2001;78:1168-78.

[25] Gao Y, Pimplikar SW. The gamma -secretase-cleaved C-terminal fragment of amyloid precursor protein mediates signaling to the nucleus. Proc Natl Acad Sci U S A. 2001;98:14979-84.

[26] Kimberly WT, Zheng JB, Guenette SY, Selkoe DJ. The intracellular domain of the beta-amyloid precursor protein is stabilized by Fe65 and translocates to the nucleus in a notch-like manner. The Journal of biological chemistry. 2001;276:40288-92.

[27] Cao X, Sudhof TC. A transcriptionally [correction of transcriptively] active complex of APP with Fe65 and histone acetyltransferase Tip60. Science. 2001;293:115-20.

[28] Guenette SY. A role for APP in motility and transcription? Trends in pharmacological sciences. 2002;23:203-5; discussion 5-6.

[29] Nakayama K, Ohkawara T, Hiratochi M, Koh CS, Nagase H. The intracellular do-
      main of amyloid precursor protein induces neuron-specific apoptosis. Neurosci Lett.
      2008;444:127-31.

[30] Ohkawara T, Nagase H, Koh CS, Nakayama K. The amyloid precursor protein intra-
      cellular domain alters gene expression and induces neuron-specific apoptosis. Gene.
      2011;475:1-9.

[31] Wharton KA, Johansen KM, Xu T, Artavanis-Tsakonas S. Nucleotide sequence from
      the neurogenic locus notch implies a gene product that shares homology with pro-
      teins containing EGF-like repeats. Cell. 1985;43:567-81.

[32] Rebay I, Fleming RJ, Fehon RG, Cherbas L, Cherbas P, Artavanis-Tsakonas S. Specific
      EGF repeats of Notch mediate interactions with Delta and Serrate: implications for
      Notch as a multifunctional receptor. Cell. 1991;67:687-99.

[33] Logeat F, Bessia C, Brou C, LeBail O, Jarriault S, Seidah NG, et al. The Notch1 recep-
      tor is cleaved constitutively by a furin-like convertase. Proc Natl Acad Sci U S A.
      1998;95:8108-12.

[34] Kopczynski CC, Alton AK, Fechtel K, Kooh PJ, Muskavitch MA. Delta, a Drosophila
      neurogenic gene, is transcriptionally complex and encodes a protein related to blood
      coagulation factors and epidermal growth factor of vertebrates. Genes Dev.
      1988;2:1723-35.

[35] Fleming RJ, Scottgale TN, Diederich RJ, Artavanis-Tsakonas S. The gene Serrate enc-
      odes a putative EGF-like transmembrane protein essential for proper ectodermal de-
      velopment in Drosophila melanogaster. Genes Dev. 1990;4:2188-201.

[36] Bettenhausen B, Hrabe de Angelis M, Simon D, Guenet JL, Gossler A. Transient and
      restricted expression during mouse embryogenesis of Dll1, a murine gene closely re-
      lated to Drosophila Delta. Development. 1995;121:2407-18.

[37] Dunwoodie SL, Henrique D, Harrison SM, Beddington RS. Mouse Dll3: a novel di-
      vergent Delta gene which may complement the function of other Delta homologues
      during   early   pattern   formation   in   the   mouse   embryo.   Development.
      1997;124:3065-76.

[38] Shutter JR, Scully S, Fan W, Richards WG, Kitajewski J, Deblandre GA, et al. Dll4, a
      novel Notch ligand expressed in arterial endothelium. Genes Dev. 2000;14:1313-8.

[39] Lindsell CE, Shawber CJ, Boulter J, Weinmaster G. Jagged: a mammalian ligand that
      activates Notch1. Cell. 1995;80:909-17.

[40] Shawber C, Boulter J, Lindsell CE, Weinmaster G. Jagged2: a serrate-like gene ex-
      pressed during rat embryogenesis. Dev Biol. 1996;180:370-6.

[41] Tax FE, Yeargers JJ, Thomas JH. Sequence of C. elegans lag-2 reveals a cell-signalling
      domain shared with Delta and Serrate of Drosophila. Nature. 1994;368:150-4.

[42] Henderson ST, Gao D, Christensen S, Kimble J. Functional domains of LAG-2, a putative signaling ligand for LIN-12 and GLP-1 receptors in Caenorhabditis elegans. Mol Biol Cell. 1997;8:1751-62.

[43] Brown MS, Ye J, Rawson RB, Goldstein JL. Regulated intramembrane proteolysis: a control mechanism conserved from bacteria to humans. Cell. 2000;100:391-8.

[44] Pan D, Rubin GM. Kuzbanian controls proteolytic processing of Notch and mediates lateral inhibition during Drosophila and vertebrate neurogenesis. Cell. 1997;90:271-80.

[45] Brou C, Logeat F, Gupta N, Bessia C, LeBail O, Doedens JR, et al. A novel proteolytic cleavage involved in Notch signaling: the role of the disintegrin-metalloprotease TACE. Mol Cell. 2000;5:207-16.

[46] Kopan R, Schroeter EH, Weintraub H, Nye JS. Signal transduction by activated mNotch: importance of proteolytic processing and its regulation by the extracellular domain. Proc Natl Acad Sci U S A. 1996;93:1683-8.

[47] Schroeter EH, Kisslinger JA, Kopan R. Notch-1 signalling requires ligand-induced proteolytic release of intracellular domain. Nature. 1998;393:382-6.

[48] Okochi M, Steiner H, Fukumori A, Tanii H, Tomita T, Tanaka T, et al. Presenilins mediate a dual intramembranous gamma-secretase cleavage of Notch-1. EMBO J. 2002;21:5408-16.

[49] Roehl H, Bosenberg M, Blelloch R, Kimble J. Roles of the RAM and ANK domains in signaling by the C. elegans GLP-1 receptor. EMBO J. 1996;15:7002-12.

[50] Wu L, Aster JC, Blacklow SC, Lake R, Artavanis-Tsakonas S, Griffin JD. MAML1, a human homologue of Drosophila mastermind, is a transcriptional co-activator for NOTCH receptors. Nat Genet. 2000;26:484-9.

[51] Wallberg AE, Pedersen K, Lendahl U, Roeder RG. p300 and PCAF act cooperatively to mediate transcriptional activation from chromatin templates by notch intracellular domains in vitro. Mol Cell Biol. 2002;22:7812-9.

[52] Kageyama R, Ohtsuka T, Kobayashi T. The Hes gene family: repressors and oscillators that orchestrate embryogenesis. Development. 2007;134:1243-51.

[53] Kang J, Lemaire HG, Unterbeck A, Salbaum JM, Masters CL, Grzeschik KH, et al. The precursor of Alzheimer's disease amyloid A4 protein resembles a cell-surface receptor. Nature. 1987;325:733-6.

[54] Yoshikai S, Sasaki H, Doh-ura K, Furuya H, Sakaki Y. Genomic organization of the human amyloid beta-protein precursor gene. Gene. 1990;87:257-63.

[55] Sisodia SS, Koo EH, Hoffman PN, Perry G, Price DL. Identification and transport of full-length amyloid precursor proteins in rat peripheral nervous system. J Neurosci. 1993;13:3136-42.

[56] Coulson EJ, Paliga K, Beyreuther K, Masters CL. What the evolution of the amyloid protein precursor supergene family tells us about its function. Neurochem Int. 2000;36:175-84.

[57] Dahms SO, Hoefgen S, Roeser D, Schlott B, Guhrs KH, Than ME. Structure and biochemical analysis of the heparin-induced E1 dimer of the amyloid precursor protein. Proc Natl Acad Sci U S A.107:5381-6.

[58] Wang Y, Ha Y. The X-ray structure of an antiparallel dimer of the human amyloid precursor protein E2 domain. Mol Cell. 2004;15:343-53.

[59] Hung AY, Koo EH, Haass C, Selkoe DJ. Increased expression of beta-amyloid precursor protein during neuronal differentiation is not accompanied by secretory cleavage. Proc Natl Acad Sci U S A. 1992;89:9439-43.

[60] Leyssen M, Ayaz D, Hebert SS, Reeve S, De Strooper B, Hassan BA. Amyloid precursor protein promotes post-developmental neurite arborization in the Drosophila brain. EMBO J. 2005;24:2944-55.

[61] McGowan E, editor. Alzheimer animal models: models of Abeta deposition in transgenic mice. Basel: ISN Neuropath Press; 2003.

[62] Soba P, Eggert S, Wagner K, Zentgraf H, Siehl K, Kreger S, et al. Homo- and heterodimerization of APP family members promotes intercellular adhesion. EMBO J. 2005;24:3624-34.

[63] Ho A, Sudhof TC. Binding of F-spondin to amyloid-beta precursor protein: a candidate amyloid-beta precursor protein ligand that modulates amyloid-beta precursor protein cleavage. Proc Natl Acad Sci U S A. 2004;101:2548-53.

[64] Park JH, Gimbel DA, GrandPre T, Lee JK, Kim JE, Li W, et al. Alzheimer precursor protein interaction with the Nogo-66 receptor reduces amyloid-beta plaque deposition. J Neurosci. 2006;26:1386-95.

[65] Lorenzo A, Yuan M, Zhang Z, Paganetti PA, Sturchler-Pierrat C, Staufenbiel M, et al. Amyloid beta interacts with the amyloid precursor protein: a potential toxic mechanism in Alzheimer's disease. Nat Neurosci. 2000;3:460-4.

[66] Hardy J, Selkoe DJ. The amyloid hypothesis of Alzheimer's disease: progress and problems on the road to therapeutics. Science. 2002;297:353-6.

[67] Jarrett JT, Berger EP, Lansbury PT, Jr. The carboxy terminus of the beta amyloid protein is critical for the seeding of amyloid formation: implications for the pathogenesis of Alzheimer's disease. Biochemistry. 1993;32:4693-7.

[68] Lippa CF, Smith TW, Swearer JM. Alzheimer's disease and Lewy body disease: a comparative clinicopathological study. Ann Neurol. 1994;35:81-8.

[69] Askanas V, Engel WK, Alvarez RB. Light and electron microscopic localization of beta-amyloid protein in muscle biopsies of patients with inclusion-body myositis. Am J Pathol. 1992;141:31-6.

[70] Haan J, Roos RA. Amyloid in central nervous system disease. Clin Neurol Neurosurg. 1990;92:305-10.

[71] Miners JS, Baig S, Palmer J, Palmer LE, Kehoe PG, Love S. Abeta-degrading enzymes in Alzheimer's disease. Brain Pathol. 2008;18:240-52.

[72] Miners JS, Van Helmond Z, Chalmers K, Wilcock G, Love S, Kehoe PG. Decreased expression and activity of neprilysin in Alzheimer disease are associated with cerebral amyloid angiopathy. J Neuropathol Exp Neurol. 2006;65:1012-21.

[73] Cook DG, Leverenz JB, McMillan PJ, Kulstad JJ, Ericksen S, Roth RA, et al. Reduced hippocampal insulin-degrading enzyme in late-onset Alzheimer's disease is associated with the apolipoprotein E-epsilon4 allele. Am J Pathol. 2003;162:313-9.

[74] Turner AJ, Murphy LJ. Molecular pharmacology of endothelin converting enzymes. Biochem Pharmacol. 1996;51:91-102.

[75] Erdos EG, Skidgel RA. The angiotensin I-converting enzyme. Lab Invest. 1987;56:345-8.

[76] Lee MK, Slunt HH, Martin LJ, Thinakaran G, Kim G, Gandy SE, et al. Expression of presenilin 1 and 2 (PS1 and PS2) in human and murine tissues. J Neurosci. 1996;16:7513-25.

[77] Yu G, Nishimura M, Arawaka S, Levitan D, Zhang L, Tandon A, et al. Nicastrin modulates presenilin-mediated notch/glp-1 signal transduction and betaAPP processing. Nature. 2000;407:48-54.

[78] Shah S, Lee SF, Tabuchi K, Hao YH, Yu C, LaPlant Q, et al. Nicastrin functions as a gamma-secretase-substrate receptor. Cell. 2005;122:435-47.

[79] Struhl G, Adachi A. Requirements for presenilin-dependent cleavage of notch and other transmembrane proteins. Mol Cell. 2000;6:625-36.

[80] Esch FS, Keim PS, Beattie EC, Blacher RW, Culwell AR, Oltersdorf T, et al. Cleavage of amyloid beta peptide during constitutive processing of its precursor. Science. 1990;248:1122-4.

[81] Vassar R, Bennett BD, Babu-Khan S, Kahn S, Mendiaz EA, Denis P, et al. Beta-secretase cleavage of Alzheimer's amyloid precursor protein by the transmembrane aspartic protease BACE. Science. 1999;286:735-41.

[82] Buxbaum JD, Liu KN, Luo Y, Slack JL, Stocking KL, Peschon JJ, et al. Evidence that tumor necrosis factor alpha converting enzyme is involved in regulated alpha-secretase cleavage of the Alzheimer amyloid protein precursor. The Journal of biological chemistry. 1998;273:27765-7.

[83] Lammich S, Kojro E, Postina R, Gilbert S, Pfeiffer R, Jasionowski M, et al. Constitutive and regulated alpha-secretase cleavage of Alzheimer's amyloid precursor protein by a disintegrin metalloprotease. Proc Natl Acad Sci U S A. 1999;96:3922-7.

[84] Farzan M, Schnitzler CE, Vasilieva N, Leung D, Choe H. BACE2, a beta -secretase ho-molog, cleaves at the beta site and within the amyloid-beta region of the amyloid-beta precursor protein. Proc Natl Acad Sci U S A. 2000;97:9712-7.

[85] Ikeuchi T, Sisodia SS. The Notch ligands, Delta1 and Jagged2, are substrates for pre-senilin-dependent "gamma-secretase" cleavage. The Journal of biological chemistry. 2003;278:7751-4.

[86] LaVoie MJ, Selkoe DJ. The Notch ligands, Jagged and Delta, are sequentially process-ed by alpha-secretase and presenilin/gamma-secretase and release signaling frag-ments. The Journal of biological chemistry. 2003;278:34427-37.

[87] Hiratochi M, Nagase H, Kuramochi Y, Koh CS, Ohkawara T, Nakayama K. The Delta intracellular domain mediates TGF-beta/Activin signaling through binding to Smads and has an important bi-directional function in the Notch-Delta signaling pathway. Nucleic Acids Res. 2007;35:912-22.

[88] Edbauer D, Willem M, Lammich S, Steiner H, Haass C. Insulin-degrading enzyme rapidly removes the beta-amyloid precursor protein intracellular domain (AICD). The Journal of biological chemistry. 2002;277:13389-93.

[89] Schulz JG, Annaert W, Vandekerckhove J, Zimmermann P, De Strooper B, David G. Syndecan 3 intramembrane proteolysis is presenilin/gamma-secretase-dependent and modulates cytosolic signaling. The Journal of biological chemistry. 2003;278:48651-7.

[90] Ni CY, Murphy MP, Golde TE, Carpenter G. gamma -Secretase cleavage and nuclear localization of ErbB-4 receptor tyrosine kinase. Science. 2001;294:2179-81.

[91] Buoso E, Lanni C, Schettini G, Govoni S, Racchi M. beta-Amyloid precursor protein metabolism: focus on the functions and degradation of its intracellular domain. Phar-macol Res. 2011;62:308-17.

[92] Ando K, Iijima KI, Elliott JI, Kirino Y, Suzuki T. Phosphorylation-dependent regula-tion of the interaction of amyloid precursor protein with Fe65 affects the production of beta-amyloid. The Journal of biological chemistry. [Research Support, Non-U.S. Gov't]. 2001;276:40353-61.

[93] Kimberly WT, Zheng JB, Town T, Flavell RA, Selkoe DJ. Physiological regulation of the beta-amyloid precursor protein signaling domain by c-Jun N-terminal kinase JNK3 during neuronal differentiation. J Neurosci. 2005;25:5533-43.

[94] Belyaev ND, Nalivaeva NN, Makova NZ, Turner AJ. Neprilysin gene expression re-quires binding of the amyloid precursor protein intracellular domain to its promoter: implications for Alzheimer disease. EMBO reports. [Research Support, Non-U.S. Gov't]. 2009;10:94-100.

[95] Ryan KA, Pimplikar SW. Activation of GSK-3 and phosphorylation of CRMP2 in transgenic mice expressing APP intracellular domain. J Cell Biol. 2005;171:327-35.

[96] Ghosal K, Vogt DL, Liang M, Shen Y, Lamb BT, Pimplikar SW. Alzheimer's disease-like pathological features in transgenic mice expressing the APP intracellular domain. Proc Natl Acad Sci U S A. 2009;106:18367-72.

[97] Vogt DL, Thomas D, Galvan V, Bredesen DE, Lamb BT, Pimplikar SW. Abnormal neuronal networks and seizure susceptibility in mice overexpressing the APP intracellular domain. Neurobiol Aging. 2009.

[98] Vazquez MC, Vargas LM, Inestrosa NC, Alvarez AR. c-Abl modulates AICD dependent cellular responses: transcriptional induction and apoptosis. J Cell Physiol. 2009;220:136-43.

[99] DeGiorgio LA, DeGiorgio N, Milner TA, Conti B, Volpe BT. Neurotoxic APP C-terminal and beta-amyloid domains colocalize in the nuclei of substantia nigra pars reticulata neurons undergoing delayed degeneration. Brain research. [Research Support, Non-U.S. Gov't Research Support, U.S. Gov't, P.H.S.]. 2000;874:137-46.

[100] Klein WL, Krafft GA, Finch CE. Targeting small Abeta oligomers: the solution to an Alzheimer's disease conundrum? Trends Neurosci. 2001;24:219-24.

[101] Selkoe DJ. Alzheimer's disease is a synaptic failure. Science. 2002;298:789-91.

[102] Terry RD KR, Bick KL, Sisodia SS. Alzheimer's disease. Philadelphia: Lippincott, Williams & Wilkins; 1999.

[103] Abbot A. The plaque plan. Nature. 2008;456:161-4.

[104] Holmes C, Boche D, Wilkinson D, Yadegarfar G, Hopkins V, Bayer A, et al. Long-term effects of Abeta42 immunisation in Alzheimer's disease: follow-up of a randomised, placebo-controlled phase I trial. Lancet. [Research Support, Non-U.S. Gov't]. 2008;372:216-23.

[105] Schnabel J. Alzheimer's theory makes a splash. Nature. 2009;459:310.

[106] Nikolaev A, McLaughlin T, O'Leary DD, Tessier-Lavigne M. APP binds DR6 to trigger axon pruning and neuron death via distinct caspases. Nature. 2009;457:981-9.

[107] Iijima K, Ando K, Takeda S, Satoh Y, Seki T, Itohara S, et al. Neuron-specific phosphorylation of Alzheimer's beta-amyloid precursor protein by cyclin-dependent kinase 5. Journal of neurochemistry. [Research Support, Non-U.S. Gov'tResearch Support, U.S. Gov't, P.H.S.]. 2000;75:1085-91.

Chapter 5

Pin1 Protects Against Alzheimer's Disease: One Goal, Multiple Mechanisms

Lucia Pastorino, Asami Kondo, Xiao Zhen Zhou and Kun Ping Lu

Additional information is available at the end of the chapter

1. Introduction

1.1. Plaque and tangle pathology in AD

Alzheimer's disease (AD] is the most common form of dementia, and it accounts for more than 60% of all cases of dementia. Although many factors may increase the risk for AD, the only cause so far known is aging [1]. Most of the cases are sporadic, as only less than 0.1% of the cases occur because of inherited mutations on genes directly involved in the disease (familial AD, FAD] [2].

AD is caused by progressive and irreversible neurodegeneration. At the moment, there is no cure for AD. Therapies available are only aimed at lessening the progression of the cognitive decline and neurodegeneration and do not target pathways directly causative of the disease [3]. These include the acetylcholinesterase inhibitors (Aricept] [4] or inhibitors of the glutamatergic NMDA receptor (Namenda] [5] and were shown to be mostly effective when administered at early stages [6-8]. However, a proper diagnostic approach able to identify AD early in the development is still missing, and this reduces the efficacy of the treatments available. Therefore, there is the need to develop both diagnostic tools able to detect early stages of the disease, and to generate effective treatments targeting the early pathogenic events in AD. This is becoming increasingly important also considering that the population affected by AD will dramatically increase in the years to come. Numbers are in fact dramatic: 10 million baby boomers may develop AD within the next 10-20 years [9]. Currently, in the United States alone there are more than 5 million AD patients, and the costs to the US government exceeds the 200 billion/year.These numbers are expected to quadruple in the next 40 years, causing unsustainable costs for the care of these patients and their caregivers, who could not receive support and care and would then have to face undignified life conditions.

Studying the molecular mechanisms responsible for the neurodegeneration in AD can help identify new effective therapeutic targets. Two main pathways are identified in AD. They involve two proteins, the amyloid precursor protein APP and the microtubule-associated protein tau, as they are responsible for the formation of the two characteristic lesions, the extracellular plaques and the intracellular neurofibrillary tangles (NFTs], respectively [10, 11]. Both plaques and tangles are considered causative of the disease; they deposit following the progression of the disease, and they could contribute to alter neuronal morphology leading to neuronal death [12-16].

The origin and composition of plaques and tangles are quite different. Plaques are forms of aggregated, fibrillar material called amyloid, insoluble fibrous protein aggregations organized in β-sheet strands that deposits in the outer part of the brain [17-19]. Their core is mainly composed of Abeta (beta-amyloid], a peptide of small molecular weight deriving from APP, which tends to form small size aggregates called oligomers with known toxic properties [20]. Oligomers are found intracellularly, but can be secreted to the extracellular space, where they will aggregate into larger structures called fibrils, forming the core of the plaque [18, 21, 22].

Similarly, tangles are formed by insoluble structures organized into fibrils, the pair helical filaments (PHFs], which eventually organize and aggregate into larger structures, the tangles [19]. The main component is hyperphosphorylated protein tau, which in this form becomes insoluble and tends to form aggregates [13, 23].

The biological functions of APP and tau are very different [13, 24], but during the disease both the beta amyloid product and the hyperphosphorylated tau become toxic to the neuron, causing neurodegeneration. However, the mechanisms by which tau and Abeta may be toxic differ. In fact, as a microtubule stabilizing protein, tau can become toxic to the cytoskeleton when hyperphosphorylated, as in this form it would detach from the microtubules destabilizing them. Hyperphosphorylated tau would also tend to aggregate into NFTs, impairing cellular functions [23]. As to the plaques, their mechanism of toxicity is still under debate. Although they cause the formation of dystrophic neuritis [18], it is still unclear whether they are really toxic or rather protecting, by sequestering Abeta oligomers from the environment. In facts, Abeta is sequestered from the extracellular space to form the plaque [25]. Indeed, oligomers are considered toxic: they form early in the pathology [26], associate with impaired cognitive functions in mice [27] and in AD patients [28], and impair neurotransmission [29-33]. Therefore, identifying the pathways that lead to both increased Abeta production and/or tau hyperphosphorylation and also regulate their aggregation into organized insoluble structure may dramatically help find a cure to treat AD.

1.2. Pin1–regulated protein isomerization as a mechanism to control tangle and plaque pathologies

Protein phosphorylation seems to be a common feature of both plaque and tangle pathologies. In fact, changes in the levels of phosphorylated APP seems to influence APP function and toxicity in the pathology, as increased phosphorylation of APP at specific domains positively regulates Abeta production [34-36]. Of note, both APP and tau can be phosphorylated by the same kinases, such as cdc2, CDK5 and GSK3, and such kinases seem to be particularly active during the disease [23, 37-40]. Hence, the identification of molecular pathways that can control non physiologic phosphorylation of both tau and APP in the disease could help identify targets to tackle at the same time both tangle and plaque pathologies.

We found that the enzyme Pin1 protects from both tangle and Abeta pathology, since a genetically modified animal model lacking Pin1 (Pin1KO] developed age-dependent tauopathy and was characterized by increased production of Abeta, deposited in form of intracellular aggregates [41, 42]. This seems to be due to the capability of Pin1 to regulate the conformation of cis and trans isomers of both phosphorylated tau and APP, as shown using conformation specific antibodies for tau, and by means of NMR.

Pin1 (Protein interacting with NIMA (never in mitosis A]-1] is a prolyl isomerase, which regulates the function of phosphorylated protein substrates by regulating their cis/trans isomerization [43, 44]. Pin1 belongs to the family of PPIase (peptidyl prolyl cis trans isomerase], enzymes that are evolutionary conserved. Unlike other PPIases, Pin1 specifically regulates the conformation of substrates phosphorylated at specific serine or threonine residues preceding a proline (S/T-P motifs] [45-47]. The stereochemistry of Proline allows the protein to undergo two different conformations (cis and trans], which could be determined by the presence of a phospho group on the S or T residue [43, 48]. Since Proline-directed phosphorylation regulates key cellular mechanisms, by maintaining the equilibrium between the two conformations, Pin1 may dramatically contribute to the maintenance of vital cellular functions.

The structure of Pin1 consists of two domains, an N-terminal WW domain comprised of the first 40 aminoacids which is responsible for Pin1 binding to its substrates, and a larger PPIase domain that spans the remaining part of the protein and catalyzes the substrate's isomerization [49]. Of note, although mostly in the nucleus, Pin1 subcellular localization is driven by the presence of its substrates [50], to extranuclear compartments, with obvious expression in the plasma membrane, cytosol and cytosolic organelles involved in endocytosis [41, 51]. The ubiquitous expression of Pin1 allows the protein to control the isomerization of multiple substrates in different cellular compartments, including cytosolic proteins like NF-KappaB [52], p53 [53], beta-catenin [54], IRAK1 [55] and others [46], or protein that localize at different compartments like APP [41, 51] and tau [42, 56]. This determines a crucial role for Pin1 in controlling the physiological activity of proteins involved in diverse functions, such as protein transcription and stability, and protein interaction, by regulating the aforementioned substrates [43].

Notably, Pin1 function is highly regulated and its aberration affects Pin1's ability to isomerize its substrates with consequences on their function, contributing to an increasing number of pathological conditions, including Alzheimer's disease, cancer and immunologic disorders and aging. Lack of Pin1 function was found to impair immune responses in Pin1KO animal models [55], due to lack of activation of IRAK1, which is involved in the regulation of the TLR signaling [57]. In cancer, Pin1 levels are increased due to transcriptional activation and loss of inhibitory phosphorylation and other mechanisms [45, 58]. This leads to up-regulated isomerization of substrates involved in hyperproliferative processes, activating two dozens of oncogenes and inactivating a dozen of tumor suppressors [46, 59, 60]. On the contrary, in AD brain Pin1 activity is reduced due to decreased protein level and to oxidation [56, 61, 62]. Some genetic polymorphisms on the Pin1 gene were found to associate with forms of late onset AD [63-65]. Interestingly, a polymorphism that associated with increased Pin1 levels by regulating AP-4 mediated transcription, was found to be protective as it correlates with delayed disease onset in a Chinese cohort [66]. In AD, the changes in Pin1 levels and activity prevent from an effective isomerization of the phosphorylated APP and tau [41, 56]. As a consequence, the equilibrium between the cis and trans conformation is not maintained and the proteins exist in the pathogenic cis conformation: APP will generate more Abeta and tau will lose normal microtubule function and become toxic, leading to both plaque and tangle pathologies.

In this book chapter we will discuss findings from our and other labs that point to a crucial role of Pin1 in protecting against AD by regulating diverse cellular pathways using multiple mechanisms. We will specifically highlight how Pin1 regulates protein conformation of APP and tau to control APP trafficking, APP stability and Abeta production as well as tau phosphorylation, microtubule function, stabilization and aggregation in vivo and in vitro. We will also emphasize the importance of Pin1-mediated regulation of APP and tau conformation as a modulator of pathogenic mechanisms that might occur early in the development of the disease. Finally, we will also discuss how Pin1 is emerging as a novel diagnostic and therapeutic tool for early intervention to tackle both tau and Abeta pathologies in AD.

2. Pin1 as a crucial regulator of APP trafficking and stabilization to protect from Abeta pathology in AD

Although both tau and Abeta pathologies define AD, only Abeta is the characteristic feature that distinguishes AD from other forms of dementia. In fact, only the presence of plaques containing Abeta peptide allows a definite AD diagnosis [10,67-69], whereas the presence of PHF alone could be related also to other forms of tauopathies, like FTPD, Pick disease and others [13]. The specificity of Abeta pathology to AD makes of Abeta and its precursor APP ideal therapeutic targets. Here we will review the role of APP in AD, the molecular mechanisms that regulate Abeta formation, focusing on the role of Pin1 as a post-phosphorylative event to regulate both APP intracellular localization and trafficking, and also turnover, preventing Abeta formation. These topics are of particular relevance for the understanding of the mechanisms underlying Abeta production in AD. In fact, the intracellular localization of APP will determine whether APP will be toxic influencing the production of beta-amyloid peptides. Moreover, impaired APP turnover will cause APP stabilization, which will lead to increased levels of both APP and beta-amyloid peptides. This phenomenon is particularly consistent with pathologies associated with higher levels of APP and development of AD, such as Down syndrome.

2.1. APP trafficking and processing pathways

APP is a type 1 transmembrane protein that is ubiquitously expressed. APP is characterized by a long extracellular domain, a short transmembrane domain and a small intracellular domain that regulates APP phosphorylation and trafficking [68, 70]. The domain that contains the sequence for Abeta spans a region of approximately 40 aminoacids across the N-terminal portion of the trasmembrane domain [71]. Three isoforms of APP exists characterized by different molecular weight, the result of alternative RNA splicing, APP751, APP750 and APP695 [72]. Since the splicing occurs in the most N-terminal region of the protein, all the three isoforms express the domains for both Abeta and the intracellular domain [72]. APP isoforms may be differently expressed in the various organs. AP770 is for example mostly present in the heart and in peripheral cells, whereas APP695 is the only form expressed in the brain and therefore linked to Abeta generation in AD [72]. For this reason, the APP isoform considered in AD studies is APP695, and the numbering of the aminoacids follows this sequence.

Within the cell, APP localization is not limited to a single part, as it undergoes trafficking through different compartments. Upon synthesis in the ER, APP travels through the Golgi compartment where it undergoes glycosylation, to finally reach the plasma membrane. It eventually will recycle to the Golgi, following internalization from the plasma membrane and trafficking through the endosomal pathway [70, 73, 74]. Of note, the significance of APP physiological function may depend on the compartment where APP localizes during the life of the cell. In fact, depending on whether APP is retained at the plasma membrane or it is internalized to the endosomes, it will generate different metabolites with diverse function, either neurotrophic and therefore protective from AD, or toxic. More in details, at the plasma membrane APP will undergo a processing pathway called non-amyloidogenic [75, 76], in which metalloproteases of the ADAMs family and others (ADAM10, ADAM17 and TACE [77-81]], called alpha secretase, will cleave APP in the middle of the sequence for Abeta, generating the extracellular stub alphaAPPs with known neurotrophic properties [82], and a C-terminal stub called C83. C83 will be further cleaved in the late endosomes by a complex of four proteins called gamma-secretase, to generate a small fragment called p3 with no amyloidogenic properties. This pathway is called non-amyloidogenic, as it prevents the formation of intact Abeta peptides. The amount of APP at the plasma membrane that does not undergo alpha-secretase cleavage will internalize in the cell through the endocytic pathway [70, 73, 74]. This occurs thanks to the binding of proteins such as Fe65 to the 682YNPTY687 motif at the intracellular, C-terminal domain of APP [83-85]. Once in the early endosomes, full length APP is cleaved by BACE or beta secretase [86, 87], an aspartyl protease that cuts APP at the beginning of the sequence for Abeta. Such cleavage generates a soluble stub called betaAPPs with known apoptotic properties in the neuron [88], and a C-terminal stub called C99 which still contains the intact sequence for Abeta. C99 will traffic to the late endosomes, where it will be cleaved by gamma-secretase to generate intact Abeta [17, 89]. This pathway is called amyloidogenic as it produces Abeta peptides, and is increased in AD [90, 91].

It is clear that the intracellular localization of APP will determine whether APP will be amyloidogenic or not. Therefore, any mechanism that may help APP stay retained at the plasma membrane will protect from Abeta production and AD, whereas those that help APP internalize to the endosomes will favor the amyloidogenic processing and Abeta formation.

2.2. APP phosphorylation and conformation to regulate APP processing

One such mechanism is APP phosphorylation. In fact, it was shown that the Y682 residue can be phosphorylated by different kinases such as abl and TrkA [92, 93]. Phosphorylation at this level can regulate the association of APP to binding partners such as Fe65, X11/MINTs and Shc [94-97], ultimately controlling APP trafficking, processing and function also associated with cell movement and axonal branching [98, 99], and with NGF activity [100]. Tyr phosphorylation at Y682 motif has also been associated with increased Abeta production and amyloidogenic processing in vitro [101], in vivo [102] and in AD [103].

Interestingly, APP can be phosphorylated at a further N-terminal part of the intracellular domain, the 668Thr-669Pro residue [104], and phosphorylation at this domain has been associated with increased amyloidogenic processing of APP, both in vivo [39, 40] and in vitro [34]. The kinases involved in such phosphorylation are GSK3beta, CDK5, cdc2, known to be overactive in AD and responsible also for tau phosphorylation [23, 38, 39, 104, 105]. Of note, T668 phosphorylation was found to be elevated in AD brain [34], suggesting that it might induce toxic mechanisms linked to Abeta production. Such mechanisms seemed to relate to conformational changes affecting the 682YNPTY687 motif and therefore its ability to interact with binding partners [106, 107]. In support of this hypothesis, T668 has been linked to specific isomer formation. In fact, by means of NMR studies, it was observed that phosphorylation at the Thr668 residue causes an isomerization of APP from trans to cis. In fact, non-phosphorylated APP retains 100% trans conformation, and upon phosphorylation at T668 approximately 10% of the population turns to cis [108, 109].

Altogether, these findings draw attention to the role of T668 phosphorylation as an initiator of molecular pathways that lead to Abeta production by regulating APP conformation, trafficking and processing. They also suggest that different cis and trans APP isomers may contribute to shift the processing of APP towards either the amyloidogenic or the non-amyloidogenic processing, and therefore T668 phosphorylation may emerge as a potential target to halt amyloidogenic pathways in AD.

2.3. Pin1 to protect from Abeta pathology in animal models

Based on these findings and on the capability of Pin1 to protect from tau pathology by regulating tau conformation [42, 56], we hypothesized that Pin1 might regulate also the conformation of APP protecting from Abeta pathology. We found that Pin1 can bind to phosphorylated APP at T668, maintains the equilibrium between cis and trans conformation, ultimately shifting the processing of APP from the toxic amyloidogenic to the protective non-amyloidogenic [41].

More in detail, by means of pull down experiments, we observed that Pin1 can bind to APP only if phosphorylated at T668 [41]. Such interaction regulates APP isomerization. In fact, using a pentapeptide containing part of the C-terminal domain and the T668-P motif, we observed that Pin1 isomerizes the conformation of this peptide from cis to trans 1000 times faster than the reversed equilibrium, suggesting that shifting the isomerization towards the trans conformation may be crucial for APP function, and that Pin1 might be key to regulate APP physiologic activity. We then tested whether altering the equilibrium between cis and trans conformation might result in changes of APP functions. For this purpose, we manipulated Pin1 cellular levels either by knocking Pin1 out in genetically modified animals (Pin1KO], or by overexpressing Pin1 in cultured cells. Our in vitro experiments showed that when levels of

Pin1 were elevated beyond physiologic, APP amyloidogenic processing would be reduced, as Abeta levels were decreased in the media of the cultured cells. On the contrary, lack of Pin1 expression in cultured Pin1KO breast cancer cells resulted in decreased alphaAPPs secretion and increased Abeta production. Similarly, in the brain of Pin1KO mice we could observe age-dependent increase of Abeta production, since levels of aggregated insoluble Abeta were elevated in 18 months old mice when compared to 5 months old mice.

We then crossed PinKO animals to APPtg2576 and studied the processing of APP. We observed an age-dependent shift in the processing of APP that would result in an increase of the amyloidogenic versus the non-amyloidogenic, paralleled by the accumulation of Abeta42 deposits in multivesicular bodies, a form of deposited Abeta associated with early stages of AD [32, 33]. This led us to hypothesize a model in which Pin1 would protect against neuro-degeneration possibly by maintaining the equilibrium between the cis and the trans confor-mation of APP. In particular, in physiological conditions, Pin1 would favor the trans conformation of APP, increasing the non-amylodogenic processing. Vice versa in the absence of Pin1, the cis form would accumulate as the isomerization between the two forms would be lost, ultimately favoring the amyloidogenic processing.

2.4. Pin1 inhibits APP trafficking and internalization

Because Pin1 was found to localize with full length APP at the plasma membrane, we specu-lated that Pin1 may be involved in APP trafficking and internalization, regulating the amount of APP that undergoes amyloidogenic processing. We therefore tested the hypothesis whether Pin1 protects from Abeta formation by inhibiting APP internalization to amyloidogenic compartments [51]. For this purpose we used brain derived human H4 neuroglioma cells expressing APP either at endogenous level or stably overexpressing it, and Pin1 expression was knocked down by RNAi. We found that lower Pin1 levels associated with i) decreased levels of APP at the plasma membrane, ii) increased levels of betaAPPs and decreased alphaAPPs and iii) increased kinetic of internalization, as evidenced by means of immunocy-tochemistry in both fixed and living cells [51]. Levels of APP phosphoryated at T668 seemed to be elevated too. These data are in agreement with data from other groups that propose a toxic role of T688 phosphorylated APP [34], and may suggest that reduced Pin1 levels could be toxic in the same pathways. Interestingly, Ando and colleagues suggested that phosphor-ylation at T668 may affect APP conformation to ultimately alter the capability of APP to bind to partners such as Fe65 regulating APP trafficking, even if such interaction occurs at the 682YNPTY687 domain, further C-terminal than T668 [106]. This effect could be related to Pin1-mediated changes in APP conformation that could change the 682YNPTY687 stereochemistry. Of note, in Pin1 KD treated cells that were also overexpressing Fe65, we found that higher amounts of Fe65 associated with APP and that C99 accumulated, as compared to wild type cells. This was probably due to stabilization of Fe65 under these conditions, since Fe65 levels were elevated at the steady state in Pin1KD cells. Together with our immunocytochemistry data, under conditions that promote Fe65/APP interaction, these results suggest that reduced Pin1 expression may be linked to fastened internalization of APP to amyloidogenic compart-ments, where C99 is produced and accumulates (Fig. 1).

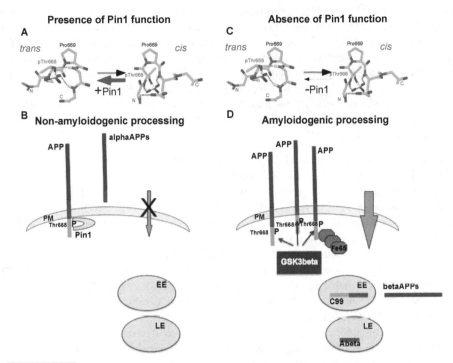

Our hypothesis is that Pin1 binds to and isomerizes the phosphorylated T668-Pro motif in full length APP, resulting in protein conformational changes that ultimately affect APP intracellular trafficking. (A, B). In the presence of proper Pin1 function, the equilibrium between the cis and the trans form of phosphorylated APP is maintained [41] (A), and this may help APP stay anchored at the plasma membrane where it will undergo the non-amyloidogenic processing (B). On the contrary, when Pin1 function is reduced, as in AD, the equilibrium between the cis and the trans form of phosphorylated APP will be disrupted, as the cis form of phosphorylated APP would not be isomerized to trans in a timely manner (C), and the levels of Fe65 will be stabilized. Moreover, reduced Pin1 function will enhance GSK3beta activity, leading to overall increase of phosphorylated APP at T668 and inhibiting APP turnover. These effects may lead to overall increased levels of APP undergoing internalization, trafficking and amyloidogenic processing (D). PM: Plasma membrane. EE: Early Endosomes. LE: Late Endosomes.

Figure 1. A model for the role of Pin1 in inhibiting APP accumulation and amyloidogenic processing.

We had previously observed that reduced Pin1 expression is linked to Abeta production [41], and we found that Pin1KD may increase gamma-secretase cleavage of APP to generate AICD [51]. Hence, we could assume that AD-associated reduced Pin1 expression is linked to increased amyloidogenic processing, promoting both internalization and gamma-secretase dependent cleavage of APP.

2.5. Pin1 increases APP protein turnover

Recent findings from our lab link Pin1 deficit and amyloidogenic processing in AD to increased APP stabilization [110]. This is particularly relevant to a role of increased APP in the disease, as it is known that higher APP levels correlate with AD. In fact, genetic modifications causing either duplication of the APP gene [111] or increased expression [112] were found to cause familial early onset AD. In addition, in Down syndrome patients, the triplication of the APP gene associates with the development of AD after age 40 [113], with the exception of those individuals affected by partial trisomy excluding the APP region [114]. In our experimental paradigm, such APP stabilization is caused by the lack of GSK3beta inhibition under conditions of impaired Pin1 activity. This may suggest that lack of Pin1 in AD impacts Abeta pathology by targeting multiple pathways, from APP trafficking to APP stabilization via GSK3beta activation.

More in details, we found that GSK3beta inhibitory mechanism was decreased in Pin1KO mice [110], since phoshorylation at S9, a mechanism that inhibits the kinase's activity, was decreased in these mice. We speculated that GSK3beta, which contains several Ser-Pro motifs, might serve as a substrate of Pin1 and that, by regulating GSK3beta conformation, Pin1 could control GSK3beta activity. This mechanism would contribute to the understanding of a link between loss of Pin1 activity and APP and tau pathologies in AD. GSK3beta in fact is responsible for the phosphorylation of both T668 in APP and T231 in tau, crucial in determining toxic conformations of both proteins in the disease. We found that Pin1 binds to GSK3beta at the T330 residue, and that lack of phosphorylation at this site using a T330A mutant would prevent such interaction. Of note, changes in Pin1 levels would affect GSK3beta activity, in vivo and in vitro. In fact, in crude brain lysates from Pin1Tg mice, GSK3beta activity was decreased, whereas it increased in Pin1KO mice. Similarly, overexpression of a wild type form of Pin1 reduced GSK3beta activity in H4 cells, whereas overexpression of mutants in regulatory regions of Pin1 such as the WW (W34A) or at the PPIase (K63A) domains, or at the Pin1 binding site (T330A) would not induce any change in the kinase activity, suggesting that by binding to T330, Pin1 is a crucial negative regulator of GSK3beta activity.

We then tested the hypothesis whether the Pin1-mediated control of GSK3beta activity could help prevent APP from entering the amyloidogenic processing. We found that lack of Pin1-mediated regulation of GSK3beta activity in T330A mutant expressing H4 cells reduced the levels of the non-amyloidogenic alphaAPPs, whereas it increased overall T668 APP phosphorylation. Of note, under these conditions, levels of APP were elevated at the steady state in cells, as well as in mice Pin1 concentration regulated APP levels. In fact, APP was reduced in Pin1Tg mice, whereas it accumulated in the brain of Pin1KO mice, similarly to what we had previously observed [41]. We found that APP accumulation in Pin1KO mice or in Pin1KD cells is the result of a failed physiologic degradation of APP, which is stabilized under these conditions. In fact, by means of cycloheximide treatment, we tested APP turnover under conditions of either reduced Pin1 expression (Pin1KD cells) or in absence of Pin1-mediated regulation of GSK3beta activity, in cells overexpressing the T330A mutant. We found not only that APP was stabilized in Pin1 KD cells as compared to wild type cells, also such stabilization seemed to depend on Pin1-mediated regulation of GSK3beta activity, since APP was stabilized in cells overexpressing the GSK3beta mutant T330A as compared to cells GSK3beta wild type.

Altogether, these data suggest that Pin1 regulates APP turnover by inhibiting GSK3beta activation and therefore contributes to lower T668 phosphorylation, which is responsible for toxic conformations of APP, as previously discussed in this chapter. These evidences suggest that in the pathology, mechanisms that favor the accumulation of APP will be toxic by increasing the amount of APP that will undergo amyloidogenic processing, and lack of Pin1 function could be one of these (Fig.1). Therefore, Pin1-mediated GSK3beta activity is an additional mechanism that Pin1 uses to protect from Abeta pathology, and strengthen the possibility to consider Pin1 as a valid tool to target Abeta pathologies in AD.

3. Role of T668 phosphorylation and APP conformation in AD: Pin1 as a molecular switch to regulate APP function

The question how increased APP phosphorylation at T668 is linked to AD has raised a real debate in the field. Many evidences point to a role in the disease. In fact, not only phospho-T668 levels were increased in AD brains [34], also many studies in vitro and in vivo point to a role of T668 phosphorylation by different kinases in altered protein transport in neurons [115, 116], also associated with increased amyloidogenic processing and Abeta production in cellular and animal models [34, 36, 39, 117]. In these studies, a non-phosphorylatable mutant T668A was used as an experimental paradigm to compare the effects of phosphorylated endogenous APP to the non-phosphorylated T668A form. Interestingly, a knock-in T668A animal model did not show any age-dependent alteration in APP processing [118], since in this study levels of Abeta, alphaAPPs and betaAPPs were comparable in both T668A and wild type mice during aging. Although at a first glance these data seem to challenge the hypothesis that regulation of T668 phosphorylation might be involved in AD, from these data it cannot be concluded that such phosphorylation is irrelevant to AD progression. It is not by abolishing APP phosphorylation at T668 by either knocking out APP or knocking in a non-phosphory-latable version of it that we can exclude a role for such pathway in the disease. APP KO mice are viable and their development and aging does not rely on alterations of APP processing [119, 120], and yet a role for APP in the development of AD is not disputed. Similarly, tau KO mice develop properly, reach adulthood and age normally [121-123], however a role for hyperphosphorylated tau in AD is quite clear.

It is possible that the controversy around the role of T668 phosphorylation in AD lies in the fact that physiologic phosphorylation at this domain is low, and it is only elevated in AD. This would explain why the T668A knock in mice did not show any difference from the wild type [118], because basal levels of phosphorylated T668 APP are very low, and phosphorylation-mediated regulation of APP activity in wild type mice was therefore comparable to the T668A mutant mice in this study.

Based on our data in vivo in Pin1KO mice and in vitro in Pin1KD cells [41, 51], we could hypothesize that the relevance of physiological T668 phosphorylation could be to maintain allow the equilibrium between cis and trans conformation. We could also assume that reduced Pin1 levels or increased T668 phosphorylation, both conditions associated with AD [34, 56], may disturb such equilibrium leading to increased Abeta production. Of note, the overexpression in Pin1KO breast cancer cells of a T668A APP mutant, which retains 100% trans conformation, rescued the amount of APP anchored at the plasma membrane, and also the levels of alphaAPPs [51]. These data may suggest that the protective non-amyloidogenic processing of APP is maintained only if APP is in the trans conformation, a conditions that associates with physiologic low levels of phosphorylated T668 and to physiologic levels of Pin1. This poses attention on protein isomerization and Pin1 as a fine post-phosphorylative tool to regulate a protein function, bypassing the regulation of the kinases. Targeting abnormal protein isomerization and Pin1 function may therefore offer a preferred approach in AD to halt the toxic effects of hyperphosphorylated proteins, such as phosphorylated T668 APP and T231 tau, instead of the pharmacological inhibition of the many kinases responsible for their phosphorylation.

Altogether, the data discussed here emphasize a role for Pin1-mediated isomerization of APP and GSK3beta as a mechanism to control APP physiologic function, shifting APP processing toward the non-amyloidogenic pathway (Fig. 1). Such regulation prevents the formation of toxic species produced downstream the amyloidogenic pathway, such as Abeta and betaAPPs, by regulating both APP trafficking and stabilization, and occurs as a post-phosphorylative event to maintain the equilibrium between cis and trans conformations. Therefore, Pin1 and regulation of APP conformation emerge as ideal candidates in the search of therapeutic targets for AD.

4. Pin1 and tau pathology in animal models and in AD

Tau-mediated neurodegeneration may result from the combination of toxic gains-of-function acquired by the aggregates or their precursors and the detrimental effects that arise from the loss of the normal function(s) of tau in the disease state [15]. The toxic gains-of-function includes sequestration of normal tau function by NFTs made of hyperphosphorylated tau. NFTs also become physical obstacles to the transport of vesicles and other cargos[15]. The loss of the normal function of tau includes detachment of tau from microtubules that causes loss of microtubule-stabilizing function [124]. Although dynamic tau phosphorylation occurs during embryonic development [125], aberrant tau phosphorylation in mature neurons is harmful to the neuron [126]. Tau hyperphosphorylation is a key regulatory mechanism that leads to both such toxic gains-of-function and the loss of the normal function(s) of tau [15].

4.1. Prolyl isomerization of tau

A high proportion of prolines residues are common to intrinsically disordered proteins, and tau is no exception [127]. Nearly 10% of full-length tau is composed of proline residues and around 20% of the residues between I151 and Q244 are proline. Many functions of tau are mediated through microtubule (MT) binding domains distal to this proline-rich domain. Interestingly, many disease-associated phosphorylation events that seed tau tangle formation occur at proline-directed serine (S) and threonine (T) residues in this proline-rich region. This indicates that important structural changes in the proline-rich region of tau are regulating tangle formation. In particular, cis-trans isomerization around these prolines modulates protein phosphatase binding and activity at specific S/T sites. We discovered that Pin1 regulates tau phosphorylation in concert with protein phosphatase 2A (PP2A) especially at T231 [42, 56, 128-130]. Findings by Dickey's group suggest that FKBP51 has a similar activity to Pin1; but unlike Pin1, FKBP51 coordinates with Hsp90 to isomerize tau [131].

4.2. Deletion of Pin1 causes tauopathy in mice

Pin1 knockout (KO) mice [42] serve as a good model to investigate the effect of Pin1 on endogenous tau *in vivo*. Pin1-deficient mice showed progressive age-dependent motor and behavioral deficits including abnormal limb-clasping reflexes, hunched postures and reduced mobility [42] similar to tau transgenic mice [132, 133]. These phenotypes in Pin1 mutant mice are significant because the total level of NFTs correlates with the degree of cognitive impairment [134, 135]. Pioneering studies that used immunohistochemical techniques to determine the level of both NFTs and senile plaques in different brain regions of AD patients, as well as non-demented elderly individuals, demonstrated that the number of NFTs, but not the numbers of senile plaques, correlates with the degree of cognitive impairment [134, 135].

4.3. Pin1 acts on the pT231–P motif in p–tau to protect against tauopathy in AD

It is increasingly evident that tauopathy in AD may result from the combination of toxic gains-of function acquired by phosphorylated tau (p-tau) aggregates, and the malignant effects from loss of tau normal function, including the failure of p-tau to bind and promote microtubule (MT) assembly [15]. Interestingly, a common characteristic event that disrupts tau MT function and precedes tangle formation is increased phosphorylation of tau especially on S/T-P motifs [11, 126, 136-141]. Indeed, tau kinases, such as mitogen-activated protein (MAP) kinases, cyclin-dependent protein kinase 5 (CDK5) and glycogen synthase 3 (GSK3) [142-144] or phosphatases, such as protein phosphatase 2A (PP2A) [145, 146] are deregulated in AD and modulating these enzymes can affect tauopathy [23, 39, 147-155]. Moreover, recent GWAS studies identify several new AD genes that might modulate tau phosphorylation and/or cytoskeleton, including MARK4 (pro-directed tau kinase) and BIN1 [156], and CD2AP [157, 158]. Notably, T231 phosphorylation in tau is reported to be the first of a number of tau phosphoepitopes appearing sequentially during early stages in pretangle AD neurons: pT231 → TG3 → AT8 → AT100 → Alz50 → → NFTs. However, it is still unclear how this phosphorylation leads to tau misfolding, aggregation and tangle formation [130, 159-161]. The results from our group and others support a critical role for Pin1 in protecting against tauopathy in AD by acting on the phosphorylated T231-P (pT231-P)motif (Fig.2). We discovered that pT231-P motif in tau exists in distinct cis and trans conformations, and that the cis to trans conversion is accelerated by a unique isomerase, Pin1 [44, 56, 128, 162], thereby protecting against tangle formation in AD [42, 48, 56, 163, 164]. pT231 is the first of sequential tau phosphoepitopes appearing in pretangle neurons in prodromal AD [159, 160] and its cerebrospinal fluid (CSF) level is an early biomarker that tracks MCI (mild cognitive impairment) conversion to AD, albeit with wide interindividual variations [165, 166]. Pin1 acts on the pT231-P motif in tau (i) to restore the ability of p-tau to promote MT assembly [56], (ii) to facilitate p-tau dephosphorylation because PP2A is trans-specific [42, 128], and (iii) to promote p-tau degradation [164] (Fig.2). Indeed, Pin1 overexpression promotes tau dephosphorylation selectively on pT231 in neurons and mouse brains [167, 168]. Pin1 has no effect on T231A mutant tau in vitro or vivo [56, 128, 139, 164]. Furthermore, Pin1 deficiency (Pin1-KO) mice display age-dependent tauopathy [42], whereas Pin1 overexpression in postnatal neurons effectively suppresses tauopathy induced by human wild-type (WT) tau in mice, albeit it enhances tauopathy induced by the P301L mutant tau [164].

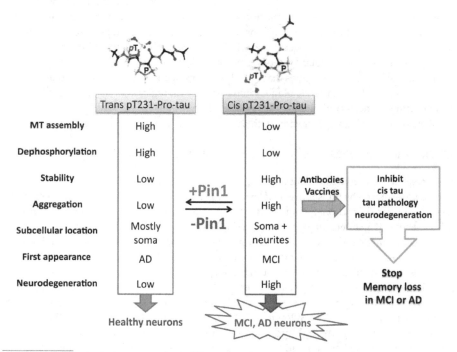

pT231-tau protein exists in the two completely different cis and trans conformations, as depicted in cartoons of the primary backbone structures. Cis, but not trans, pT231-tau loses normal function and also gains toxic function. Pin1 inhibits the accumulation of the pathogenic cis pT231-tau conformation in AD by converting it to the nonpathogenic trans form. Conformation-specific antibody and/or vaccines against the pathogenic cis pT231-tau might be developed for the diagnosis and treatment of AD, especially during its early stages.

Figure 2. Pin1 inhibits the accumulation of the pathogenic cis pT231-tau conformation in AD by converting it to the nonpathogenic trans form

These findings are highly relevant to human AD. We found that Pin1 localize to tangle and is depleted in AD brains [56], which has been confirmed and expanded to other tauopathies including FTD [61, 62, 169-172]. Furthermore, Pin1 is induced by neuron differentiation and highly expressed in most normal neurons, but inhibited by various mechanisms in AD neurons [44, 54, 56, 59, 62, 167, 169, 171-175]. For example, Pin1 expression is especially low in AD vulnerable neurons or actual degenerated neurons in AD [42]. Pin1 can be inactivated by oxidation in mild cognitive impairment (MCI) and AD neurons [61, 169, 170]. Pin1 is sequestered into tangles [56] or tangle or Ab-free granulovacuolar bodies with increasing tauopaty [176]. The human Pin1 gene is located at 19p13.2, a new late onset AD locus distinct from ApoE4 [173] and Pin1 promoter SNPs that reduce Pin1 expression [177] are associated with increased risk for AD in some cohorts [174], although not in others [65, 178]. A different Pin1 promoter SNP that prevents its suppression by AP4 is associated with delayed onset of AD [178]. Our findings of the opposite effects of Pin1 on cancer and AD [43, 45] have been supported by genetic association studies [174, 177, 179] and epidemiological studies [180-182]. Our analysis of the Framingham Study has further shown that cancer patients have decreased risk of AD, that AD patients have reduced cancer risk, and importantly, that this inverse relationship in not due to selective mortality or underdiagnosis [183]. Thus, we recently proposed that lack of sufficient Pin1 to catalyze cis to trans isomerization of pT231-tau might be a pathogenic mechanism leading to tauopathy in AD [48, 163].

5. Regulation of tau conformation as an early change in AD pathology: Implications for Pin1–catalyzed protein conformational regulation as a therapeutic and diagnostic tool

5.1. Cis pT231–tau is extremely early pathogenic conformation that is accumulated in MCI and AD

To analysis Pin1-catalyzed cis/trans protein conformational regulation and conformation-specific function or regulation, we have developed a novel technology to generate the first cis and trans-specific antibodies. We discovered that cis, but not trans, pT231-tau is extremely early pathogenic conformation in AD due to lack of Pin1 convert it to the physiological trans [129].

We found that replacing the five membered ring of Pro232 with the six membered ring homoproline (Pip) increases cis to 74%, since ~90% of pT231-P motif in a synthetic peptide in trans. Polyclonal antibodies raised against a pT231-Pip tau peptide recognize human and mouse p-tau. Resulting cis-specific antibody recognize regular pT231-Pro tau and cis pT231-5,5-demethylproline (Dmp) tau peptide, whereas trans-specific antibody recognizes regular pT231-Pro and trans pT231-Ala tau peptide. Neither antibody recognizes the non-phosphopeptide. Furthermore, both antibodies recognize tau, but not its T231A mutant expressed in SY5Y cells. Thus, cis- or trans- antibodies are highly specific [129]. Antibodies against cis pT231-tau might provide opportunity for efficient immunotherapy and diagnostic tools against early pathogenic tau conformation, raising the possibility of preventing tauopathy in AD patients at early stages.

5.2. Cis pT231–tau not only loses normal MT functions, but also gains toxic functions

As we and other groups had been shown [56, 184-186], phosphorylation of tau on T231 by Ccd2 abolishes its ability to promote MT assembly, which can be restored after dephosphorylation by PP2A or Pin1 [129]. Importantly, the ability of Pin1 to restore p-tau MT function is fully blocked by incubation of Pin1-treated p-tau with trans antibodies, but not cis antibodies. Furthermore, trans pT231-tau peptide is readily dephosphorylated by the tau phosphatase PP2A, which dephosphorylate on trans pS/T-P motifs [128]. Moreover, cis pT231-tau is much more stable than the trans both in cells and in Tau-transgenic (Tg) mouse brain slice cultures. Finally cis pT231-tau is much more prone to aggregation than the trans in Tau-Tg mouse brains and human MCI brains, as detected by sarcosyl fractionation experiments [42, 164, 187]. Thus, cis, but not trans, p-tau loses normal MT functions, and gains toxic functions.

5.3. Pin1 overexpression increases cis to trans pT231–P conversion in WT tau–Tg mice

To detect the ability of Pin1 to increase cis to trans isomerization, we showed that Pin1 reduces cis, but increases trans pT231-tau in vitro [129]. Moreover, Pin1 overexpression in Tau-Tg mice (Tau+Pin1) reduces the cis content, but increases the trans content, whereas Pin1 deficiency in Tau-Tg mice (Tau+Pin1-KO) has the opposite effects, as shown by immunoblots and immunostains [129]. In contrast to Wt tau-Tg mice, Pin1 overexpression increased cis, but decreased trans pT231-tau in P301L tau Tau-Tg mice because the P301L tau mutation greatly reduced cis, but not trans, pT231-tau, as we hypothesized [164]. These results explain why Pin1 has the opposite effects on WT tau and P301L tau [164] and are consistent with that CSF pT231-tau can differentiate AD form frontotemporal dementia[165, 166].

5.4. Cis, but not trans, pT231–tau is significantly elevated and localized to dystrophic neurites in MCI and further accumulated in AD

To examine p-tau conformational changes during the development of AD, we analyzed different Braak brain tissues with *cis* or *trans*-specific tau antibodies. There is little *cis* or *trans* pT231-tau in normal brains [129]. In AD cortex, *trans* pT231-tau is very low, but the *cis* is readily detected, even at Braak stages III and IV (MCI), and further accumulates as the Braak stage increases [129]. Notably, *cis*, but not *trans*, is localized to the dystrophic neurites [129], an early hallmark change highly correlating with synaptic and cognitive loss in AD [188-194]. Given Pin1 inhibition by oxidation in MCI brains [169, 170, 195], Pin1 might act at a very early step to inhibit tauopathy in AD.

5.5. Cis pT231–tau fully overlaps with neurofibrillary degeneration and correlates with reduced Pin1 levels in the AD hippocampus

As shown [42, 134, 196, 197], Pin1 is highly expressed in the CA2 region of the hippocampus, but dramatically reduced in the CA1 region, whereas PHF-1, a solid neurofibrillary neurodegeneration marker [161], is prevalent in the CA1, but not in CA2 region [129]. Importantly, trans-positive neurons are dominant in the CA2 region. However, in the CA region, cis-positive neurons are greatly increased. All cis-positive neurons are also positive for PHF-1 in both CA2 and CA1 regions. However, 74% of trans-positive cells in the CA2 region are negative for PHF-1. Thus, cis, but not trans, pT231-tau is fully overlapped with neurofibrillary degeneration.

5.6. Potential novel cis and trans conformation–specific disease diagnoses and therapies

Our exciting new insight into the role and regulation of p-tau conformations in AD might have important and novel therapeutic implications. For example, it has been shown that Thr231 phosphorylation is the earliest detectable tau phosphorylation event in human AD [130, 159, 160, 198] and its levels are elevated in cerebrospinal fluids and tracks AD progression, but with large individual variations [199, 200], making it difficult to become a standardized test. Our findings that the *cis* conformation appears earlier in MCI and is pathologically more relevant suggest that *cis* pThr231-tau and especially its ratio with *trans* might be a better and easier standardized diagnostic marker, especially for early diagnosis and patient comparison. Furthermore, the findings that Pin1 overexpression converts *cis* to *trans*, promotes tau degradation and inhibits tau pathology and neurodegeneration in AD mouse models [201] and that Pin1 SNPs preventing its inhibition by brain-specific transcription factor AP-4 is associated with delayed onset of AD [202] suggest that overexpressing Pin1 or preventing Pin1 inhibition might be a new approach to reduce the *cis* to *trans* pThr231-tau ratio to block tau pathology at early stages. Finally, active or passive immunization against some pSer/Thr-Pro motifs in tau including the pThr231-Pro motif has been shown to reduce tau aggregates and improve memory deficits in mouse models [203-209]. However, we have here shown that only ~10% of regular synthetic pThr231-tau peptides is in the pathologically relevant *cis* conformation and the remaining 90% is in *trans*, which can still promote MT assembly and is not related to neurofibrillary degeneration. Therefore, immunotherapies either using conformation-specific vaccines or antibodies specifically against the pathological-ly relevant *cis* pT231-tau conformation might be more specific and effective and safer in treating AD. Given the critical role of Pin1 and other isomerases in controlling the function of many other key regulators in the pathogenesis of human disease, notable Alzheimer's disease, cancer, viral infection, inflammation and autoimmune disorders [210-213], it would be interesting to deter-mine whether prolyl isomerization regulates the cellular function of these proteins and whether these conformational switches might be explored for developing novel diagnoses and therapies.

6. Finding a proper animal model to study AD: A lesson from the pin1KO mice

One of the biggest challenges when studying a disease is to develop the proper animal model that would reproduce the main features of that disease within the animal's biological envi-ronment. In the case of AD, this is not an easy goal, since mice do not spontaneously develop the features characteristic of this disease.

The only way to induce AD-like pathology with plaques and/or tangles in mice is by generating genetically altered animals. These may either overexpress aggressive mutants of APP linked to familial forms of AD (FAD) [214-218] and hence produce higher amounts of Abeta peptide, or express either wild type or aggressive mutants of tau [217, 218], leading to sustained tau hyperphosphorylation and tangle formation or may express both [217, 218]. These models may recapitulate plaque (APPTg) or tangle (tauTg) pathologies, or both (APPtg crossed to tauTg) [217, 218], and are extremely useful to understand the molecular pathways involved in AD, however they may [216] or may not [219] undergo neurodegeneration, which is a feature of AD. Moreover, they may not be representative of the way the disease progresses in sporadic AD, which affects the vast majority of AD patients, as they may represent only those familial cases of AD caused by those same mutations. Furthermore, these models may not be all specific for AD, since tau hyperphosphorylation and tangle formation occur also in other neurodegenerative diseases, and some of the tau mutations used to generate animal models for AD do not associate with AD, but with other neurodegenerative diseases, such as frontotemporal dementia associated with parkinsonism FTDP [17, 220, 221].

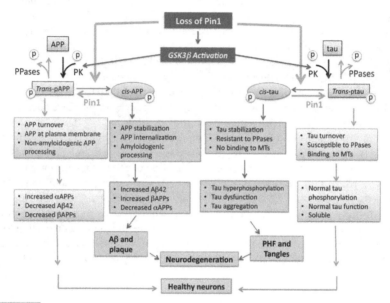

Both APP and tau are phosphorylated by protein kinase (PKs) as part of their normal function. The trans-conformation of phosphorylated APP and tau may present the physiological conformation that promotes their normal function (green boxes). Pin1 expression is induced during neuron differentiation and necessary to maintain normal neuronal function by preventing the unscheduled activation of mitotic events and/or controlling the function of phosphoproteins in the event that they become abnormally phosphorylated. For example, by catalyzing isomerization of the cis to trans conformation, Pin1 might promote non-amyloidogenic APP processing reducing Abeta production, as well as promote tau dephosphorylation and restore tau function. However in AD, a loss of Pin1 function, either through downregulation of Pin1 function, oxidative inactivation, phosphorylation or possible genetic alterations, can lead to build-up of cis-pS/T –P motifs. Cis-p-tau and cis-p-APP are proposed to represent pathological conformations (red ovals). Cis-p-APP is processed by the amyloidogenic pathway, which lead to a build-up of amyloid beta-42 (Abeta42), decreased levels of neurotropic alphaAPPs and the resultant formation of amyloid plaques. Cis-p-tau is resistant to protein phosphatases, which leads to a loss of MT binding, hyperphosphorylated tau an the formation of neurofibrillary tangles. The formation of tangles and plaques might further reduce Pin1 function by sequestering Pin1 and inducing oxidative modifications, respectively, in a positive feedback loop. In addition, a lack of proper Pin1 function leads to activation of kinases such as GSK3beta, which further increases both phosphorylation of tau and APP and also inhibits APP turnover, contributing to both tau and Abeta pathologies and causing neuronal death. Therefore, Pin1 deregulation might act on multiple pathways to contribute to AD development.

Figure 3. The regulation of APP processing and tau function by Pin1 in healthy and Alzheimer's neuron.

In addition, also animal models developed to understand a specific pathway even in absence of plaques [118], show limitations in the interpretation of the results.

In contrast, the model offered by knocking out the Pin1 gene in our Pin1KO model may recapitulate some of the features characteristic of both tau and Abeta pathology in sporadic AD, and therefore could serve as a valid tool to investigate the pathways that can be targeted to prevent or halt the disease progression. In fact, Pin1KO mice 1) develop age-dependent Abeta pathology associated with early neuronal deficit that leads to neurodegeneration (elevated Abeta levels associated with increased intracellular deposition) [41], 2) are characterized by age-dependent tau hyperphosphorylation, stabilization and PHF formation [42], and 3) show age-dependent neurodegeneration in selected areas [42]. Because genetic and proteomic findings link decreased Pin1 levels and/or activity to AD [56, 61], we could speculate that the Pin1KO animal model be very close to recapitulating the features that characterize AD in humans, and therefore may serve as a valid model to study the molecular pathways involved in AD.

7. Conclusion

We have here reviewed studies showing how Pin1 is an essential regulator of APP, tau and GSK3beta conformations, maintaining their physiological functions, and how loss of Pin1 in AD contributes to the accumulation of toxic conformations that turn the proteins' function pathologic. Moreover, the data here discussed present Pin1 as a link between both Abeta and tau pathology that could be exploited to tackle both pathologies in AD, even at early stages. The emerging new concept is that protein conformation might be a key regulatory element in toxic pathways in AD, and that Pin1 regulation of protein conformations might be a promising avenue to fight AD.

The debate about Abeta and tau pathology, which occurs first, which causes the other, is still unsolved, and clarifying it would help identify the correct therapeutic target to successfully prevent AD progression. Although studies in animal models in vivo showed that Abeta pathology occurs first and may be causative of tau pathology [222, 223], they were performed in animal models genetically modified to develop both tau and Abeta pathologies, and therefore may not be representative of the molecular mechanisms underlying sporadic forms of AD. In fact, it is still unclear which pathology occurs first in human AD, and only fine diagnostic tools able to identify early modification on both APP and tau that may render the proteins toxic would be of help.

As appropriate early diagnostic tools are still missing, the evidences here presented highlight Pin1 as an ideal therapeutic target to block the toxicity of both APP and tau in AD. In fact, the data here discussed show that equilibrium between cis and trans conformation of APP and tau is crucial to maintain their physiological function, and that this is disrupted either by hyperphosphorylation at S/T-P or by lower Pin1 levels or both in AD. In addition, we show here evidences that, in tau, alteration in the equilibrium between cis and trans conformation is an event that precedes massive cognitive decline, since the cis form of phosphorylated tau accumulates in MCI patients [129]. These results directly link conformational changes to pathologic protein functions, and highlight Pin1 as a successful regulator of such toxic conformations, opening new avenues in the medical field of AD. In fact, if a therapeutic target, Pin1 could block both tau and Abeta pathologies early in the disease, also resolving the eternal and unsolvable conflict: What happens first?

Author details

Lucia Pastorino, Asami Kondo, Xiao Zhen Zhou and Kun Ping Lu

*Address all correspondence to: lpastori@bidmc.harvard.edu

*Address all correspondence to: klu@bidmc.harvard.edu

Department of Medicine, Beth Israel Deaconess Medical Center, Harvard Medical School, Boston, USA

References

[1] Holtzman DM, Morris JC, Goate AM. Alzheimer's disease: the challenge of the second century. Sci Transl Med. 2011 Apr 6;3(77):77sr1.

[2] Bateman RJ, Aisen PS, De Strooper B, Fox NC, Lemere CA, Ringman JM, et al. Autosomal-dominant Alzheimer's disease: a review and proposal for the prevention of Alzheimer's disease. Alzheimers Res Ther. 2011;3(1):1.

[3] Aisen PS, Cummings J, Schneider LS. Symptomatic and nonamyloid/tau based pharmacologic treatment for Alzheimer disease. Cold Spring Harb Perspect Med. 2012 Mar;2(3):a006395.

[4] Winblad B, Engedal K, Soininen H, Verhey F, Waldemar G, Wimo A, et al. A 1-year, randomized, placebo-controlled study of donepezil in patients with mild to moderate AD. Neurology. 2001 Aug 14;57(3):489-95.

[5] Winblad B, Poritis N. Memantine in severe dementia: results of the 9M-Best Study (Benefit and efficacy in severely demented patients during treatment with memantine). Int J Geriatr Psychiatry. 1999 Feb;14(2):135-46.

[6] Tariot PN, Farlow MR, Grossberg GT, Graham SM, McDonald S, Gergel I. Memantine treatment in patients with moderate to severe Alzheimer disease already receiving donepezil: a randomized controlled trial. JAMA. 2004 Jan 21;291(3):317-24.

[7] Schneider LS, Insel PS, Weiner MW. Treatment with cholinesterase inhibitors and memantine of patients in the Alzheimer's Disease Neuroimaging Initiative. Arch Neurol. 2011 Jan;68(1):58-66.

[8]   Whitehead A, Perdomo C, Pratt RD, Birks J, Wilcock GK, Evans JG. Donepezil for the symptomatic treatment of patients with mild to moderate Alzheimer's disease: a meta-analysis of individual patient data from randomised controlled trials. Int J Geriatr Psychiatry. 2004 Jul;19(7):624-33.

[9]   Holtzman DM, Goate A, Kelly J, Sperling R. Mapping the road forward in Alzheimer's disease. Sci Transl Med. 2011 Dec 21;3(114):114ps48.

[10] Glenner GG, Wong CW, Quaranta V, Eanes ED. The amyloid deposits in Alzheimer's disease: their nature and pathogenesis. Appl Pathol. 1984;2(6):357-69.

[11] Goedert M, Spillantini MG, Cairns NJ, Crowther RA. Tau proteins of Alzheimer paired helical filaments: abnormal phosphorylation of all six brain isoforms. Neuron. 1992 Jan;8(1):159-68.

[12] Meyer-Luehmann M, Spires-Jones TL, Prada C, Garcia-Alloza M, de Calignon A, Rozkalne A, et al. Rapid appearance and local toxicity of amyloid-beta plaques in a mouse model of Alzheimer's disease. Nature. 2008 Feb 7;451(7179):720-4.

[13] Buee L, Bussiere T, Buee-Scherrer V, Delacourte A, Hof PR. Tau protein isoforms, phosphorylation and role in neurodegenerative disorders. Brain Res Brain Res Rev. 2000 Aug;33(1):95-130.

[14] Gomez-Isla T, Hollister R, West H, Mui S, Growdon JH, Petersen RC, et al. Neuronal loss correlates with but exceeds neurofibrillary tangles in Alzheimer's disease. Ann Neurol. 1997 Jan;41(1):17-24.

[15] Ballatore C, Lee VM, Trojanowski JQ. Tau-mediated neurodegeneration in Alzheimer's disease and related disorders. Nat Rev Neurosci. 2007 Sep;8(9):663-72.

[16] Parvathy S, Davies P, Haroutunian V, Purohit DP, Davis KL, Mohs RC, et al. Correlation between Abetax-40-, Abetax-42-, and Abetax-43-containing amyloid plaques and cognitive decline. Arch Neurol. 2001 Dec;58(12):2025-32.

[17] De Strooper B. Proteases and proteolysis in Alzheimer disease: a multifactorial view on the disease process. Physiol Rev. 2010 Apr;90(2):465-94.

[18] Masters CL, Selkoe DJ. Biochemistry of Amyloid beta-Protein and Amyloid Deposits in Alzheimer Disease. Cold Spring Harb Perspect Med. 2012 Jun;2(6):a006262.

[19] Jucker M, Walker LC. Pathogenic protein seeding in Alzheimer disease and other neurodegenerative disorders. Ann Neurol. 2011 Oct;70(4):532-40.

[20] Benilova I, Karran E, De Strooper B. The toxic Abeta oligomer and Alzheimer's disease: an emperor in need of clothes. Nat Neurosci. 2012 Mar;15(3):349-57.

[21] Larson ME, Lesne SE. Soluble Abeta oligomer production and toxicity. J Neurochem. 2012 Jan;120 Suppl 1:125-39.

[22] Haass C, Selkoe DJ. Soluble protein oligomers in neurodegeneration: lessons from the Alzheimer's amyloid beta-peptide. Nat Rev Mol Cell Biol. 2007 Feb;8(2):101-12.

[23] Noble W, Olm V, Takata K, Casey E, Mary O, Meyerson J, et al. Cdk5 is a key factor in tau aggregation and tangle formation in vivo. Neuron. 2003 May 22;38(4):555-65.

[24] Reinhard C, Hebert SS, De Strooper B. The amyloid-beta precursor protein: integrating structure with biological function. EMBO J. 2005 Dec 7;24(23):3996-4006.

[25] Hong S, Quintero-Monzon O, Ostaszewski BL, Podlisny DR, Cavanaugh WT, Yang T, et al. Dynamic analysis of amyloid beta-protein in behaving mice reveals opposing changes in ISF versus parenchymal Abeta during age-related plaque formation. J Neurosci. 2011 Nov 2;31(44):15861-9.

[26] Walsh DM, Selkoe DJ. Deciphering the molecular basis of memory failure in Alzheimer's disease. Neuron. 2004 Sep 30;44(1):181-93.

[27] Cleary JP, Walsh DM, Hofmeister JJ, Shankar GM, Kuskowski MA, Selkoe DJ, et al. Natural oligomers of the amyloid-beta protein specifically disrupt cognitive function. Nat Neurosci. 2005 Jan;8(1):79-84.

[28] Santos AN, Ewers M, Minthon L, Simm A, Silber RE, Blennow K, et al. Amyloid-beta oligomers in cerebrospinal fluid are associated with cognitive decline in patients with Alzheimer's disease. J Alzheimers Dis. 2012 Jan 1;29(1):171-6.

[29] Walsh DM, Klyubin I, Fadeeva JV, Cullen WK, Anwyl R, Wolfe MS, et al. Naturally secreted oligomers of amyloid beta protein potently inhibit hippocampal long-term potentiation in vivo. Nature. 2002 Apr 4;416(6880):535-9.

[30] Wang Q, Walsh DM, Rowan MJ, Selkoe DJ, Anwyl R. Block of long-term potentiation by naturally secreted and synthetic amyloid beta-peptide in hippocampal slices is mediated via activation of the kinases c-Jun N-terminal kinase, cyclin-dependent kinase 5, and p38 mitogen-activated protein kinase as well as metabotropic glutamate receptor type 5. J Neurosci. 2004 Mar 31;24(13):3370-8.

[31] Shankar GM, Li S, Mehta TH, Garcia-Munoz A, Shepardson NE, Smith I, et al. Amyloid-beta protein dimers isolated directly from Alzheimer's brains impair synaptic plasticity and memory. Nat Med. 2008 Aug;14(8):837-42.

[32] Takahashi RH, Milner TA, Li F, Nam EE, Edgar MA, Yamaguchi H, et al. Intraneuronal Alzheimer abeta42 accumulates in multivesicular bodies and is associated with synaptic pathology. Am J Pathol. 2002 Nov;161(5):1869-79.

[33] Takahashi RH, Almeida CG, Kearney PF, Yu F, Lin MT, Milner TA, et al. Oligomerization of Alzheimer's beta-amyloid within processes and synapses of cultured neurons and brain. J Neurosci. 2004 Apr 7;24(14):3592-9.

[34] Lee MS, Kao SC, Lemere CA, Xia W, Tseng HC, Zhou Y, et al. APP processing is regulated by cytoplasmic phosphorylation. J Cell Biol. 2003 Oct 13;163(1):83-95.

[35] Suzuki T, Nakaya T. Regulation of amyloid beta-protein precursor by phosphorylation and protein interactions. J Biol Chem. 2008 Oct 31;283(44):29633-7.

[36] Phiel CJ, Wilson CA, Lee VM, Klein PS. GSK-3alpha regulates production of Alzheimer's disease amyloid-beta peptides. Nature. 2003 May 22;423(6938):435-9.

[37] Lee MS, Tsai LH. Cdk5: one of the links between senile plaques and neurofibrillary tangles? J Alzheimers Dis. 2003;5(2):127-37.

[38] Mandelkow EM, Drewes G, Biernat J, Gustke N, Van Lint J, Vandenheede JR, et al. Glycogen synthase kinase-3 and the Alzheimer-like state of microtubule-associated protein tau. FEBS Lett. 1992 Dec 21;314(3):315-21.

[39] Cruz JC, Kim D, Moy LY, Dobbin MM, Sun X, Bronson RT, et al. p25/cyclin-dependent kinase 5 induces production and intraneuronal accumulation of amyloid beta in vivo. J Neurosci. 2006 Oct 11;26(41):10536-41.

[40] Cruz JC, Tsai LH. Cdk5 deregulation in the pathogenesis of Alzheimer's disease. Trends Mol Med. 2004 Sep;10(9):452-8.

[41] 41. Pastorino L, Sun A, Lu PJ, Zhou XZ, Balastik M, Finn G, et al. The prolyl isomerase Pin1 regulates amyloid precursor protein processing and amyloid-beta production. . Nature. 2006;440:528-34

[42] Liou YC, Sun A, Ryo A, Zhou XZ, Yu ZX, Huang HK, et al. Role of the prolyl isomerase Pin1 in protecting against age-dependent neurodegeneration. Nature. 2003 Jul 31;424(6948):556-61.

[43] Lu KP, Zhou XZ. The prolyl isomerase PIN1: a pivotal new twist in phosphorylation signalling and disease. Nat Rev Mol Cell Biol. 2007 Nov;8(11):904-16.

[44] Lu KP, Hanes SD, Hunter T. A human peptidyl-prolyl isomerase essential for regulation of mitosis. Nature. 1996;380(6574):544-7.

[45] Lu KP. Pinning down cell signaling, cancer and Alzheimer's disease. Trends Biochem Sci. 2004;29:200-9.

[46] Wulf G, Finn G, Suizu F, Lu KP. Phosphorylation-specific prolyl isomerization: is there an underlying theme? Nat Cell Biol. 2005 May;7(5):435-41.

[47] Yaffe MB, Schutkowski M, Shen M, Zhou XZ, Stukenberg PT, Rahfeld J, et al. Sequence-specific and phosphorylation-dependent proline isomerization: A potential mitotic regulatory mechanism. Science. 1997;278:1957-60.

[48] Lu KP, Finn G, Lee TH, Nicholson LK. Prolyl cis-trans isomerization as a molecular timer. Nat Chem Biol. 2007 Oct;3(10):619-29.

[49] Lu KP, Liou YC, Zhou XZ. Pinning down proline-directed phosphorylation signaling. Trends Cell Biol. 2002 Apr;12(4):164-72.

[50] Lu PJ, Zhou XZ, Liou YC, Noel JP, Lu KP. Critical role of WW domain phosphorylation in regulating phosphoserine binding activity and Pin1 function. J Biol Chem. 2002 Jan 25;277(4):2381-4.

[51] Pastorino L, Ma SL, Balastik M, Huang P, Pandya D, Nicholson L, et al. Alzheimer's disease-related loss of Pin1 function influences the intracellular localization and the processing of AbetaPP. J Alzheimers Dis. 2012 Jan 1;30(2):277-97.

[52] Ryo A, Suizu F, Yoshida Y, Perrem K, Liou YC, Wulf G, et al. Regulation of NF-kappaB signaling by Pin1-dependent prolyl isomerization and ubiquitin-mediated proteolysis of p65/RelA. Mol Cell. 2003;12:1413-26.

[53] Wulf GM, Liou YC, Ryo A, Lee SW, Lu KP. Role of Pin1 in the regulation of p53 stability and p21 transactivation,and cell cycle checkpoints in response to DNA damage. J Biol Chem. 2002;277:47976-9.

[54] Ryo A, Nakamura M, Wulf G, Liou YC, Lu KP. Pin1 regulates turnover and subcellular localization of beta-catenin by inhibiting its interaction with APC. Nat Cell Biol. 2001 Sep;3(9):793-801.

[55] Tun-Kyi A, Finn G, Greenwood A, Nowak M, Lee TH, Asara JM, et al. Essential role for the prolyl isomerase Pin1 in Toll-like receptor signaling and type I interferon-mediated immunity. Nat Immunol. 2011 Aug;12(8):733-41.

[56] Lu PJ, Wulf G, Zhou XZ, Davies P, Lu KP. The prolyl isomerase Pin1 restores the function of Alzheimer-associated phosphorylated tau protein. Nature. 1999 Jun 24;399(6738):784-8.

[57] Cook DN, Pisetsky DS, Schwartz DA. Toll-like receptors in the pathogenesis of human disease. Nat Immunol. 2004 Oct;5(10):975-9.

[58] Ryo A, Liou YC, Lu KP, Wulf G. Prolyl isomerase Pin1: a catalyst for oncogenesis and a potential therapeutic target in cancer. J Cell Sci. 2003 Mar 1;116(Pt 5):773-83.

[59] Wulf GM, Ryo A, Wulf GG, Lee SW, Niu T, Petkova V, et al. Pin1 is overexpressed in breast cancer and cooperates with Ras signaling in increasing the transcriptional activity of c-Jun towards cyclin D1. EMBO J. 2001 Jul 2;20(13):3459-72.

[60] Wulf G, Ryo A, Liou YC, Lu KP. The prolyl isomerase Pin1 in breast development and cancer. Breast Cancer Res. 2003;5(2):76-82.

[61] Sultana R, Boyd-Kimball D, Poon HF, Cai J, Pierce WM, Klein JB, et al. Oxidative modification and down-regulation of Pin1 in Alzheimer's disease hippocampus: A redox proteomics analysis. Neurobiol Aging. 2006 Jul;27(7):918-25.

[62] Wang S, Simon BP, Bennett DA, Schneider JA, Malter JS, Wang DS. The significance of Pin1 in the development of Alzheimer's disease. J Alzheimers Dis. 2007 Mar;11(1):13-23.

[63] Lambert JC, Bensemain F, Chapuis J, Cottel D, Amouyel P. Association study of the PIN1 gene with Alzheimer's disease. Neurosci Lett. 2006 Jul 24;402(3):259-61.

[64] Poli M, Gatta LB, Dominici R, Lovati C, Mariani C, Albertini A, et al. DNA sequence variations in the prolyl isomerase Pin1 gene and Alzheimer's disease. Neurosci Lett. 2005 Dec 2;389(2):66-70.

[65] Nowotny P, Bertelsen S, Hinrichs AL, Kauwe JS, Mayo K, Jacquart S, et al. Association studies between common variants in prolyl isomerase Pin1 and the risk for late-onset Alzheimer's disease. Neurosci Lett. 2007 May 23;419(1):15-7.

[66] Ma SL, Tang NL, Tam CW, Cheong Lui VW, Lam LC, Chiu HF, et al. A PIN1 polymorphism that prevents its suppression by AP4 associates with delayed onset of Alzheimer's disease. Neurobiol Aging.Jun 24.

[67] Hardy J. A hundred years of Alzheimer's disease research. Neuron. 2006 Oct 5;52(1): 3-13.

[68] Hardy J, Selkoe DJ. The amyloid hypothesis of Alzheimer's disease: progress and problems on the road to therapeutics. Science. 2002 Jul 19;297(5580):353-6.

[69] Wong CW, Quaranta V, Glenner GG. Neuritic plaques and cerebrovascular amyloid in Alzheimer disease are antigenically related. Proc Natl Acad Sci U S A. 1985 Dec; 82(24):8729-32.

[70] Thinakaran G, Koo EH. Amyloid precursor protein trafficking, processing, and function. J Biol Chem. 2008 Oct 31;283(44):29615-9.

[71] Goldgaber D, Lerman MI, McBride OW, Saffiotti U, Gajdusek DC. Characterization and chromosomal localization of a cDNA encoding brain amyloid of Alzheimer's disease. Science. 1987 Feb 20;235(4791):877-80.

[72] Golde TE, Estus S, Usiak M, Younkin LH, Younkin SG. Expression of beta amyloid protein precursor mRNAs: recognition of a novel alternatively spliced form and quantitation in Alzheimer's disease using PCR. Neuron. 1990 Feb;4(2):253-67.

[73] Haass C, Kaether C, Thinakaran G, Sisodia S. Trafficking and Proteolytic Processing of APP. Cold Spring Harb Perspect Med. 2012 May;2(5):a006270.

[74] Rajendran L, Annaert W. Membrane trafficking pathways in Alzheimer's disease. Traffic. 2012 Jun;13(6):759-70.

[75] Parvathy S, Hussain I, Karran EH, Turner AJ, Hooper NM. The amyloid precursor protein (APP) and the angiotensin converting enzyme (ACE) secretase are inhibited by hydroxamic acid-based inhibitors. Biochem Soc Trans. 1998 Aug;26(3):S242.

[76] Parvathy S, Hussain I, Karran EH, Turner AJ, Hooper NM. Cleavage of Alzheimer's amyloid precursor protein by alpha-secretase occurs at the surface of neuronal cells. Biochemistry. 1999 Jul 27;38(30):9728-34.

[77] Lammich S, Kojro E, Postina R, Gilbert S, Pfeiffer R, Jasionowski M, et al. Constitutive and regulated alpha-secretase cleavage of Alzheimer's amyloid precursor protein by a disintegrin metalloprotease. Proc Natl Acad Sci U S A. 1999 Mar 30;96(7): 3922-7.

[78] Postina R. Activation of alpha-secretase cleavage. J Neurochem. 2012 Jan;120 Suppl 1:46-54.

[79] Postina R, Schroeder A, Dewachter I, Bohl J, Schmitt U, Kojro E, et al. A disintegrin-metalloproteinase prevents amyloid plaque formation and hippocampal defects in an Alzheimer disease mouse model. J Clin Invest. 2004 May;113(10):1456-64.

[80] Buxbaum JD, Liu KN, Luo Y, Slack JL, Stocking KL, Peschon JJ, et al. Evidence that tumor necrosis factor alpha converting enzyme is involved in regulated alpha-secretase cleavage of the Alzheimer amyloid protein precursor. J Biol Chem. 1998 Oct 23;273(43):27765-7.

[81] Asai M, Hattori C, Szabo B, Sasagawa N, Maruyama K, Tanuma S, et al. Putative function of ADAM9, ADAM10, and ADAM17 as APP alpha-secretase. Biochem Biophys Res Commun. 2003 Jan 31;301(1):231-5.

[82] Young-Pearse TL, Chen AC, Chang R, Marquez C, Selkoe DJ. Secreted APP regulates the function of full-length APP in neurite outgrowth through interaction with integrin beta1. Neural Dev. 2008;3:15.

[83] Cao X, Sudhof TC. A transcriptionally [correction of transcriptively) active complex of APP with Fe65 and histone acetyltransferase Tip60. Science. 2001 Jul 6;293(5527): 115-20.

[84] Cao X, Sudhof TC. Dissection of amyloid-beta precursor protein-dependent transcriptional transactivation. J Biol Chem. 2004 Jun 4;279(23):24601-11.

[85] Sabo SL, Lanier LM, Ikin AF, Khorkova O, Sahasrabudhe S, Greengard P, et al. Regulation of beta-amyloid secretion by FE65, an amyloid protein precursor-binding protein. J Biol Chem. 1999 Mar 19;274(12):7952-7.

[86] Vassar R, Bennett BD, Babu-Khan S, Kahn S, Mendiaz EA, Denis P, et al. Beta-secretase cleavage of Alzheimer's amyloid precursor protein by the transmembrane aspartic protease BACE. Science. 1999 Oct 22;286(5440):735-41.

[87] Hussain I, Powell D, Howlett DR, Tew DG, Meek TD, Chapman C, et al. Identification of a novel aspartic protease (Asp 2) as beta-secretase. Mol Cell Neurosci. 1999 Dec;14(6):419-27.

[88] Nikolaev A, McLaughlin T, O'Leary DD, Tessier-Lavigne M. APP binds DR6 to trigger axon pruning and neuron death via distinct caspases. Nature. 2009 Feb 19;457(7232):981-9.

[89]   De Strooper B, Vassar R, Golde T. The secretases: enzymes with therapeutic potential in Alzheimer disease. Nat Rev Neurol.Feb;6(2):99-107.

[90]   De Strooper B, Vassar R, Golde T. The secretases: enzymes with therapeutic potential in Alzheimer disease. Nat Rev Neurol. 2010 Feb;6(2):99-107.

[91]   O'Brien RJ, Wong PC. Amyloid precursor protein processing and Alzheimer's disease. Annu Rev Neurosci. 2011;34:185-204.

[92]   Zambrano N, Bruni P, Minopoli G, Mosca R, Molino D, Russo C, et al. The beta-amyloid precursor protein APP is tyrosine-phosphorylated in cells expressing a constitutively active form of the Abl protoncogene. J Biol Chem. 2001 Jun 8;276(23):19787-92.

[93]   Tarr PE, Contursi C, Roncarati R, Noviello C, Ghersi E, Scheinfeld MH, et al. Evidence for a role of the nerve growth factor receptor TrkA in tyrosine phosphorylation and processing of beta-APP. Biochem Biophys Res Commun. 2002 Jul 12;295(2):324-9.

[94]   Rogelj B, Mitchell JC, Miller CC, McLoughlin DM. The X11/Mint family of adaptor proteins. Brain Res Rev. 2006 Sep;52(2):305-15.

[95]   Schettini G, Govoni S, Racchi M, Rodriguez G. Phosphorylation of APP-CTF-AICD domains and interaction with adaptor proteins: signal transduction and/or transcriptional role--relevance for Alzheimer pathology. J Neurochem. 2010 Dec;115(6): 1299-308.

[96]   McLoughlin DM, Miller CC. The FE65 proteins and Alzheimer's disease. J Neurosci Res. 2008 Mar;86(4):744-54.

[97]   Tarr PE, Roncarati R, Pelicci G, Pelicci PG, D'Adamio L. Tyrosine phosphorylation of the beta-amyloid precursor protein cytoplasmic tail promotes interaction with Shc. J Biol Chem. 2002 May 10;277(19):16798-804.

[98]   Sabo SL, Ikin AF, Buxbaum JD, Greengard P. The Alzheimer amyloid precursor protein (APP) and FE65, an APP-binding protein, regulate cell movement. J Cell Biol. 2001 Jun 25;153(7):1403-14.

[99]   Sabo SL, Ikin AF, Buxbaum JD, Greengard P. The amyloid precursor protein and its regulatory protein, FE65, in growth cones and synapses in vitro and in vivo. J Neurosci. 2003 Jul 2;23(13):5407-15.

[100] Matrone C, Barbagallo AP, La Rosa LR, Florenzano F, Ciotti MT, Mercanti D, et al. APP is phosphorylated by TrkA and regulates NGF/TrkA signaling. J Neurosci. 2011 Aug 17;31(33):11756-61.

[101] Perez RG, Soriano S, Hayes JD, Ostaszewski B, Xia W, Selkoe DJ, et al. Mutagenesis identifies new signals for beta-amyloid precursor protein endocytosis, turnover, and the generation of secreted fragments, including Abeta42. J Biol Chem. 1999 Jul 2;274(27):18851-6.

[102] Barbagallo AP, Weldon R, Tamayev R, Zhou D, Giliberto L, Foreman O, et al. Tyr(682) in the intracellular domain of APP regulates amyloidogenic APP processing in vivo. PLoS One. 2010;5(11):e15503.

[103] Russo C, Salis S, Dolcini V, Venezia V, Song XH, Teller JK, et al. Amino-terminal modification and tyrosine phosphorylation of [corrected) carboxy-terminal fragments of the amyloid precursor protein in Alzheimer's disease and Down's syndrome brain. Neurobiol Dis. 2001 Feb;8(1):173-80.

[104] Suzuki T, Oishi M, Marshak DR, Czernik AJ, Nairn AC, Greengard P. Cell cycle-dependent regulation of the phosphorylation and metabolism of the Alzheimer amyloid precursor protein. EMBO J. 1994 Mar 1;13(5):1114-22.

[105] Vincent IJ, Davies P. A protein kinase associated with paired helical filaments in Alzheimer disease. Proc Natl Acad Sci U S A. 1992 Apr 1;89(7):2878-82.

[106] Ando K, Iijima KI, Elliott JI, Kirino Y, Suzuki T. Phosphorylation-dependent regulation of the interaction of amyloid precursor protein with Fe65 affects the production of beta-amyloid. J Biol Chem. 2001 Oct 26;276(43):40353-61.

[107] Tamayev R, Zhou D, D'Adamio L. The interactome of the amyloid beta precursor protein family members is shaped by phosphorylation of their intracellular domains. Mol Neurodegener. 2009;4:28.

[108] Ramelot TA, Gentile LN, Nicholson LK. Transient structure of the amyloid precursor protein cytoplasmic tail indicates preordering of structure for binding to cytosolic factors. Biochemistry. 2000 Mar 14;39(10):2714-25.

[109] Ramelot TA, Nicholson LK. Phosphorylation-induced structural changes in the amyloid precursor protein cytoplasmic tail detected by NMR. J Mol Biol. 2001 Mar 30;307(3):871-84.

[110] Ma SL, Pastorino L, Zhou XZ, Lu KP. Prolyl isomerase Pin1 promotes amyloid precursor protein (APP) turnover by inhibiting glycogen synthase kinase-3beta (GSK3beta) activity: novel mechanism for Pin1 to protect against Alzheimer disease. J Biol Chem. 2012 Mar 2;287(10):6969-73.

[111] Sleegers K, Brouwers N, Gijselinck I, Theuns J, Goossens D, Wauters J, et al. APP duplication is sufficient to cause early onset Alzheimer's dementia with cerebral amyloid angiopathy. Brain. 2006 Nov;129(Pt 11):2977-83.

[112] Theuns J, Brouwers N, Engelborghs S, Sleegers K, Bogaerts V, Corsmit E, et al. Promoter mutations that increase amyloid precursor-protein expression are associated with Alzheimer disease. American journal of human genetics. 2006 Jun;78(6):936-46.

[113] Mann DM. Alzheimer's disease and Down's syndrome. Histopathology. 1988 Aug; 13(2):125-37.

[114] Prasher VP, Farrer MJ, Kessling AM, Fisher EM, West RJ, Barber PC, et al. Molecular mapping of Alzheimer-type dementia in Down's syndrome. Ann Neurol. 1998 Mar; 43(3):380-3.

[115] Muresan Z, Muresan V. c-Jun NH2-terminal kinase-interacting protein-3 facilitates phosphorylation and controls localization of amyloid-beta precursor protein. J Neurosci. 2005 Apr 13;25(15):3741-51.

[116] Muresan Z, Muresan V. Coordinated transport of phosphorylated amyloid-beta precursor protein and c-Jun NH2-terminal kinase-interacting protein-1. J Cell Biol. 2005 Nov 21;171(4):615-25.

[117] Parr C, Carzaniga R, Gentleman S, Van Leuven F, Walter J, Sastre M. GSK3 inhibition promotes lysosomal biogenesis and the autophagic degradation of the Amyloid-beta Precursor Protein. Mol Cell Biol. 2012 Aug 27.

[118] Sano Y, Nakaya T, Pedrini S, Takeda S, Iijima-Ando K, Iijima K, et al. Physiological mouse brain Abeta levels are not related to the phosphorylation state of threonine-668 of Alzheimer's APP. PLoS One. 2006;1:e51.

[119] Zheng H, Jiang M, Trumbauer ME, Sirinathsinghji DJ, Hopkins R, Smith DW, et al. beta-Amyloid precursor protein-deficient mice show reactive gliosis and decreased locomotor activity. Cell. 1995 May 19;81(4):525-31.

[120] Heber S, Herms J, Gajic V, Hainfellner J, Aguzzi A, Rulicke T, et al. Mice with combined gene knock-outs reveal essential and partially redundant functions of amyloid precursor protein family members. J Neurosci. 2000 Nov 1;20(21):7951-63.

[121] Harada A, Oguchi K, Okabe S, Kuno J, Terada S, Ohshima T, et al. Altered microtubule organization in small-calibre axons of mice lacking tau protein. Nature. 1994 Jun 9;369(6480):488-91.

[122] Dawson HN, Ferreira A, Eyster MV, Ghoshal N, Binder LI, Vitek MP. Inhibition of neuronal maturation in primary hippocampal neurons from tau deficient mice. J Cell Sci. 2001 Mar;114(Pt 6):1179-87.

[123] Gomez de Barreda E, Perez M, Gomez Ramos P, de Cristobal J, Martin-Maestro P, Moran A, et al. Tau-knockout mice show reduced GSK3-induced hippocampal degeneration and learning deficits. Neurobiol Dis. 2010 Mar;37(3):622-9.

[124] Stoothoff WH, Johnson GV. Tau phosphorylation: physiological and pathological consequences. Biochim Biophys Acta. 2005 Jan 3;1739(2-3):280-97.

[125] Mawal-Dewan M, Henley J, Van de Voorde A, Trojanowski JQ, Lee VM. The phosphorylation state of tau in the developing rat brain is regulated by phosphoprotein phosphatases. J Biol Chem. 1994 Dec 9;269(49):30981-7.

[126] Matsuo ES, Shin RW, Billingsley ML, Van deVoorde A, O'Connor M, Trojanowski JQ, et al. Biopsy-derived adult human brain tau is phosphorylated at many of the

same sites as Alzheimer's disease paired helical filament tau. Neuron. 1994 Oct;13(4): 989-1002.

[127]   Romero PR, Zaidi S, Fang YY, Uversky VN, Radivojac P, Oldfield CJ, et al. Alternative splicing in concert with protein intrinsic disorder enables increased functional diversity in multicellular organisms. Proc Natl Acad Sci U S A. 2006 May 30;103(22): 8390-5.

[128]   Zhou XZ, Kops O, Werner A, Lu PJ, Shen M, Stoller G, et al. Pin1-dependent prolyl isomerization regulates dephosphorylation of Cdc25C and tau proteins. Mol Cell. 2000 Oct;6(4):873-83.

[129]   Nakamura K, Greenwood A, Binder L, Bigio EH, Denial S, Nicholson L, et al. Proline isomer-specific antibodies reveal the early pathogenic tau conformation in Alzheimer's disease. Cell. 2012 Mar 30;149(1):232-44.

[130]   Jicha GA, Lane E, Vincent I, Otvos L, Jr., Hoffmann R, Davies P. A conformation- and phosphorylation-dependent antibody recognizing the paired helical filaments of Alzheimer's disease. J Neurochem. 1997 Nov;69(5):2087-95.

[131]   Pei H, Li L, Fridley BL, Jenkins GD, Kalari KR, Lingle W, et al. FKBP51 affects cancer cell response to chemotherapy by negatively regulating Akt. Cancer cell. 2009 Sep 8;16(3):259-66.

[132]   Allen B, Ingram E, Takao M, Smith MJ, Jakes R, Virdee K, et al. Abundant tau filaments and nonapoptotic neurodegeneration in transgenic mice expressing human P301S tau protein. J Neurosci. 2002 Nov 1;22(21):9340-51.

[133]   Lewis J, McGowan E, Rockwood J, Melrose H, Nacharaju P, Van Slegtenhorst M, et al. Neurofibrillary tangles, amyotrophy and progressive motor disturbance in mice expressing mutant (P301L) tau protein. Nat Genet. 2000 Aug;25(4):402-5.

[134]   Arriagada PV, Growdon JH, Hedley-Whyte ET, Hyman BT. Neurofibrillary tangles but not senile plaques parallel duration and severity of Alzheimer's disease. Neurology. 1992 Mar;42(3 Pt 1):631-9.

[135]   Arriagada PV, Marzloff K, Hyman BT. Distribution of Alzheimer-type pathologic changes in nondemented elderly individuals matches the pattern in Alzheimer's disease. Neurology. 1992 Sep;42(9):1681-8.

[136]   Vincent I, Zheng JH, Dickson DW, Kress Y, Davies P. Mitotic phosphoepitopes precede paired helical filaments in Alzheimer's disease. Neurobiol Aging. 1998 Jul-Aug; 19(4):287-96.

[137]   Preuss U, Mandelkow EM. Mitotic phosphorylation of tau protein in neuronal cell lines resembles phosphorylation in Alzheimer's disease. European journal of cell biology. 1998 Jul;76(3):176-84.

[138] Bancher C, Brunner C, Lassmann H, Budka H, Jellinger K, Wiche G, et al. Accumulation of abnormally phosphorylated tau precedes the formation of neurofibrillary tangles in Alzheimer's disease. Brain Res. 1989 Jan 16;477(1-2):90-9.

[139] Lu KP, Liou YC, Vincent I. Proline-directed phosphorylation and isomerization in mitotic regulation and in Alzheimer's Disease. Bioessays. 2003 Feb;25(2):174-81.

[140] Lee VM, Balin BJ, Otvos L, Jr., Trojanowski JQ. A68: a major subunit of paired helical filaments and derivatized forms of normal Tau. Science. 1991 Feb 8;251(4994):675-8.

[141] Greenberg SG, Davies P, Schein JD, Binder LI. Hydrofluoric acid-treated tau PHF proteins display the same biochemical properties as normal tau. J Biol Chem. 1992 Jan 5;267(1):564-9.

[142] Pelech SL. Networking with proline-directed protein kinases implicated in tau phosphorylation. Neurobiol Aging. 1995 May-Jun;16(3):247-56; discussion 57-61.

[143] Dolan PJ, Johnson GV. The role of tau kinases in Alzheimer's disease. Current opinion in drug discovery & development. 2010 Sep;13(5):595-603.

[144] Illenberger S, Zheng-Fischhofer Q, Preuss U, Stamer K, Baumann K, Trinczek B, et al. The endogenous and cell cycle-dependent phosphorylation of tau protein in living cells: implications for Alzheimer's disease. Mol Biol Cell. 1998 Jun;9(6):1495-512.

[145] Goedert M, Satumtira S, Jakes R, Smith MJ, Kamibayashi C, White CL, 3rd, et al. Reduced binding of protein phosphatase 2A to tau protein with frontotemporal dementia and parkinsonism linked to chromosome 17 mutations. J Neurochem. 2000 Nov; 75(5):2155-62.

[146] Sontag E, Nunbhakdi-Craig V, Lee G, Bloom GS, Mumby MC. Regulation of the phosphorylation state and microtubule-binding activity of Tau by protein phosphatase 2A. Neuron. 1996 Dec;17(6):1201-7.

[147] Ishiguro K, Shiratsuchi A, Sato S, Omori A, Arioka M, Kobayashi S, et al. Glycogen synthase kinase 3 beta is identical to tau protein kinase I generating several epitopes of paired helical filaments. FEBS Lett. 1993 Jul 5;325(3):167-72.

[148] Sperber BR, Leight S, Goedert M, Lee VM. Glycogen synthase kinase-3 beta phosphorylates tau protein at multiple sites in intact cells. Neurosci Lett. 1995 Sep 8;197(2):149-53.

[149] Patrick GN, Zukerberg L, Nikolic M, de la Monte S, Dikkes P, Tsai LH. Conversion of p35 to p25 deregulates Cdk5 activity and promotes neurodegeneration. Nature. 1999 Dec 9;402(6762):615-22.

[150] James ND, Davis DR, Sindon J, Hanger DP, Brion JP, Miller CC, et al. Neurodegenerative changes including altered tau phosphorylation and neurofilament immunoreactivity in mice transgenic for the serine/threonine kinase Mos. Neurobiol Aging. 1996 Mar-Apr;17(2):235-41.

[151] Brownlees J, Irving NG, Brion JP, Gibb BJ, Wagner U, Woodgett J, et al. Tau phos-
       phorylation in transgenic mice expressing glycogen synthase kinase-3beta trans-
       genes. Neuroreport. 1997 Oct 20;8(15):3251-5.

[152] Ahlijanian MK, Barrezueta NX, Williams RD, Jakowski A, Kowsz KP, McCarthy S, et
       al. Hyperphosphorylated tau and neurofilament and cytoskeletal disruptions in mice
       overexpressing human p25, an activator of cdk5. Proc Natl Acad Sci U S A. 2000 Mar
       14;97(6):2910-5.

[153] Kins S, Crameri A, Evans DR, Hemmings BA, Nitsch RM, Gotz J. Reduced protein
       phosphatase 2A activity induces hyperphosphorylation and altered compartmentali-
       zation of tau in transgenic mice. J Biol Chem. 2001 Oct 12;276(41):38193-200.

[154] Bian F, Nath R, Sobocinski G, Booher RN, Lipinski WJ, Callahan MJ, et al. Axonop-
       athy, tau abnormalities, and dyskinesia, but no neurofibrillary tangles in p25-trans-
       genic mice. The Journal of comparative neurology. 2002 May 6;446(3):257-66.

[155] Plattner F, Angelo M, Giese KP. The roles of cyclin-dependent kinase 5 and glycogen
       synthase kinase 3 in tau hyperphosphorylation. J Biol Chem. 2006 Sep 1;281(35):
       25457-65.

[156] Seshadri S, Fitzpatrick AL, Ikram MA, DeStefano AL, Gudnason V, Boada M, et al.
       Genome-wide analysis of genetic loci associated with Alzheimer disease. JAMA.
       2010 May 12;303(18):1832-40.

[157] Hollingworth P, Harold D, Sims R, Gerrish A, Lambert JC, Carrasquillo MM, et al.
       Common variants at ABCA7, MS4A6A/MS4A4E, EPHA1, CD33 and CD2AP are as-
       sociated with Alzheimer's disease. Nat Genet. 2011 May;43(5):429-35.

[158] Naj AC, Jun G, Beecham GW, Wang LS, Vardarajan BN, Buros J, et al. Common var-
       iants at MS4A4/MS4A6E, CD2AP, CD33 and EPHA1 are associated with late-onset
       Alzheimer's disease. Nat Genet. 2011 May;43(5):436-41.

[159] Luna-Munoz J, Chavez-Macias L, Garcia-Sierra F, Mena R. Earliest stages of tau con-
       formational changes are related to the appearance of a sequence of specific phospho-
       dependent tau epitopes in Alzheimer's disease. J Alzheimers Dis. 2007 Dec;12(4):
       365-75.

[160] Luna-Munoz J, Garcia-Sierra F, Falcon V, Menendez I, Chavez-Macias L, Mena R. Re-
       gional conformational change involving phosphorylation of tau protein at the
       Thr231, precedes the structural change detected by Alz-50 antibody in Alzheimer's
       disease. J Alzheimers Dis. 2005 Sep;8(1):29-41.

[161] Augustinack JC, Schneider A, Mandelkow EM, Hyman BT. Specific tau phosphoryla-
       tion sites correlate with severity of neuronal cytopathology in Alzheimer's disease.
       Acta Neuropathol. 2002 Jan;103(1):26-35.

[162] Yaffe MB, Schutkowski M, Shen M, Zhou XZ, Stukenberg PT, Rahfeld JU, et al. Sequence-specific and phosphorylation-dependent proline isomerization: a potential mitotic regulatory mechanism. Science. 1997 Dec 12;278(5345):1957-60.

[163] Lee TH, Pastorino L, Lu KP. Peptidyl-prolyl cis-trans isomerase Pin1 in ageing, cancer and Alzheimer disease. Expert reviews in molecular medicine. 2011;13:e21.

[164] Lim J, Balastik M, Lee TH, Nakamura K, Liou YC, Sun A, et al. Pin1 has opposite effects on wild-type and P301L tau stability and tauopathy. J Clin Invest. 2008 May; 118(5):1877-89.

[165] Hampel H, Blennow K, Shaw LM, Hoessler YC, Zetterberg H, Trojanowski JQ. Total and phosphorylated tau protein as biological markers of Alzheimer's disease. Experimental gerontology. 2010 Jan;45(1):30-40.

[166] Blennow K, Hampel H, Weiner M, Zetterberg H. Cerebrospinal fluid and plasma biomarkers in Alzheimer disease. Nat Rev Neurol. 2010 Mar;6(3):131-44.

[167] Hamdane M, Dourlen P, Bretteville A, Sambo AV, Ferreira S, Ando K, et al. Pin1 allows for differential Tau dephosphorylation in neuronal cells. Mol Cell Neurosci. 2006 May-Jun;32(1-2):155-60.

[168] Galas MC, Dourlen P, Begard S, Ando K, Blum D, Hamdane M, et al. The peptidyl-prolyl cis/trans-isomerase Pin1 modulates stress-induced dephosphorylation of Tau in neurons. Implication in a pathological mechanism related to Alzheimer disease. J Biol Chem. 2006 Jul 14;281(28):19296-304.

[169] Butterfield DA, Poon HF, St Clair D, Keller JN, Pierce WM, Klein JB, et al. Redox proteomics identification of oxidatively modified hippocampal proteins in mild cognitive impairment: insights into the development of Alzheimer's disease. Neurobiol Dis. 2006 May;22(2):223-32.

[170] Butterfield DA, Abdul HM, Opii W, Newman SF, Joshi G, Ansari MA, et al. Pin1 in Alzheimer's disease. J Neurochem. 2006 Sep;98(6):1697-706.

[171] Thorpe JR, Morley SJ, Rulten SL. Utilizing the peptidyl-prolyl cis-trans isomerase pin1 as a probe of its phosphorylated target proteins. Examples of binding to nuclear proteins in a human kidney cell line and to tau in Alzheimer's diseased brain. The journal of histochemistry and cytochemistry : official journal of the Histochemistry Society. 2001 Jan;49(1):97-108.

[172] Thorpe JR, Mosaheb S, Hashemzadeh-Bonehi L, Cairns NJ, Kay JE, Morley SJ, et al. Shortfalls in the peptidyl-prolyl cis-trans isomerase protein Pin1 in neurons are associated with frontotemporal dementias. Neurobiol Dis. 2004 Nov;17(2):237-49.

[173] Wijsman EM, Daw EW, Yu CE, Payami H, Steinbart EJ, Nochlin D, et al. Evidence for a novel late-onset Alzheimer disease locus on chromosome 19p13.2. American journal of human genetics. 2004 Sep;75(3):398-409.

[174] Segat L, Milanese M, Crovella S. Pin1 promoter polymorphisms in hepatocellular carcinoma patients. Gastroenterology. 2007 Jun;132(7):2618-9; author reply 9-20.

[175] Ramakrishnan P, Dickson DW, Davies P. Pin1 colocalization with phosphorylated tau in Alzheimer's disease and other tauopathies. Neurobiol Dis. 2003 Nov;14(2): 251-64.

[176] Dakson A, Yokota O, Esiri M, Bigio EH, Horan M, Pendleton N, et al. Granular expression of prolyl-peptidyl isomerase PIN1 is a constant and specific feature of Alzheimer's disease pathology and is independent of tau, Abeta and TDP-43 pathology. Acta Neuropathol. 2011 May;121(5):635-49.

[177] Lu J, Hu Z, Wei S, Wang LE, Liu Z, El-Naggar AK, et al. A novel functional variant (-842G>C) in the PIN1 promoter contributes to decreased risk of squamous cell carcinoma of the head and neck by diminishing the promoter activity. Carcinogenesis. 2009 Oct;30(10):1717-21.

[178] Ma SL, Tang NL, Tam CW, Lui VW, Lam LC, Chiu HF, et al. A PIN1 polymorphism that prevents its suppression by AP4 associates with delayed onset of Alzheimer's disease. Neurobiol Aging. 2012 Apr;33(4):804-13.

[179] Han CH, Lu J, Wei Q, Bondy ML, Brewster AM, Yu TK, et al. The functional promoter polymorphism (-842G>C) in the PIN1 gene is associated with decreased risk of breast cancer in non-Hispanic white women 55 years and younger. Breast cancer research and treatment. 2010 Jul;122(1):243-9.

[180] Roe CM, Behrens MI, Xiong C, Miller JP, Morris JC. Alzheimer disease and cancer. Neurology. 2005 Mar 8;64(5):895-8.

[181] Roe CM, Fitzpatrick AL, Xiong C, Sieh W, Kuller L, Miller JP, et al. Cancer linked to Alzheimer disease but not vascular dementia. Neurology. 2010 Jan 12;74(2):106-12.

[182] Behrens MI, Lendon C, Roe CM. A common biological mechanism in cancer and Alzheimer's disease? Curr Alzheimer Res. 2009 Jun;6(3):196-204.

[183] Driver JA, Beiser A, Au R, Kreger BE, Splansky GL, Kurth T, et al. Inverse association between cancer and Alzheimer's disease: results from the Framingham Heart Study. Bmj. 2012;344:e1442.

[184] Bramblett GT, Goedert M, Jakes R, Merrick SE, Trojanowski JQ, Lee VM. Abnormal tau phosphorylation at Ser396 in Alzheimer's disease recapitulates development and contributes to reduced microtubule binding. Neuron. 1993 Jun;10(6):1089-99.

[185] Yoshida H, Ihara Y. Tau in paired helical filaments is functionally distinct from fetal tau: assembly incompetence of paired helical filament-tau. J Neurochem. 1993 Sep; 61(3):1183-6.

[186] Alonso AC, Zaidi T, Grundke-Iqbal I, Iqbal K. Role of abnormally phosphorylated tau in the breakdown of microtubules in Alzheimer disease. Proc Natl Acad Sci U S A. 1994 Jun 7;91(12):5562-6.

[187] Ishihara T, Hong M, Zhang B, Nakagawa Y, Lee MK, Trojanowski JQ, et al. Age-dependent emergence and progression of a tauopathy in transgenic mice overexpressing the shortest human tau isoform. Neuron. 1999 Nov;24(3):751-62.

[188] Davies CA, Mann DM, Sumpter PQ, Yates PO. A quantitative morphometric analysis of the neuronal and synaptic content of the frontal and temporal cortex in patients with Alzheimer's disease. Journal of the neurological sciences. 1987 Apr;78(2):151-64.

[189] Scheff SW, DeKosky ST, Price DA. Quantitative assessment of cortical synaptic density in Alzheimer's disease. Neurobiol Aging. 1990 Jan-Feb;11(1):29-37.

[190] DeKosky ST, Scheff SW. Synapse loss in frontal cortex biopsies in Alzheimer's disease: correlation with cognitive severity. Ann Neurol. 1990 May;27(5):457-64.

[191] Terry RD, Masliah E, Salmon DP, Butters N, DeTeresa R, Hill R, et al. Physical basis of cognitive alterations in Alzheimer's disease: synapse loss is the major correlate of cognitive impairment. Ann Neurol. 1991 Oct;30(4):572-80.

[192] Masliah E, Ellisman M, Carragher B, Mallory M, Young S, Hansen L, et al. Three-dimensional analysis of the relationship between synaptic pathology and neuropil threads in Alzheimer disease. J Neuropathol Exp Neurol. 1992 Jul;51(4):404-14.

[193] Coleman PD, Yao PJ. Synaptic slaughter in Alzheimer's disease. Neurobiol Aging. 2003 Dec;24(8):1023-7.

[194] Thies E, Mandelkow EM. Missorting of tau in neurons causes degeneration of synapses that can be rescued by the kinase MARK2/Par-1. J Neurosci. 2007 Mar 14;27(11): 2896-907.

[195] Sultana R, Boyd-Kimball D, Poon HF, Cai J, Pierce WM, Klein JB, et al. Oxidative modification and down-regulation of Pin1 in Alzheimer's disease hippocampus: A redox proteomics analysis. Neurobiol Aging. 2006;27:918-25.

[196] Davies DC, Horwood N, Isaacs SL, Mann DM. The effect of age and Alzheimer's disease on pyramidal neuron density in the individual fields of the hippocampal formation. Acta Neuropathol. 1992;83(5):510-7.

[197] Hof PR, Morrison JH. Neocortical neuronal subpopulations labeled by a monoclonal antibody to calbindin exhibit differential vulnerability in Alzheimer's disease. Exp Neurol. 1991 Mar;111(3):293-301.

[198] Augustinack JC, Schneider A, Mandelkow EM, Hyman BT. Specific tau phosphorylation sites correlate with severity of neuronal cytopathology in Alzheimer's disease. Acta Neuropathol (Berl). 2002 Jan;103(1):26-35.

[199] Ewers M, Buerger K, Teipel SJ, Scheltens P, Schroder J, Zinkowski RP, et al. Multicenter assessment of CSF-phosphorylated tau for the prediction of conversion of MCI. Neurology. 2007 Dec 11;69(24):2205-12.

[200] Hampel H, Buerger K, Kohnken R, Teipel SJ, Zinkowski R, Moeller HJ, et al. Tracking of Alzheimer's disease progression with cerebrospinal fluid tau protein phosphorylated at threonine 231. Ann Neurol. 2001 Apr;49(4):545-6.

[201] Lim J, Balastik M, Lee TH, Liou YC, Sun A, Finn G, et al. Pin1 has opposite effects on wild-type and P301L tau stability and tauopathy. J Clin Invest. 2008;118:1877-89.

[202] Ma SL, Tang NLS, Tam CWC, Lui VWC, Lam LCW, Chiu HFK, et al. A functional polymorphism in Pin1 thatprevents its suppression by AP4 Is associated with delayed onset of Alzheimer's disease. Neurobiol Aging. 2010:(in press).

[203] Asuni AA, Boutajangout A, Quartermain D, Sigurdsson EM. Immunotherapy targeting pathological tau conformers in a tangle mouse model reduces brain pathology with associated functional improvements. J Neurosci. 2007 Aug 22;27(34):9115-29.

[204] Boutajangout A, Quartermain D, Sigurdsson EM. Immunotherapy targeting pathological tau prevents cognitive decline in a new tangle mouse model. J Neurosci. 2010 Dec 8;30(49):16559-66.

[205] Boimel M, Grigoriadis N, Lourbopoulos A, Haber E, Abramsky O, Rosenmann H. Efficacy and safety of immunization with phosphorylated tau against neurofibrillary tangles in mice. Exp Neurol. 2010 Aug;224(2):472-85.

[206] Kayed R, Jackson GR. Prefilament tau species as potential targets for immunotherapy for Alzheimer disease and related disorders. Current opinion in immunology. 2009 Jun;21(3):359-63.

[207] Wisniewski T, Boutajangout A. Vaccination as a therapeutic approach to Alzheimer's disease. The Mount Sinai journal of medicine, New York. 2010 Jan-Feb;77(1):17-31.

[208] Ubhi K, Masliah E. Recent advances in the development of immunotherapies for tauopathies. Exp Neurol. 2011 Oct 21;230.

[209] Boutajangout A, Ingadottir J, Davies P, Sigurdsson EM. Passive immunization targeting pathological phospho-tau protein in a mouse model reduces functional decline and clears tau aggregates from the brain. J Neurochem. 2011 Jun 3;118:658-67.

[210] Lu KP, Zhou XZ. The prolyl isomerase Pin1: a pivotal new twist in phosphorylation signalling and human disease. Nat Rev Mol Cell Biol. 2007;8:904-16.

[211] Lu KP, Finn G, Lee TH, Nicholson LK. Prolyl cis-trans isomerization as a molecular timer. Nature Chem Biol. 2007;3:619-29.

[212] Liou YC, Zhou XZ, Lu KP. The prolyl isomerase Pin1 as a molecular switch to determine the fate of phosphoproteins. Trends Biochem Sci. 2011:(Accepted).

[213] Theuerkorn M, Fischer G, Schiene-Fischer C. Prolyl cis/trans isomerase signalling pathways in cancer. Curr Opin Pharmacol. 2011 Apr 13:Epub 2011/04/19.

[214] Hsiao K, Chapman P, Nilsen S, Eckman C, Harigaya Y, Younkin S, et al. Correlative memory deficits, Abeta elevation, and amyloid plaques in transgenic mice. Science. 1996 Oct 4;274(5284):99-102.

[215] Duff K, Eckman C, Zehr C, Yu X, Prada CM, Perez-tur J, et al. Increased amyloid-beta42(43) in brains of mice expressing mutant presenilin 1. Nature. 1996 Oct 24;383(6602):710-3.

[216] Games D, Adams D, Alessandrini R, Barbour R, Berthelette P, Blackwell C, et al. Alzheimer-type neuropathology in transgenic mice overexpressing V717F beta-amyloid precursor protein. Nature. 1995 Feb 9;373(6514):523-7.

[217] Hall AM, Roberson ED. Mouse models of Alzheimer's disease. Brain Res Bull. 2012 May 1;88(1):3-12.

[218] Gotz J, Ittner LM. Animal models of Alzheimer's disease and frontotemporal dementia. Nat Rev Neurosci. 2008 Jul;9(7):532-44.

[219] Irizarry MC, Soriano F, McNamara M, Page KJ, Schenk D, Games D, et al. Abeta deposition is associated with neuropil changes, but not with overt neuronal loss in the human amyloid precursor protein V717F (PDAPP) transgenic mouse. J Neurosci. 1997 Sep 15;17(18):7053-9.

[220] Poorkaj P, Bird TD, Wijsman E, Nemens E, Garruto RM, Anderson L, et al. Tau is a candidate gene for chromosome 17 frontotemporal dementia. Ann Neurol. 1998 Jun; 43(6):815-25.

[221] Spillantini MG, Murrell JR, Goedert M, Farlow MR, Klug A, Ghetti B. Mutation in the tau gene in familial multiple system tauopathy with presenile dementia. Proc Natl Acad Sci U S A. 1998 Jun 23;95(13):7737-41.

[222] Gotz J, Chen F, van Dorpe J, Nitsch RM. Formation of neurofibrillary tangles in P301l tau transgenic mice induced by Abeta 42 fibrils. Science. 2001 Aug 24;293(5534): 1491-5.

[223] Lewis J, Dickson DW, Lin WL, Chisholm L, Corral A, Jones G, et al. Enhanced neurofibrillary degeneration in transgenic mice expressing mutant tau and APP. Science. 2001 Aug 24;293(5534):1487-91.

Chapter 6

Phosphorylation of Tau Protein Associated as a Protective Mechanism in the Presence of Toxic, C-Terminally Truncated Tau in Alzheimer's Disease

José Luna-Muñoz, Charles R. Harrington,
Claude M. Wischik, Paola Flores-Rodríguez,
Jesús Avila, Sergio R. Zamudio, Fidel De la Cruz,
Raúl Mena, Marco A. Meraz-Ríos and
Benjamin Floran-Garduño

Additional information is available at the end of the chapter

1. Introduction

Alzheimer's disease (AD) is the most common cause of dementia in the elderly and is characterized by progressive memory loss leading to a gradual and irreversible deterioration of cognitive function. The neuropathology of AD is characterized by the accumulation of fibrillary lesions in the form of neuritic plaques (NPs, Fig. 1A), neurofibrillary tangles (NFTs, Fig. 1C,D; small arrow) and dystrophic neurites (DNs, Fig. 1; arrows) in neocortex, amygdala and hippocampus [1]. The density of the NPs and NFTs correlate with the degree of dementia in AD [2]. The accumulation of these lesions does not occur at random; the presence of NFTs is associated with vulnerability of the perforant pathway [3]. NPs are comprised of extracellular deposits of amyloid-β peptide fibrils that are associated with DNs of dendritic and axonal origin (Fig. 1A; arrows). Intracellular NFTs selectively kill neurons in specific brain areas. In AD, the distribution of NFTs follows a stereotypical profile arising first in layer II of the entorhinal cortex, hippocampal region and CA1/subicular layer IV of the entorhinal cortex and then neocortex (mainly in fronto-temporal and parietal areas). This pattern of distribution was first described by Braak and Braak in 1991 [4], and provides the most important neuropathological criteria for a definite diagnosis of AD (Fig. 2) [5]. Ultrastructurally, NFTs are composed of dense accumulations of structures known as paired helical filaments (PHFs) [6, 7], which are mainly distributed in the perinuclear area of the neuron and in proximal processes (Fig. 1C). Tau protein is the major structural constituent of the PHF subunits [7-9]. Normally, tau protein exists as a family of microtubule-associated protein (MAPs) that are found predominantly in axons. Through repeated domains located toward the carboxy-terminus of the protein, tau provides stability to the microtubule and this process can be regulated through a balance in the phosphorylation/dephosphorylation process of tau protein [10]. In AD, tau protein accumulates as PHFs in the somatodendritic compartment, with consequent destabilization of axonal microtubules. Tau is further posttranslationally in AD, with modifications of ubiquitination [11, 12], glycation [13, 14], glycosylation [15], nitration [16], polyamination [17], hyperphosphorylation [18, 19] and proteolysis [7, 20-24]. The latter two changes occur throughout the tau molecule [25-27].

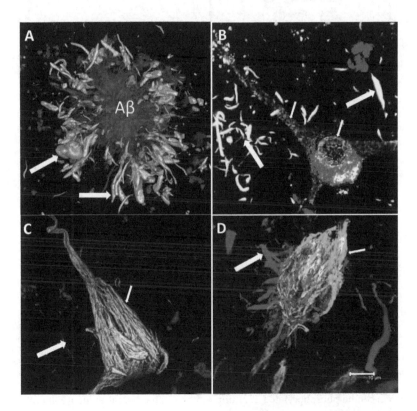

Figure 1. Neuropathological hallmarks of Alzheimer's disease. Double labelling with tau antibody (green channel) counterstained with thiazine red (red channel). A) A classical neuritic plaquein which an amyloid fibrillar plaque (Aβ), recognized by thiazine red, is associated with dystrophic neurites (arrows). B). Pre-tangle cells are characterized by diffuse granular deposits throughout the perinuclear area (small arrow) and proximal processes. C) A neurofibrillary tangle that is strongly labeled by tau antibody and colocalized with tiazine red. (A,B) projection of 20 and 9 confocal microscopy sections, respectively, each of 1.0 μm thickness.

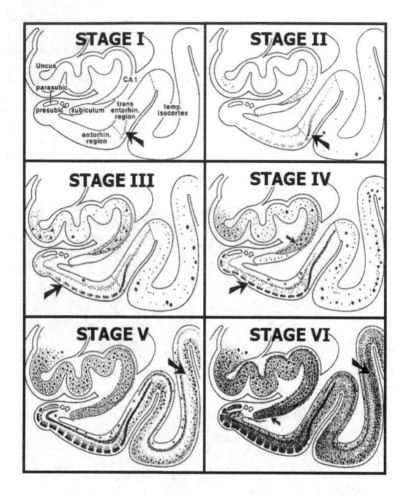

Figure 2. Braak stages of AD neuropathology base on the pattern of neurofibrillary change (NFT, Neuropil threads and plaques dystrofic neurites) [4], Although clinic-pathological correlations were not made, Braak and Braak did speculate that the entorhinal stage (I-II) represents clinically silent periods of the disease with NFT involvement confined to trans-entorhinal layer pre-alpha. Limbic stages (III/IV) correspond with clinically incipient AD, and NFT involvement of CA1, and neocortical stages (V/VI) represent fully developed AD, with NFT involvement of all areas of association cortex.

Tau protein can be phosphorylated at multiple sites. While there is evidence that phosphorylation of tau protein promotes its assembly into PHFs [18, 19, 28, 29], the role of phosphorylation in the genesis of PHFs has been limited to the analysis of "mature", intracellular NFTs (NFT-I). By this stage in the disease, tau protein will have been affected by many different pathological processes, several of which may be associated with the hyperphosphorylation process [25, 26, 30].

Another post-translational modification found in AD is the proteolytic truncation of the C-terminal portion of tau protein [7, 20, 21, 23, 31, 32]. It has been proposed that such truncation unlike hyperphosphorylation, favours polymerisation of tau [33, 34][35].

In recent years, evidence from both *in vitro* and *in vivo* studies[36, 37], suggests that hyperphosphorylation of tau protein has a protective role. In this review, we analyze the protective effects of hyperphosphorylated species of tau protein and their relationship to toxicity, and the participation of truncated species of tau in the formation of PHFs.

2. Tau protein

The cytoskeleton is formed by three types of filaments: microfilaments, intermediate filaments and microtubules [38]. The cytoskeleton provides a dynamic scaffold to proteins, vesicles and organelles, essential for proper cell function and changes in the state of its polymerization, play an important role in neuronal process such as polarization, axonal transport, maintenance of neuronal extensions, synaptic plasticity and protein sorting [39]. Tau protein functions as a regulator of microtubule assembly [40]. Tau protein participates in microtubule polymerization [41], regulation of axonal diameter [42], regulation of axonal transport [43], neurogenesis and the establishment of neuronal polarity in development [44]. Furthermore, tau participates in the regulation of signaling pathways by acting as a protein scaffold.

The gene that encodes for tau consists of 16 exons and is located at the chromosomal locus 17q21 [45]. Through alternative splicing, six tau isoforms are generated in the CNS, varying from 352-441 amino acids in length (Fig. 3). Tau protein can be divided into three domains: an acidic region in the N-terminal projection, a proline-rich domain and a microtubule-binding domain (Fig. 4) [46]. The alternative transcription of exons 2, 3 and 10 modifies the presence of repeats in the N-terminus of tau (0-2N) and the number of microtubule-binding repeat domains (3R or 4R), respectively.

3. Tau protein metabolism

The *MAPT* (tau) gene is transcribed mainly in neurons and a promoter that confers neuronal specificity has been described [47]. It has been reported that the presence of a tau promoter lacking neuronal specificity might account for the expression of tau in peripheral tissue [48]. In both cases, sequences containing binding sites for transcription factors AP2 and Sp1 were described. Whereas tau protein synthesis is unaffected by microtubule polymerization or depolymerization, degradation of tau is stimulated by microtubule depolymerization [49].

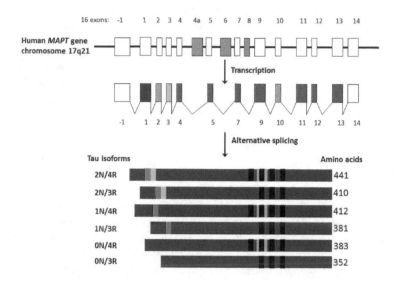

Figure 3. Schematic representation of the human *MAPT* (tau) gene, the primary tau transcript and the six CNS tau protein isoforms. The *MAPT* gene is located over 100kb of the long arm of chromosome 17 at position 17q21. It contains 16 exons, with exon −1 is a part of the promoter (upper panel). The tau primary transcript contains 13 exons. Exons −1 and 14 are transcribed but not translated. Exons 1, 4, 5, 7, 9, 11, 12, 13 are constitutive, and exons 2, 3, and 10 are alternatively spliced, giving rise to six different mRNAs, translated in six different CNS tau isoforms (lower panel). These isoforms differ by the absence or presence of one or two N-terminal inserts of 29 amino acids encoded by exon 2 (yellow box) and 3 (green box), in combination with either three (R1, R3 and R4) or four (R1–R4) C-terminal repeat-regions (black boxes). The additional microtubule-binding domain is encoded by exon 10 (pink box) (lower panel). Adult tau includes all six tau isoforms, including the largest isoform of 441-amino acids containing all inserts and other isoforms as indicated. The shortest 352-amino acids isoform is the only one found only in fetal brain.

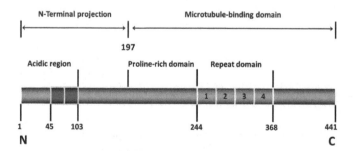

Figure 4. Schematic representation of the functional domains of the largest tau isoform (441 amino acids). The projection domain, including an acidic and a proline-rich region, interacts with cytoskeletal elements to determine the spacing between microtubules in axons. The N-terminal part is also involved in signal transduction pathways by interacting with proteins such as PLC-γ and Src-kinases. The C-terminal part, referred to as the microtubule-binding domain, regulates the rate of microtubules polymerization and is involved in binding with functional proteins such as protein phosphatase 2A (PP2A) or presenilin 1(PS1).

It is technically difficult to determine the half life of the different tau isoforms and several factors may regulate tau degradation such as, for example, the extent of phosphorylation and acetylation of tau (see below). The half life of tau decreases in rats by neonatal period P20 and there is less demand for tau in non-dividing, mature neurons [50].

Two main mechanisms for tau protein degradation have been documented: 1) the proteasomal ubiquitin pathway and 2) the lysosomal autophagic pathway. Proteasomal degradation of tau protein has been described by 20S proteasomal processing [51], although there have also been reports suggesting that tau is not normally degraded by the proteasome [52]. Tau, modified by phosphorylation, can be ubiquitinated by the CHIP-hsc70 complex and degraded by the proteasome [53]. Furthermore, acetylation of tau can regulate its proteasomal degradation by modifying those lysine residues needed for ubiquitination. In this way, acetylation of tau inhibits its degradation through a competition between ubiquitination and acetylation [54].

On the other hand, tau may get processed through a lysosomal autophagic mechanism. It has been reported that tau can be degraded by lysosomal proteases [55] and, more recently, it was shown that tau fragmentation and clearance can occur by lysosomal processing [56].

Tau protein is a microtubule-associated protein. It's mostly abundant in neurons in the Central Nervous System (CNS). The main function of Tau protein is to interact with tubulin to stabilize microtubules and promote tubulin assembly into microtubules. Tau protein controls microtubule stability in two different ways : isoforms and phosphorylation.

Normally, the tau protein is very important, as it manages the transport of materials within soma and other cellular regions through the myelin sheaths. Once it spotted something suspicious or irrelevant, it stops the information sending process automatically. However, in Alzheimer's disease, the tau proteins started to perform uncommon reaction, where it transmitting the information to the brain simultaneously, regardless of its validity.

Once the above problem happening, it causes the brain overloading with information and might lead to inflammation, clumps or tangles, which kill most of the brain cells (Fig. 5).

4. Phosphporylation of tau protein

Protein phosphorylation is the addition of a phosphate group, by esterification, to one of three different amino acids: serine, threonine and tyrosine. Phosphorylation is the most common post-translational modification of tau described and increased tau phosphorylation reduces its affinity for microtubules leading to cytoskeletal destabilization. Eighty-five putative phosphorylation sites on tau protein have been described in AD brain tissue (Fig. 6). The formation of fibrillar aggregates of post-translationally modified tau protein in the brain are characteristic of AD and other tauopathies. The phosphorylation of tau protein affects its solubility, localization, function, interaction with partners and susceptibility to other post-translational modifications. However, the role of specific sites of tau phosphorylation in early neurodegenerative mechanisms is unknown. The molecular mechanisms of aggregation of tau into insoluble forms may help to account for the different dementias in which both clinical symptoms and age of onset differ.

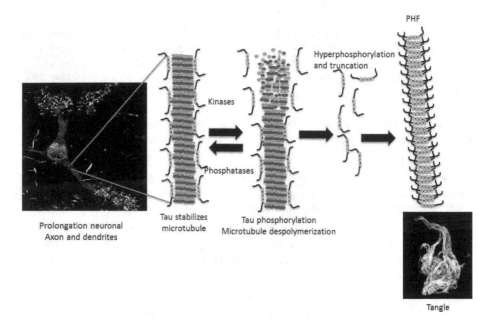

Figure 5. tau protein, which forms part of a microtubule. The microtubule helps transpot nutrients and other important substances from one part of the nerve cells to another. Axon are long threadlike extensions that conduct nerve impulses away from the nerve cells; dendrites are short branched threadlike extensions that conduct nerve impulses toward the verve cell body. In Alzheimer´s disease the tau protein is abnormal and the microtubule structures collapse.

5. C-terminal truncation of tau protein in AD

5.1. PHF-core concept

In 1988, Wischik et al, [7, 22] identified tau protein as the major constituent of Pronase-resistant PHFs and tau was characterized by a specific C-terminal truncation of the protein at Glu-391. This truncation is identified by the monoclonal antibody (mAb) 423 [23, 31], and the acid-reversible occlusion of the intact core tau domain. PHFs are labeled by the fluorescent dye, thiazin-red, a dye which can be used to differentiate between amorphous and fibrillar states of tau and amyloid proteins in AD. The minimum tau fragment in the PHF [20, 24] corresponds to the tandem repeat region in the C-terminal domain of tau protein, a species having a molecular weight of 12.5 kDa. Characteristically, this fragment is highly stable to proteolysis, insoluble and toxic and is referred to as PHF-core tau [22, 57, 58]. PHF-core tau and mAb 423 immunoreactivity of NFTs, have a close clinical-pathological relationship; the density of NFTs immunolabelled with mAb 423 is correlated with the progression of neurofibrilary pathology, as determined by Braak staging criteria (Fig. 2). Most significantly, there is a correlation between mAb 423 immunoreactivity and both clinical severity and progression to dementia [3]. On the other hand, over-expression of PHF-core tau, in cell culture, favors a programmed cell death or apoptosis, which shows that it is highly toxic[59]. Recombinant tau protein truncated at Glu-391 also shows increased rates of polymerization compared with recombinant full-length tau. From confocal microscopy studies, it has been shown that this fragment of tau is hidden within the PHF-core and exposed by formic acid treatment [57]. In the cytoplasm of susceptible neurons, this truncated tau triggers an auto-catalytic process in which the fragment has a high affinity for full length tau and, once bound, leads to cycles of proteolysis and further tau binding to form a proto-filament [60]. In this scenario, the initiating tau species that gave rise to the filament is hidden within a large number of covering tau molecules, some of which become hyperphosphorylated. This would correspond to the early aggregation of tau protein associated with PHF in small NFT. Tau molecules of the NFT would become exposed on death of the neuron to reveal the extracellular NFT, or "ghost tangle" (Fig. 1D, small arrow) which shares the properties of being stable, insoluble and immunoreactive with mAb 423 [57, 61]. The proteases responsible for truncation at Glu-391 are not known.

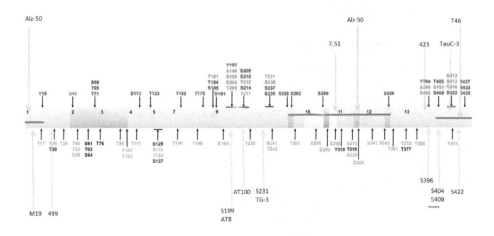

Figure 6. Location of tau phosphorylation sites and epitopes for tau antibodies. Multiple amino acids are phosphorylated with some those observed in AD brain [5], normal brain (green) and both normal and AD brains (blue). Putative phosphorylation sites that have not yet been demonstrated *in vitro* or *in vivo* (black). Localization of antibody epitopes are indicated arrows. Residues are numbered according to the longest tau isoform.

6. Truncation of tau protein at Asp-421

In 2003, a second truncation of tau protein was found to be associated with PHFs [62-65]. This truncation is found at position Asp-421 in the C-terminus of the tau molecule and its presence can be detected specifically by using mAb TauC-3[25, 63]. Unlike truncation at Glu-391, for which the protease responsible is unknown, caspase-3 (an enzyme involved in the apoptotic pathway) is responsible for the truncation at Asp-421 *in vitro* [59, 62, 63]. This suggests that cleavage of the carboxyl terminus of tau protein, could result as a neuronal response to prevent or control the polymerization of tau in PHF [58]. In 2005, Binder and colleagues discovered a truncation at the amino terminus of the tau protein associated with PHFs. This cut corresponds to Asp-13, which is produced by caspase-6, another enzyme involved in the apoptotic pathway [66]. An antibody to detect this cleavage site of the amino terminus of tau protein has not yet been generated.

Tau-C3 has an affinity for NFTs, NDs and neuropil threads in AD brains. Immunohistochemical studies indicated that truncation at Asp-421 occurs after conformational change; the antibody binds with greatest affinity when the amino terminus of tau molecule contacts the third microtubule binding repeat (MTBR), as recognized by mAb Alz-50 [26]. However, other studies have shown Tau-C3 immunoreactivity in pre-tangle cells before they become Alz-50 immunoreactive and in the absence of PHFs [64, 67].

7. Impact of phosphorylation and truncation on the abnormal processing of tau protein in AD

7.1. A neuroprotective mechanism for the phosphorylation of tau protein in the AD brain

During neurodegeneration in AD, tau protein is abnormally phosphorylated in the proline-rich region at Ser and Thr residues [68], and such phosphorylation sites can be identified using highly specific antibodies such as: AT8 (Ser-202/Thr-205) AT100 (Ser-212 and Ser-214), TG3 (Thr-231/Ser-235) and PHF-1 (Ser-396/Ser-404), among others (Fig. 6). However, NFTs are found in viable neurons at late stages of the disease, and they persist in neuronal cells for decades with a significant number of NFTs being found in the cognitively intact elderly [69, 70]. Such NFT-bearing neurons contain normal content and structure of microtubules [68]. The findings from studies in transgenic mice and human data, suggest that tau accumulation in the somatodendritic compartment may represent the manifestation of a protective mechanism or a cellular adaptation that arises with advancing age. An increase in tau phosphorylation in AD brain has been associated with a protective mechanism against oxidative stress [71]. In another study, intact microtubules were found in NFT-bearing neurons [8], calling into question whether accumulation of phosphorylated tau and destabilization of microtubules are necessarily linked. Although microtubules are depolymerized in neurons with fibrillary degeneration, one study found evidence that the reduction of microtubules in AD is marked and specifically limited to vulnerable pyramidal neurons, and that even these alterations were observed in the absence of PHF [72]. This finding is also consistent with previous work by one of the authors noting a microtubule decrease of nearly 50% in dendrites that did not correlate with either PHFs or age [73], suggesting that a proportion of phosphorylated tau protein is associated with microtubules [71]. In animal models, it has been confirmed that axonal transport is not affected by either over-expression or reduction of tau protein *in vivo* [42, 74]. Another study found evidence that axonopathy precedes the formation of NFTs in a transgenic mouse [75]. A transgenic mouse expressing a human tau isoform developed NFTs, neuronal loss and behavioral impairments [58]. After suppression of tau expression, the behavioral deficits stabilized yet NFTs continued to accumulate, suggesting that NFTs are not sufficient to cause cognitive decline or neuronal death.

Within NFTs, different species of tau protein associated with phosphorylation are observed, but the neurodegenerating neurons still appear to be functional [75]. These observations suggest that the cytoplasmic accumulation of hyperphosphorylated tau protein is non-toxic, similar to the accumulation of lipofuscin that does not alter cellular metabolism[68]. It is generally assumed that disintegration of microtubules is associated with an imbalance between kinase and phosphatase activities, which lead to an alteration in the stability of microtubules, disruption of cell function and culminate in neuronal death. The data, however, suggest that, at least, a subpopulation of hyperphosphorylated NFTs may be not toxic. This is controversial, given the fact that the hyperphosphorylation of tau and NFTs are considered to be toxic. However, the ability of tau protein fractions, purified from AD brains, to alter microtubule assembly, *in vitro*, has been attributed to sequestration of normal tau molecules [18]. Alonso and colleagues [28] demonstrated that recombinant hyperphosphorylated tau, *in vitro*, decreases the breakdown of the recombinant microtubule when assembled into small aggregates [19, 28]. On this basis, the authors suggested that hyperphosphorylated tau protein plays a protective role against the disintegration of the microtubule.

Tau that has been hyperphosphorylated with GSK3-β kinase becomes immunoreactive with mAbs AT8, PHF1 and TG-3, antibodies whose epitopes are very closely related to AD [29, 76]. The fact that GSK3-β is capable of creating epitopes considered pathological in AD suggests that there are other participants that require to be considered. These data suggest the possible existence of a toxic species of non-phosphorylated tau protein, which would be responsible for capturing further molecules of tau in PHFs, yet would not be exposed on the filament [7, 57, 61]. It is possible that, by hiding the toxic form in PHFs could protect the neuron [77]. It is important to note that the presumed "intermediaries" are present in the cytoplasm of the neuron when it is still viable. Another study showed that NFTs (and presumably tau oligomers) could remain in the cytoplasm of the neuron for decades [78], an observation that would further argue against a primary toxicity of phosphorylated tau protein in AD.

7.2. Hyperphosphorylation of tau protein protecting neurons from apoptosis

It is also proposed that apoptosis plays an important role in neuronal damage in AD. This proposal is based on the detection of fragmented DNA and expression of apoptosis signaling proteins such as caspases 3, 6, 8 and 9, Bax, Fas and Fas-L, in the cortex and hippocampus, in postmortem brain tissue [79, 80] and observations that amyloid-β can induce neuronal apoptosis [81]. Apoptosis is a process that usually occurs over a period of hours, whereas the accumulation of tangles found in AD brains occurs over a period of years or decades [78]. It has been suggested that hyperphosphorylation of tau protein is a mechanism used to evade cell death by apoptosis. Cells over-expressing hyperphosphorylated tau appear to avoid the apoptotic process [82].

8. Participation of hyperphosphorylated and truncated tau species in the early formation of PHFs

8.1. Model for the mechanism of assembly

Despite suggestions of a neuroprotective role for tau protein in AD, links between phosphorylated species (that are presumed to be protective) and the complex assembly of toxic, truncated tau into insoluble PHFs is not clear. In recent years, we have characterized the early stages of tau protein processing in neurons (pre-tangle state) (Fig. 1B, small arrows) and have described accumulations of tau that possess pathological species present in NFT, yet which do not show the presence of assembled structures in PHFs [67, 83]. The pre-tangle (Fig. 1B) is the first step in non-fibrillar aggregation of tau protein in AD and one in which at least 5 different changes take place (Fig 1 C,D). These events include: a) the presence of a C-terminally truncated and toxic tau species (Glu-391); b) a cascade of specific phosphorylation of tau protein in the N-terminus; c) C-terminal truncation via the action of caspase-3; d) oligomerization and aggregation of tau species and e) assembly of tau into PHFs.

A model to accommodate the observations are represented schematically in Fig. 7. In this model, the first event to occur would be the emergence of tau oligomers or a PHF subunit (Fig. 7 A,B). The mechanism whereby this is initiated is unknown, but its toxicity and high affinity for binding to intact tau molecules would trigger an immediate need for the cell to protect itself. That would be reflected by hyperphosphorylation of the molecule in a failed attempt to hide the PHF and prevent the capture of further intact tau molecules (Fig. 7 B,C). In AD, this protective function of the phosphorylated species favors more molecules becoming available for sequestration and formation into PHFs (Fig. 7D). Gradually, phosphorylated tau will be affected by exogenous proteolysis to re-expose the PHF-core (Fig. 7E). These steps follow as a molecular consequence of the catastrophic fragmentation of the microtubule, synaptic dysfunction, oxidative stress and post-translational modifications of tau. This model emphasizes that polymerization and neuroprotective mechanisms are both involved in the development of PHFs. The phosphorylated species of tau protein play a role in the initial protective response of the neuron to prevent the assembly of these filaments [35]. Thus NFTs, in which externally available tau is hyperphosphorylated, represents a mechanism whereby the neuron may try to protect itself from neurofibrillary degeneration and further studies to confirm this hypothesis are warranted.

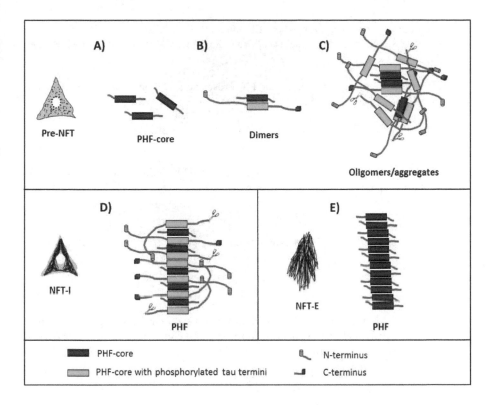

Figure 7. Scheme illustrating the early steps of aggregation and polymerization of tau protein in Alzheimer's disease. (A) The model starts with the appearance of PHF-core tau in cytoplasm of susceptible neurons. (B) The high binding capacity of PHF-tau results in the assembly of dimers of PHF-core and intact tau molecules in the cytoplasm. (C) The phosphorylation of intact tau would be an early event to hide the toxic soluble aggregates of molecules. (D). The high affinity and stability of the proto-filaments that make up the mature intracellular NFT allows tau molecules to form PHFs. (E) With the death of the neuron, the PHF-core subunit becomes exposed again in the extracellular space following proteolysis. Further details are described in the text.

Acknowledgements

Authors express their gratitude to the Mexican families for the donation of brain tissue from their beloved and without which these studies would not be possible. Amparo Viramontes Pintos for the handling of brain tissue. This work was financially supported by CONACyT grants, No. 142293 (to B.F.).

Author details

José Luna-Muñoz[1], Charles R. Harrington[2], Claude M. Wischik[2], Paola Flores-Rodríguez[1], Jesús Avila[3], Sergio R. Zamudio[4], Fidel De la Cruz[4], Raúl Mena[1], Marco A. Meraz-Ríos[5] and Benjamin Floran-Garduño[1]

1 Departments of Physiology, Biophysics and Neurosciences, National Laboratory of experimental services (LaNSE), CINVESTAV-IPN, Mexico

2 Division of Applied Health Sciences, School of Medicine and Dentistry, University of Aberdeen, USA

3 Centro de Biología Molecular "Severo Ochoa", CSIC/UAM, Universidad Autónoma de Madrid, Madrid, Spain

4 Department of Physiology, ENCB-IPN, Mexico

5 Molecular Biomedicine, CINVESTAV-IPN, Mexico

References

[1] Arnold, S.E., et al., The topographical and neuroanatomical distribution of neurofibrillary tangles and neuritic plaques in the cerebral cortex of patients with Alzheimer's disease. Cerebral cortex, 1991. 1(1): p. 103-16.

[2] Arriagada, P.V., et al., Neurofibrillary tangles but not senile plaques parallel duration and severity of Alzheimer's disease. Neurology, 1992. 42(3 Pt 1): p. 631-9.

[3] Garcia-Sierra, F., et al., The extent of neurofibrillary pathology in perforant pathway neurons is the key determinant of dementia in the very old. Acta Neuropathol, 2000. 100(1): p. 29-35.

[4] Braak, H. and E. Braak, Neuropathological stageing of Alzheimer-related changes. Acta Neuropathol, 1991. 82(4): p. 239-59.

[5] Braak, H., et al., Staging of Alzheimer disease-associated neurofibrillary pathology using paraffin sections and immunocytochemistry. Acta Neuropathol, 2006. 112(4): p. 389-404.

[6] Kidd, M., Paired helical filaments in electron microscopy of Alzheimer's disease. Nature, 1963. 197: p. 192-3.

[7] Wischik, C.M., et al., Structural characterization of the core of the paired helical filament of Alzheimer disease. Proc Natl Acad Sci U S A, 1988. 85(13): p. 4884-8.

[8] Crowther, R.A. and C.M. Wischik, Image reconstruction of the Alzheimer paired helical filament. Embo J, 1985. 4(13B): p. 3661-5.

[9]   Kondo, J., et al., The carboxyl third of tau is tightly bound to paired helical filaments. Neuron, 1988. 1(9): p. 827-34.

[10] Lee, G., R.L. Neve, and K.S. Kosik, The microtubule binding domain of tau protein. Neuron, 1989. 2(6): p. 1615-24.

[11] Perry, G., et al., Ubiquitin is detected in neurofibrillary tangles and senile plaque neurites of Alzheimer disease brains. Proc Natl Acad Sci U S A, 1987. 84(9): p. 3033-6.

[12] Mori, H., J. Kondo, and Y. Ihara, Ubiquitin is a component of paired helical filaments in Alzheimer's disease. Science, 1987. 235(4796): p. 1641-4.

[13] Ledesma, M.D., P. Bonay, and J. Avila, Tau protein from Alzheimer's disease patients is glycated at its tubulin-binding domain. J Neurochem, 1995. 65(4): p. 1658-64.

[14] Ledesma, M.D., et al., Analysis of microtubule-associated protein tau glycation in paired helical filaments. J Biol Chem, 1994. 269(34): p. 21614-9.

[15] Wang, J.Z., I. Grundke-Iqbal, and K. Iqbal, Glycosylation of microtubule-associated protein tau: an abnormal posttranslational modification in Alzheimer's disease. Nat Med, 1996. 2(8): p. 871-5.

[16] Horiguchi, T., et al., Nitration of tau protein is linked to neurodegeneration in tauopathies. Am J Pathol, 2003. 163(3): p. 1021-31.

[17] Tucholski, J., J. Kuret, and G.V. Johnson, Tau is modified by tissue transglutaminase in situ: possible functional and metabolic effects of polyamination. J Neurochem, 1999. 73(5): p. 1871-80.

[18] Alonso, A.C., I. Grundke-Iqbal, and K. Iqbal, Alzheimer's disease hyperphosphorylated tau sequesters normal tau into tangles of filaments and disassembles microtubules. Nat Med, 1996. 2(7): p. 783-7.

[19] Alonso Adel, C., et al., Polymerization of hyperphosphorylated tau into filaments eliminates its inhibitory activity. Proc Natl Acad Sci U S A, 2006. 103(23): p. 8864-9.

[20] Novak, M., J. Kabat, and C.M. Wischik, Molecular characterization of the minimal protease resistant tau unit of the Alzheimer's disease paired helical filament. Embo J, 1993. 12(1): p. 365-70.

[21] Wischik, C.M., et al., Quantitative analysis of tau protein in paired helical filament preparations: implications for the role of tau protein phosphorylation in PHF assembly in Alzheimer's disease. Neurobiol Aging, 1995. 16(3): p. 409-17; discussion 418-31.

[22] Wischik, C.M., et al., Isolation of a fragment of tau derived from the core of the paired helical filament of Alzheimer disease. Proc Natl Acad Sci U S A, 1988. 85(12): p. 4506-10.

[23] Novak, M., Truncated tau protein as a new marker for Alzheimer's disease. Acta Virol, 1994. 38(3): p. 173-89.

[24] Novak, M., et al., Difference between the tau protein of Alzheimer paired helical filament core and normal tau revealed by epitope analysis of monoclonal antibodies 423
and 7.51. Proc Natl Acad Sci U S A, 1991. 88(13): p. 5837-41.

[25] Guillozet-Bongaarts, A.L., et al., Tau truncation during neurofibrillary tangle evolution in Alzheimer's disease. Neurobiol Aging, 2005. 26(7): p. 1015-22.

[26] Garcia-Sierra, F., et al., Conformational changes and truncation of tau protein during
tangle evolution in Alzheimer's disease. J Alzheimers Dis, 2003. 5(2): p. 65-77.

[27] Garcia-Sierra, F., S. Mondragon-Rodriguez, and G. Basurto-Islas, Truncation of tau
protein and its pathological significance in Alzheimer's disease. J Alzheimers Dis,
2008. 14(4): p. 401-9.

[28] Alonso, A., et al., Hyperphosphorylation induces self-assembly of tau into tangles of
paired helical filaments/straight filaments. Proc Natl Acad Sci U S A, 2001. 98(12): p.
6923-8.

[29] Iqbal, K. and I. Grundke-Iqbal, Discoveries of tau, abnormally hyperphosphorylated
tau and others of neurofibrillary degeneration: a personal historical perspective. J
Alzheimers Dis, 2006. 9(3 Suppl): p. 219-42.

[30] Augustinack, J.C., et al., Specific tau phosphorylation sites correlate with severity of
neuronal cytopathology in Alzheimer's disease. Acta Neuropathol, 2002. 103(1): p.
26-35.

[31] Novak, M., et al., Characterisation of the first monoclonal antibody against the pro-
nase resistant core of the Alzheimer PHF. Prog Clin Biol Res, 1989. 317: p. 755-61.

[32] Garcia-Sierra, F., et al., Accumulation of C-terminally truncated tau protein associated with vulnerability of the perforant pathway in early stages of neurofibrillary pathology in Alzheimer's disease. J Chem Neuroanat, 2001. 22(1-2): p. 65-77.

[33] Wischik, C.M., Lay R.Y., Harrington C.R. , Modelling prion-like processing of tau
protein in Alzheimer's disease for pharmaceutical development., in Modifications in
Alzheimer's disease, B.R. Avila J., Kosik K.S., Editor 1997, Harwood Academic: Am-
sterdam. p. 185-241.

[34] Guillozet-Bongaarts, A.L., et al., Pseudophosphorylation of tau at serine 422 inhibits
caspase cleavage: in vitro evidence and implications for tangle formation in vivo. J
Neurochem, 2006. 97(4): p. 1005-14.

[35] Schneider, A., et al., Phosphorylation that detaches tau protein from microtubules
(Ser262, Ser214) also protects it against aggregation into Alzheimer paired helical filaments. Biochemistry, 1999. 38(12): p. 3549-58.

[36] Arendt, T., et al., Reversible paired helical filament-like phosphorylation of tau is an
adaptive process associated with neuronal plasticity in hibernating animals. J Neurosci, 2003. 23(18): p. 6972-81.

[37] Su, B., et al., Physiological regulation of tau phosphorylation during hibernation. J Neurochem, 2008. 105(6): p. 2098-108.

[38] Doherty, G.J. and H.T. McMahon, Mediation, modulation, and consequences of membrane-cytoskeleton interactions. Annu Rev Biophys, 2008. 37: p. 65-95.

[39] Morris, M., et al., The many faces of tau. Neuron, 2011. 70(3): p. 410-26.

[40] Weingarten, M.D., et al., A protein factor essential for microtubule assembly. Proc Natl Acad Sci U S A, 1975. 72(5): p. 1858-62.

[41] Witman, G.B., et al., Tubulin requires tau for growth onto microtubule initiating sites. Proc Natl Acad Sci U S A, 1976. 73(11): p. 4070-4.

[42] Harada, A., et al., Altered microtubule organization in small-calibre axons of mice lacking tau protein. Nature, 1994. 369(6480): p. 488-91.

[43] Dixit, R., et al., Differential regulation of dynein and kinesin motor proteins by tau. Science, 2008. 319(5866): p. 1086-9.

[44] Caceres, A. and K.S. Kosik, Inhibition of neurite polarity by tau antisense oligonucleotides in primary cerebellar neurons. Nature, 1990. 343(6257): p. 461-3.

[45] Neve, R.L., et al., Identification of cDNA clones for the human microtubule-associated protein tau and chromosomal localization of the genes for tau and microtubule-associated protein 2. Brain Res, 1986. 387(3): p. 271-80.

[46] Mandelkow, E.M., et al., Structure, microtubule interactions, and phosphorylation of tau protein. Ann N Y Acad Sci, 1996. 777: p. 96-106.

[47] Heicklen-Klein, A. and I. Ginzburg, Tau promoter confers neuronal specificity and binds Sp1 and AP-2. J Neurochem, 2000. 75(4): p. 1408-18.

[48] Andreadis, A., et al., A tau promoter region without neuronal specificity. J Neurochem, 1996. 66(6): p. 2257-63.

[49] Drubin, D., et al., Regulation of microtubule protein levels during cellular morphogenesis in nerve growth factor-treated PC12 cells. J Cell Biol, 1988. 106(5): p. 1583-91.

[50] Vila-Ortiz, G.J., et al., The rate of Tau synthesis is differentially regulated during postnatal development in mouse cerebellum. Cell Mol Neurobiol, 2001. 21(5): p. 535-43.

[51] David, D.C., et al., Proteasomal degradation of tau protein. J Neurochem, 2002. 83(1): p. 176-85.

[52] Delobel, P., et al., Proteasome inhibition and Tau proteolysis: an unexpected regulation. FEBS Lett, 2005. 579(1): p. 1-5.

[53] Dickey, C.A., et al., The high-affinity HSP90-CHIP complex recognizes and selectively degrades phosphorylated tau client proteins. J Clin Invest, 2007. 117(3): p. 648-58.

[54] Min, S.W., et al., Acetylation of tau inhibits its degradation and contributes to tauopathy. Neuron, 2010. 67(6): p. 953-66.

[55] Kenessey, A., et al., Degradation of tau by lysosomal enzyme cathepsin D: implication for Alzheimer neurofibrillary degeneration. J Neurochem, 1997. 69(5): p. 2026-38.

[56] Wang, Y., et al., Tau fragmentation, aggregation and clearance: the dual role of lysosomal processing. Hum Mol Genet, 2009. 18(21): p. 4153-70.

[57] Mena, R., et al., Staging the pathological assembly of truncated tau protein into paired helical filaments in Alzheimer's disease. Acta Neuropathol, 1996. 91(6): p. 633-41.

[58] Mena R., L.-M.J., Stages of pathological tau-protein processing in Alzheimer's disease: From soluble aggregation to polymetization into insoluble tau-PHFs, in Currents Hypotheses and Research Milestones, R.B.M.a.G. Perry, Editor 2009. p. 79-91.

[59] Fasulo, L., Visintin M., Novak M., Cattaneo A., Tau truncation in Alzheimer's disease: encompassing PHF core tau induces apoptosis ina COS cells. Alzheimes's reports, 1998. 1: p. 25-32.

[60] Wischik, C.M., et al., Selective inhibition of Alzheimer disease-like tau aggregation by phenothiazines. Proceedings of the National Academy of Sciences of the United States of America, 1996. 93(20): p. 11213-8.

[61] Mena, R., et al., Monitoring pathological assembly of tau and beta-amyloid proteins in Alzheimer's disease. Acta Neuropathol, 1995. 89(1): p. 50-6.

[62] Fasulo, L., et al., The neuronal microtubule-associated protein tau is a substrate for caspase-3 and an effector of apoptosis. J Neurochem, 2000. 75(2): p. 624-33.

[63] Gamblin, T.C., et al., Caspase cleavage of tau: linking amyloid and neurofibrillary tangles in Alzheimer's disease. Proc Natl Acad Sci U S A, 2003. 100(17): p. 10032-7.

[64] Rissman, R.A., et al., Caspase-cleavage of tau is an early event in Alzheimer disease tangle pathology. J Clin Invest, 2004. 114(1): p. 121-30.

[65] Gamblin, T.C., et al., In vitro polymerization of tau protein monitored by laser light scattering: method and application to the study of FTDP-17 mutants. Biochemistry, 2000. 39(20): p. 6136-44.

[66] Horowitz, P.M., et al., N-terminal fragments of tau inhibit full-length tau polymerization in vitro. Biochemistry, 2006. 45(42): p. 12859-66.

[67] Luna-Munoz, J., et al., Earliest stages of tau conformational changes are related to the appearance of a sequence of specific phospho-dependent tau epitopes in Alzheimer's disease. J Alzheimers Dis, 2007. 12(4): p. 365-75.

[68] Castellani, R.J., et al., Phosphorylated tau: toxic, protective, or none of the above. J Alzheimers Dis, 2008. 14(4): p. 377-83.

[69] Nelson, P.T., H. Braak, and W.R. Markesbery, Neuropathology and cognitive impairment in Alzheimer disease: a complex but coherent relationship. Journal of neuropathology and experimental neurology, 2009. 68(1): p. 1-14.

[70] Abner, E.L., et al., "End-stage" neurofibrillary tangle pathology in preclinical Alzheimer's disease: fact or fiction? Journal of Alzheimer's disease : JAD, 2011. 25(3): p. 445-53.

[71] Lee, H.G., et al., Tau phosphorylation in Alzheimer's disease: pathogen or protector? Trends Mol Med, 2005. 11(4): p. 164-9.

[72] Cash, A.D., et al., Microtubule reduction in Alzheimer's disease and aging is independent of tau filament formation. Am J Pathol, 2003. 162(5): p. 1623-7.

[73] Paula-Barbosa, M., M.A. Tavares, and A. Cadete-Leite, A quantitative study of frontal cortex dendritic microtubules in patients with Alzheimer's disease. Brain research, 1987. 417(1): p. 139-42.

[74] Yuan, A., et al., Axonal transport rates in vivo are unaffected by tau deletion or overexpression in mice. J Neurosci, 2008. 28(7): p. 1682-7.

[75] Leroy, K., et al., Early axonopathy preceding neurofibrillary tangles in mutant tau transgenic mice. Am J Pathol, 2007. 171(3): p. 976-92.

[76] Jicha, G.A., et al., A conformation- and phosphorylation-dependent antibody recognizing the paired helical filaments of Alzheimer's disease. J Neurochem, 1997. 69(5): p. 2087-95.

[77] McMillan, P.J., et al., Truncation of tau at E391 promotes early pathologic changes in transgenic mice. Journal of neuropathology and experimental neurology, 2011. 70(11): p. 1006-19.

[78] Morsch, R., W. Simon, and P.D. Coleman, Neurons may live for decades with neurofibrillary tangles. J Neuropathol Exp Neurol, 1999. 58(2): p. 188-97.

[79] Guo, H., et al., Active caspase-6 and caspase-6-cleaved tau in neuropil threads, neuritic plaques, and neurofibrillary tangles of Alzheimer's disease. Am J Pathol, 2004. 165(2): p. 523-31.

[80] Lassmann, H., et al., Cell death in Alzheimer's disease evaluated by DNA fragmentation in situ. Acta Neuropathol, 1995. 89(1): p. 35-41.

[81] Kudo, W., et al., Inhibition of Bax protects neuronal cells from oligomeric Abeta neurotoxicity. Cell death & disease, 2012. 3: p. e309.

[82] Li, H.L., et al., Phosphorylation of tau antagonizes apoptosis by stabilizing beta-catenin, a mechanism involved in Alzheimer's neurodegeneration. Proc Natl Acad Sci U S A, 2007. 104(9): p. 3591-6.

[83] Luna-Munoz, J., et al., Regional conformational change involving phosphorylation of tau protein at the Thr231, precedes the structural change detected by Alz-50 antibody in Alzheimer's disease. J Alzheimers Dis, 2005. 8(1): p. 29-41.

Chapter 7

Alzheimer Disease and Metabolism: Role of Cholesterol and Membrane Fluidity

Genaro G. Ortiz, Fermín P. Pacheco-Moisés,
Luis J. Flores-Alvarado, Miguel A. Macías-Islas,
Irma E. Velázquez-Brizuela,
Ana C. Ramírez-Anguiano,
Erandis D. Tórres-Sánchez,
Eddic W. Moráles-Sánchez, José A. Cruz-Ramos,
Genaro E Ortiz-Velázquez and
Fernando Cortés-Enríquez

Additional information is available at the end of the chapter

1. Introduction

Alzheimer's disease (AD) is an age-related disorder characterized by deposition of amyloid β-peptide (Aβ) and degeneration of neurons in brain regions such as the hippocampus, resulting in progressive cognitive dysfunction. The causes of Alzheimer's disease (AD) have not been fully discovered, there are three main hypotheses to explain the phenomenon: a) The deficit of acetylcholine; b) The accumulation of beta-amyloid (Aβ and / or tau protein; and c) Metabolic disorders.

The clinical criteria for diagnosing AD were defined in 1984 by the NINCDS-ADRDA; (National Institute of Neurological and Communicative Disorders and Stroke; Alzheimer's Disease and Related Disorders). It states that for the diagnosis of disease is required to prove the existence of chronic and progressive cognitive impairment in adults or elderly patients, without other underlying causes that can explain this phenomenon. However, using this criterion, it is difficult to differentiate between AD and other causes of deterioration in early stages of the disease.

A number of recent research has been related AD with metabolic disorders, particularly hyperglycemia and insulin resistance. The expression of insulin receptors has been demonstrated in the central nervous system neurons, preferably in the hippocampus. In these neurons, when insulin binds to its cellular receptor, promotes the activation of intracellular signaling cascades that lead to change in the expression of genes related to synaptic plasticity processes and enzymes involved in clearing the same insulin and Aβ. These enzymes degrading of insulin promotes the reduction of toxicity due to amyloid in animal models.

People with neuritic plaques accumulate in brain regions that correspond to brain regions in healthy people that rise in a metabolic process called aerobic glycolysis. While some regions such as prefrontal and parietal cortex, which is thought to have a role in self-recognition and control tasks, showed high levels of aerobic glycolysis, others such as the cerebellum and the hippocampal formation, believed to affect the control motor and memory, showed low levels. Brain cells use aerobic glycolysis for energy derived quickly from small amounts of glucose while obtaining the mass of its energy through a biochemical process effective to burn glucose. Since aerobic glycolysis may help the brain generate cell constituents, toxic metabolic byproducts manage and regulate programmed cell death; the findings suggest a possible link between brain function that provides energy to aerobic glycolysis and the onset of AD.

The causes of the late AD appear to be multifactorial, and cell biology studies point to cholesterol as a key factor in protein precursor of beta Amyloid (APP) processing and Aβ production. An alteration in cholesterol metabolism is attractive hypotheses, thus the carriers of the Apolipoprotein E4 genes, which is involved in cholesterol metabolism, are at increased genetic risk for Alzheimer's disease. Cholesterol is a component of cell membranes and particularly is found in microdomains functionally linked to the proteolytic processing of APP. In sporadic AD, a marked diminution of both membrane phospholipids and cholesterol has been found.

Epidemiological studies indicate that mild hypercholesterolemia may increase the risk of AD and decreased synthesis of cholesterol through statin administration can reduce the development of AD. Moreover, high cellular cholesterol content has been shown to favor the production of Aβ. Genetic studies have suggested links between AD and cholesterol control several genes including cholesterol acceptor ApoE (ε4 polymorphism). Liver X receptors (LRXs) are ligand-activated transcription factors of the nuclear hormone receptor superfamily LXRs and also are expressed in the brain. LXRs stimulate the expression of genes involved in cellular cholesterol transport, regulation of lipid content of lipoproteins (apoE, lipoprotein lipase, cholesterol ester transfer protein, and phospholipid transfer protein), metabolism of fatty acids and triglycerides (sterol regulatory element binding protein 1-c, fatty acid synthase, stearoyl coenzyme A desaturase 1, and acyl coenzyme A carboxylase). Many questions remain, but as a master regulator of cholesterol homeostasis, LXR may be considered as a potential molecular target for the treatment of AD.

In summary, numerous studies on the role of cholesterol in AD suggest that high cholesterol is a risk factor for early and late AD development.

2. Dementia and pathological changes

Dementia is a syndrome that cause cognitive and memory alterations; problems of orientation, attention, language and solving problems. Dementia involves a progressive decline in cognition that goes above and beyond the normal changes that come with age due to injuries or brain diseases. The two most common causes of dementia are AD and vascular dementia. More than 33% of women and 20% of men aged 65 year or more will develop dementia during their lifetime, and many more develop a milder form of cognitive impairment. Worldwide, the adult population is rapidly growing; prospective epidemiological studies suggest that there will be an increase of 50% of the total number of people with cognitive disorders in the next 25 years. Dementia is associated with increased mortality and disability, health care costs they mean a huge expenditure on health systems as well as a significant increase in social and economic responsibilities for caregivers and their families. With a current affection about 10% of the population over the 65 year-old Alzheimer's disease (AD) is the most common cause of progressive dementia [1].

AD is a progressive neurological disorder resulting in irreversible loss of neurons, particularly in the cortex and hippocampus, accounting for about one third of dementia syndromes, with a range that varies from 42 to 81% of all dementias. The clinical findings are characterized by progressive loose of memory, loss of: judgment, decision making, physical orientation and language disorders. The diagnosis is based on neurological examination and differential diagnosis with other dementias, but the definitive diagnosis is made only by autopsy. The pathological findings at microscopic level are: neuronal loss, gliosis, neurofibrillary tangles, neuritic plaques, Hirano bodies, granulo-vacuolar degeneration of neurons and amyloid angiopathy [2, 3]. A very early change in AD brain is the reduced glucose metabolism [4], and a recent analysis suggests that diabetes plays a role in the acceleration of brain aging. But, although it is known that type 2-diabetes may be associated with an increased risk of dementia, the exact mechanisms and mitigating factors still are not completely understood. The public health implications of this phenomenon are enormous. Although initially the association between type 2 diabetes and vascular dementia appeared to be more consistent than the relationship between type 2 diabetes and AD, there are recent studies that have yielded more consistent evidence of the relationship between diabetes and AD [5,6].

Neuritic plaques, neurofibrillary tangles and other proteins in AD brain are glycosylated [7]. Since people with diabetes have an increased blood glucose level is plausible to suspect that they have a higher chance of having AD. Animal models of induced diabetes suggest a direct neurodegenerative effect of diabetes; most of these studies show damage in the hippocampus, an area associated with learning and memory, and first structure to be affected by the neurodegeneration of AD disease. A post-mortem study revealed that people with diabetes and ApoE 4 allele, had more neuritic plaques and neurofibrilar tangles in the hippocampus and cortex, also cerebral amyloid angiopathy, in which the associated protein AD disease is deposited on the walls of blood vessels in the brain. It has been shown that those with diabetes have a greater cortical atrophy, independent of hypertension, the blood concentration of total cholesterol, smoking, coronary heart disease and sociodemographic factors than people without the condition. Today we know that obesity increases the risk of dementia and brain atrophy. However, the molecular mechanisms that are behind metabolic disorders caused by excess body fat are not fully understood yet, especially regarding its role in neurodegenerative diseases (see Figure 1). Preliminary evidence suggests that some adipocytokines could cross the blood brain barrier, and have some function in learning and memory [8].

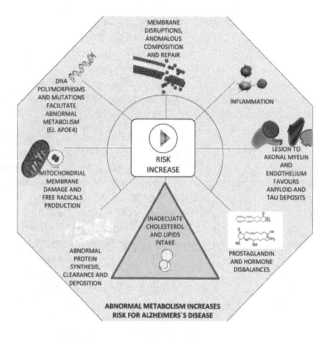

Figure 1. Abnormal metabolism increases risk for Alzheimer disease.

Recent findings from several longitudinal population studies have confirmed a link between obesity and risk of dementia. People with a body mass index (BMI) indicating obesity (≥ 30) have a greater probability of developing dementia (75%) compared with those with normal BMI (18.5 to 24.9). We must emphasize that abdominal obesity is more closely associated with dementia risk, that obesity spread throughout the body. Even for those with a healthy weight, abdominal obesity increases the risk of dementia [9].

3. Insulin-cholesterol-AD

Insulin signaling in the central nervous system has gained much interest for his participation in cognitive processes such as learning and memory and its possible relation to neurodegenerative diseases such as Alzheimer's disease. In peripheral tissues, mainly regulates insulin metabolism energetic and cell growth. The insulin receptor and several components of its signaling pathway are abundantly distributed in the mammalian brain and their activation modulates neuronal growth and synaptic plasticity [10].

It has been suggested that some alterations in the insulin signaling appear to be responsible for cognitive deficits and play an important role in the development of AD disease. Indeed, Type II diabetes is a risk factor for developing this type of dementia. Recently it has been observed that Aβ, which is overproduced in AD disease, causes alterations in the signaling pathway of insulin, supporting the causal relationships between this condition interesting and insulin [11]. In recent years the effects of insulin in the brain have drawn attention for his participation in mental processes such as memory and learning. Insulin in the brain plays an important role in the regulation of metabolism, and alterations in their activity are directly related to metabolic diseases such as obesity, diabetes or metabolic syndrome. In the mammalian brain, insulin anorexigenic effects, induces weight loss and regulates hypothalamic control of food intake. Also regulates glucose homeostasis by stimulating peripheral neurons producing pro-opiomelacortina (POMC) and agouti-related peptide (AgRP) through the IR and PI3K [12, 13].

Insulin can be generated in different brain sites. It is known that insulin is produced in the beta cells of the pancreas and can enter the brain through the blood brain barrier by active transport mediated by IR. Furthermore, the presence of messenger RNA in mammalian brain neurons, suggests that insulin can be produced locally. Likewise, there has been a strict regulation of the levels of insulin and its receptor (IR) in the brain, which may suggest that insulin level in the brain does not depend exclusively on the periphery [14]. However, if the source is local cerebral insulin, peripheral or shared has not been clarified yet. The IR is very abundant in the brains of rodents and humans with the highest concentration in the olfactory bulb, the hypothalamus, pituitary gland, hippocampus, cerebral cortex and cerebellum [15,16]. In addition, most of the proteins of the insulin signaling pathway have expression patterns that overlap with the IR in the brain. The IR is found abundantly in the hippocampus and its expression is increased after spatial learning tasks in rodents. The IR is widely found in the synapses of the dendritic trees which regulate the release of neurotransmitters and receptor recruitment [17] (see Figure 2).

Insulin regulates glutamatergic and GABAergic receptors, through the activation of the PI3K and MAPK. It is also known that the processes of long-term potentiation (LTP) and long-term depression (LTD), are associated with the molecular events underlying the establishment of memory and learning are regulated by the activation of PI3K through Complex formation with NMDA receptors, which regulates PI3K NMDA receptor translocation to the membrane. The response of the IR is reduced by the action of glutamate and depolarization, probably involving calcium influx of Ca2+ and activation of Ca2+-dependent kinases (Figure 3). This suggests a possible role of insulin in the synaptic plasticity and modulation of neuronal activity [18-20].

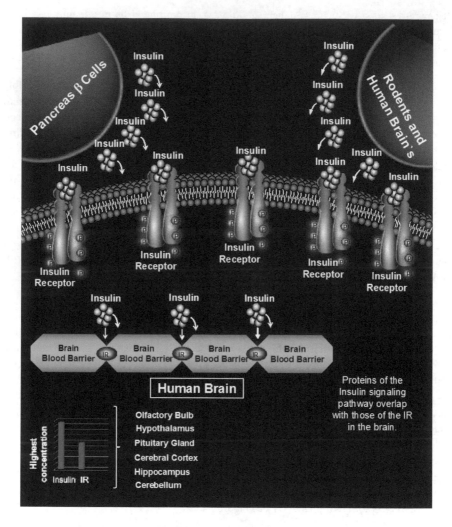

Figure 2. Insulin is produced in the Beta cells of the pancreasand enters the brain through the BBB (Brain Blood Barrier) via the IR (Insulin Receptor). Insulin levels on the brain do not depend exclusively on pherical levels. The IR is very abundant in the brain of rodents and humans, showing its highest concentration in the following areas (in descending order): Olfactory bulb, hypothalamus, pituitary gland, cerebral cortex, hippocampus and the cerebellum. Most of the proteins involved in the insulin signaling pathway have expression patterns that overlap with the IR in the brain [125].

The presence of components via postsynaptic regions, such as mTOR, p70S6K, eIF-4E, 4E-BP1 and 4EBP2 suggest the existence of the regulation of protein synthesis at synapses. Insulin regulates the levels of the postsynaptic density protein PSD-95, which binds to the NMDA receptors in the synaptic membrane, through mTOR activation and modulation of protein translation at synapses. Furthermore, mTOR modulates synaptic plasticity Thus, insulin not only modulates neuronal synaptic activity [21]

Different strategies can be proposed to prevent the characteristics of AD-related dysfunction of the insulin signaling pathway. An important factor is the signal transduction through Akt. Akt activity can be improved with appropriate levels of omega-3 and DHA, which can help reduce βA levels and amyloid burden, as has been observed in transgenic mice Tg2576 regulating the activity of the enzyme IDE [22]. The loss of inhibition of GSK3 is involved in the production of neurofibrillary tangles and tau aggregation, which leads to oxidative stress, damage and toxicity in the neuronal synapses, so that GSK3 inhibitors could be used to prevent hyperphosphorylation of tau and the production of neurofibrillary tangles. Insulin has been used to improve memory and learning in healthy subjects and also in behavioral tasks in rats, suggesting a role in enhancing memory in humans, however, the actual effects of insulin on the CNS are just being elucidated [23,24].

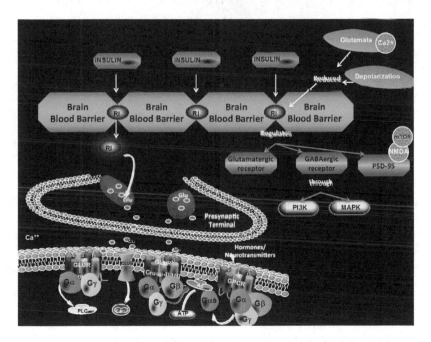

Figure 3. Insulin can enter the brain through the blood barrier by active transport mediated by IR. The IR is found abundantly in the hippocampus and synapses of dendritic trees, wich regulates the release of neurotransmitters and receptor recruitment. Insulin regulates glutamatergic and GABAergic receptors throug PI3K and MAPK [126].

Among the compounds which have been proposed as reducing agents include βA charging the statins, which lower cholesterol levels, some peptides that prevent Aβ fibril formation as PBT-531 and NC-1 (a chelating metals) and modulators of the activity of the secretases as

Bryostatin. Finally, the use of antioxidants such as vitamin E, have shown effectively to counter the effects of oxidative stress produced in the EA [25].

4. Proteins involved in cholesterol metabolism

Cholesterol, the most common steroid in humans, is a structural component of cell membranes and is a precursor of steroid hormones and bile salts. Since an excess of cholesterol is a major risk factor for the development of cardiovascular disease, it is essential a balance between cholesterol synthesis, uptake, and catabolism. Cholesterol is only synthesized in the liver and brain. The brain contains about 20% of total body cholesterol but only 2% of total body weight. The majority of this cholesterol is found in myelin membranes. Brain cholesterol is synthesized exclusively by *de novo* synthesis reaction from acetyl-CoA and acetoacetyl-CoA to form HMG-CoA. Then, is converted to mevalonate by HMG-CoA reductase, in the rate-limiting step of the process by oligodendrocytes, astrocytes and neurons [26].

After synthesis and secretion from glia via the ABCA1 transporter, cholesterol is packaged into lipoprotein particles resembling HDL. These HDL particles contain apoE. HDL is taken up into neurons through recognition of ApoE by a variety of lipoprotein receptors including the LDL receptor (LDLR); the LDL receptor related protein (LRP), the apoE receptor, as well as other lipoprotein receptors. Elimination of cholesterol from the brain occurs mainly via oxidation at the 24 and 27 positions to produce a class of compounds termed oxysterols. Water solubility of oxysterols is higher than cholesterol and diffuse across the BBB where they enter the peripheral circulation for excretion. *In vitro* studies showed a cholesterol shuttle from astrocytes to neurons that is mediated by apoE [27]. Virtually no cholesterol crosses the blood brain barrier from the peripheral circulation. Therefore, serum cholesterol levels have no effect on HMG-CoA reductase and its activity in the brain [28], and on total brain cholesterol levels [29]. The plasma half-life of cholesterol is several hours and fluctuates significantly according to intake. By contrast, cholesterol in the CNS is metabolized slowly, with a half life of 6 months in rats, and about 1 year in humans. In fact, changes in serum cholesterol have low impact on the CNS. Cholesterol metabolism in the brain is regulated by apoE4 and 24-hydroxylase. The rate-limiting enzyme 24-hydroxylase is uniquely expressed in the brain, and modulates the removal of cholesterol from the brain. The gene encoding this enzyme is called CYP46, and the CYP46 polymorphism was found to be associated with an increased Aβ deposition and tau phosphorylation, as well as with a higher risk of late-onset AD [30,31]. Cholesterol 24-hydroxylase (Cyp46) related to cytochrome P450, the ABC transporter (ABCA1), the receptor-associated protein to LDL (LRP) and the -2-macroglobulin. LRP1 is expressed mainly in neurons and activated astrocytes [32], and directly binds free Aβ, and mediates its egress from the brain [33]. Furthermore, it has been suggested that γ-secretase-mediated processing of APP plays a regulatory role in brain cholesterol and apoE metabolism through LRP1 [34]. In addition, the LRP polymorphism is negatively associated with Alzheimer. The Cyp46 is a brain specific enzyme that oxidizes cholesterol to form 24 (S)-hydroxycholesterol and its function is to remove cholesterol from the brain. Moreover, statins have been linked with AD, because the subjects medicated with them have lower prevalence of the disease [35]. The LRP-associated protein binds to LDL receptor very prominent in neurons. The α 2-macroglobulin is a protein capable of binding Aβ with high specificity and preventing its fibrillization [36]. α2M is found in neuritic plaques in AD brain [37] and it may play a role in Aβ clearance via LRP, as it is known to be able to bind other ligands and target them for internalization and degradation [38]. However, the putative role of these molecules in AD is controversial because some studies have failed to show an association between polymorphisms of α 2-macroglobulin and AD [39,40].

Studies *in vitro* showed that cholesterol depletion after treatment with both statins and methyl-β-cyclodextrin, which physically extracts membrane cholesterol, inhibits the generation of Aβ in hippocampal cells [41,42]. In transgenic AD animal models, hypercholesterolemia accelerates the development of Alzheimer's amyloid pathology [43]. Cholesterol-fed rabbits also develop changes in their brain that are typical of AD pathology [44].

Clinic-epidemiological studies suggest that increased serum cholesterol levels did not correlate substantially with AD in older ages [45,46]. However, all epidemiological studies, genetic, metabolic and laboratory show that many factors regulation of cholesterol metabolism are involved in the physiopathology of AD. The most prevalent risk factor identified to date is the Apolipoprotein E4 (Apo-E4), which is a protein carrier of cholesterol, Apo-E exists in the brain and the periphery. Although the E4 genotype appears to confer a risk for AD independent of plasma levels of cholesterol, the data do not clearly discriminate whether the polymorphism of the Apo E4 contributes to Alzheimer through a direct effect on Aβ, or an indirect effect through involving the catabolism of cholesterol (Figure 4). The levels of 24-hydroxycholesterol (24-OHC) is increased with age in subjects with AD, and recent studies suggest that genetic factors related to this molecule contribute to the pathogenesis of the disease [47].

Cholesterol catabolites also regulate the processing of the APP. Pharmacological inhibition of acyl-CoA:cholesterol acyltransferase (ACAT), which produces cholesterol esters, decreases Aβ. This is significant because the ACAT inhibitors are in development for the pharmaceutical companies for the treatment of atherosclerosis and such drugs may become useful for testing in AD. On the other hand, synthetic oxysterol, 22-hydroxycholesterol and synthetic LXR agonist reduces Aβ generation in murine models of AD via elevated apoE protein levels and increased lipidation of apoE, rather than through suppression of Aβ generation [48]. Furthermore, LXR agonist preserves cognitive function at a dose far below required to observe decreased Aβ levels [49] and AD neuropathology was exacerbated in mice lacking LXRs, providing further support for the central role of LXR target genes in the pathogenesis of AD. The enzyme that catalyzes the cleavage of β APP β-secretase is the (BACE) and their activity is particularly dependent on cholesterol levels [50] (Figure 5).

Studies on the cholesterol use in the brain of AD patients are also significant and consistent; cholesterol is removed from the brain to become 24-OHC, which appears in the plasma. The 24-OHC levels are increased in patients with AD or any other degenerative disease. The increase is probably, because cholesterol from degenerating neurons is captured and removed to maintain homeostasis. It has been shown that neurons with degenerative tangles showed increased levels of cholesterol. However, there is a striking difference between serum and brain levels of 24-OHC in AD, because the first increase; while the latter decrease. This perhaps reflects the decline in the number of neurons and synapses in the brains of subjects who died with AD [47]. Cholesterol is synthesized through a complex route that is blocked by a class of enzymes generically called statins. The clinical utility of statins has been demonstrated across multiple epidemiological studies, some of which have suggested that these drugs might be effective in treating AD disease. Advances in understanding the relationship between the biology of cholesterol and the production of Aβ peptide, crucial in the development of amyloid plaque, will lead to new therapeutic approaches for AD disease.

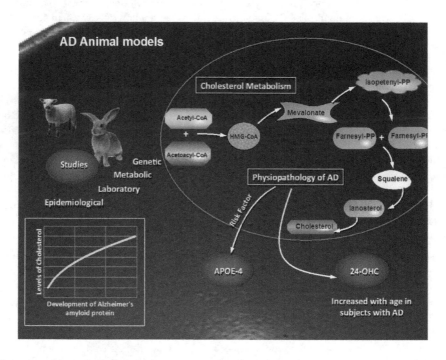

Figure 4. In Alzheimer's Disease (AD) animal models, hypercholesterolemia accelerates the development of Alzheimer's amyloid protein. Genetic, metabolic, clinical and epidemiological studies have shown that many factors involved in cholesterol's metabolism are involved in the pathophysiology of AD. The most prevalent risk factor is the APOE-4 (Apolipoprotein E4) genotype.

Statins are inhibitors of the enzyme 3-hydroxy-3-methylglutaryl coenzyme A (HMG-CoA) reductase, which converts HMG-CoA into mevalonate; this is the rate-limiting step in cholesterol biosynthesis [51]. These drugs decrease cholesterol levels about 30% and with few adverse effects. The first statin was lovastatin was synthesized, and since then have appeared fluvastatin, pravastatin, simvastatin and atorvastatin. Simvastatin and lovastatin are administered as pro-drugs and must be activated. These drugs differ in their lipid solubility; lipophilic statins, such as pravastatin, enter cells via an ATP-dependent anion transport system [52]. Pravastatin was not previously thought to cross the blood-brain barrier, however, it was recently demonstrated in mice that oral pravastatin treatment results in measurable pravastatin levels in the brain [53]. Pravastatin use is associated with a reduced risk of AD [54,55]. Statins inhibit cholesterol synthesis but also seem to affect other processes, because they can increase apoptosis and alter neuronal proliferation. Also decrease the immune response, anti-inflammatory property that has made recently has made the proposal to treat multiple sclerosis. Also appear to inhibit bone turnover and thereby reduce osteoporosis. The probable protective effects of statins in AD seem stronger than any association between plasma cholesterol and disease.

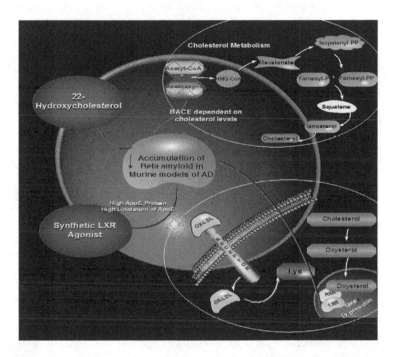

Figure 5. The inhibition of Acetyl-CoA and Acetoacyl-CoA (ACAT) produces cholesterol esters and decreases Amyloid Beta (AB). Synthetic oxysterol, 22-hydroxychoresterol and synthetic LXR agonists reduce AB generation in murine models of AD via elevated ApoE protein levels and increased lipidation of ApoE [124].

Oral administration of statins, in addition to inhibiting cholesterol synthesis, also affects gene expression the mouse brain [53]. Therefore, statins may protect the brain from AD by a mechanism independent of their effect on cholesterol. In addition to inhibition of cholesterol synthesis, statins block mevalonate formation and subsequently prevent formation of isoprenoids such as famesylpyrophosphate and geranylpyrophosphate. Statins inhibit isoprenylation of proteins, including the Rho family of small GTPases, in neuronal cells [56] and cultured microglia [57,58]. RhoA is a monomeric G-protein that is negatively coupled to cell growth; prevention of RhoA isoprenylation increases neurite extension [59]. At this regard, treatment of neurons with pravastatin enhanced neurite number, length and branching, and that this effect is mediated by inhibition of mevalonate synthesis and subsequent inhibition of isoprenylation of Rho GTPases and subsequent prevention of neuritic dystrophy and deterioration [60].

Epidemiological studies have found an inverse relationship between usage of the cholesterol-lowering drugs and risk of developing AD [54,55,61]. Statins are inhibitors of the enzyme HMG-CoA reductase, which converts HMG-CoA into mevalonate; this is the rate-limiting step in cholesterol biosynthesis [51]. However, reduction of cholesterol levels may or may not correlate with reduced risk of AD in patients taking statin drugs [62-64]. Furthermore, statin usage is associated with a decreased risk of depression and anxiety, which is not correlated with plasma cholesterol levels [65]. Oral administration of statins, in addition to inhibiting cholesterol synthesis, also affects gene expression in the mouse brain [53]. Thus, statins might prevent onset of AD by a mechanism independent of their effect on cholesterol.

Apolipoprotein E (apoE) is the major apolipoprotein in the brain and is a structural component of triglyceride-rich lipoproteins, chylomicrons, very-low-density lipoproteins (VLDL), and high-density-lipoproteins (HDL). ApoE is synthesized and secreted from astrocytes and microglia. Variation in the APOE gene sequence results in the 3 common alleles ($\varepsilon2$, $\varepsilon3$ and $\varepsilon4$), which can produce 6 different genotypes ($\varepsilon2/\varepsilon2$, $\varepsilon2/\varepsilon3$, $\varepsilon2/\varepsilon4$, $\varepsilon3/\varepsilon3$, $\varepsilon3/\varepsilon4$ and $\varepsilon4/\varepsilon4$). The $\varepsilon2$, $\varepsilon3$ and $\varepsilon4$ alleles encode three distinct forms of apoE (E2, E3 and E4) that differ in their amino acid composition at positions 112 and 158 [66]. ApoE3 seems to be the normal isoform, while apoE4 and apoE2 can each be dysfunctional [67]. Inheritance of apoE4 is associated with a greater risk of developing AD at an earlier age [68], whereas inheritance of apoE2 correlates with lower risk and later onset of AD [69]. individuals with the APOE $\varepsilon4$ allele show higher levels of plasma cholesterol, especially LDL cholesterol [70]. Subjects with APOE $\varepsilon3/\varepsilon4$ and $\varepsilon4/\varepsilon4$ genotypes absorb cholesterol effectively and have higher non-fasting serum triglyceride values than $\varepsilon4$ negative individuals [71,72]. A ApoE gene mutation (allele 4), the main risk factor for AD, may influence the risk of dementia more strongly among those with diabetes, in fact, findings from population studies show that people with diabetes and ApoE 4 are at greatest risk of AD compared with those without diabetes and without the ApoE 4. Although we know that people with diabetes are at increased risk of stroke, little is known about the effect of diabetes on the pathophysiology of neurodegeneration.

5. Membrane fluidity in Alzheimer disease

The role of the physical–chemical properties of intracellular membranous structures such as membrane fluidity in AD pathogenesis has been extensively studied. Membrane fluidity is a complex parameter, influenced both through some biophysical (temperature, electrical charges, pH) and biochemical factors (protein/phospholipids ratio, phospholipids/cholesterol ratio, degree of fatty acids unsaturation). It is a parameter that reflects the main membrane characteristic organization (gel or liquid crystal structure). Experiments provide consistent data about membrane fluidity relations to various cellular processes, especially membrane processes. Changes in the membrane composition and structure could alter the conformation and function of transmembranal ion channels, as well as affect the interaction of receptors and effectors, leading to altered signal transduction, handling of Ca", and response to exogenous stimuli [73].

Cholesterol distribution within the plasma membrane is not homogeneous: the highest level of free cholesterol inside the plasma membrane is found in cytofacial bilayer leaflet [74]. The exofacial leaflet contains substantially less cholesterol, and it is mostly condensed in lipid rafts, which are more tightly packed than nonlipid raft domains due to intermolecular hydrogen bonding involving sphingolipid and cholesterol [75]. This asymmetric distribution of cholesterol is altered by aging: it is significantly increased in exofacial leaflet with increasing age [76,77]. It has been reported that membrane fluidity of lipid membranes in the brain cortex of AD samples were significantly thinner (that is, had less microviscosity) than corresponding age-matched controls. This change in membrane width correlated with a 30% decrease in the ratio cholesterol/ phospholipid [78].

In our group of research we assessed the membrane fluidity in platelet submitochondrial particles and erythrocyte membranes from Mexican patients with Alzheimer disease. Submitochondrial particles are mainly constituted of inner mitochondrial membrane and are the site of oxidative phosphorylation and other enzymatic systems involved in the transport and utilization of metabolites. Membrane fluidity was estimated measuring the intramolecular excimer formation of the fluorescent probe 1,3 dipyrenylpropane incorporated in membranes. Similarly to the data reported from mitochondria in AD brains fluidity [79]., a reduced fluidity in the platelet inner mitochondrial membrane was found. It can partially be due to increased levels of lipid peroxidation [80]. Reduced membrane fluidity can diminish the activities of the enzymes of oxidative phosphorylation and other transport and receptor proteins, in as much as these enzymes are regulated by the physicochemical state of the lipid environment of the membrane. It may diminish significantly the ATP generation from the mitochondria. Interestingly, dysfunctional mitochondria and oxidative damage has been involved in Alzheimer's disease [81]. In agreement with previous reports, membrane fluidity from erythrocyte was not altered in AD [82], regardless of increased lipid oxidation in erythrocyte AD patients. This suggests that, in AD, mitochondrial membranes are more sensitive to oxidative stress than erythrocytes. In contrast to platelet inner mitochondrial membrane, it has been reported an increase in fluidity in whole membranes from platelets of AD patients [83]. This increase results from the elaboration of an internal membrane compartment resembling endoplasmic reticulum that is functionally abnormal [84]. At this regard, it is worth noting that the contribution of mitochondrial membranes to the whole cell membranes in platelets could be minimized since platelets contain few mitochondria [85].

On the other hand, it has been reported that using diphenil-hexatriene (DPH) and trimethylammonium-diphenyl-hexatriene (TMA-DPH) as fluorescent probes, the membrane fluidity in mitocondrial membranes was similar in platelets from AD patients and controls [86]. That discrepancy with our data may be due to intrinsic differences in the populations tested, the purity of the used mitochondrial fraction and the nature of the probes used. Additionally, it's clear that the lipophilic probes are sensitive to slightly different membrane properties. For instance, DPH and TMA-DPH are rotational probes [87] and dipyrenylpropane is a lateral diffusion sensitive probe [88]. In addition, DPH partitions into the interior of the bilayer and its average location has been shown to be about 8 Å from the center of the bilayer. TMA-DPH is oriented in the membrane bilayer with its positive charge localized at the lipid-water interface. Its DPH moiety is localized at about 11 Å from the center of the bilayer and reports the interfacial region of the membrane [89]. Whereas dipyrenylpropane is a highly hydrophobic probe which partitions into the membrane lipid bilayer [88].

As shown in figure 1, we found a significant decrease of membrane fluidity in hippocampal neurons from AD patients compared with membranes from elderly non demented controls (Figure 6). Lower membrane fluidity in AD patients was correlated with abnormal APP processing and cognitive decline [90].

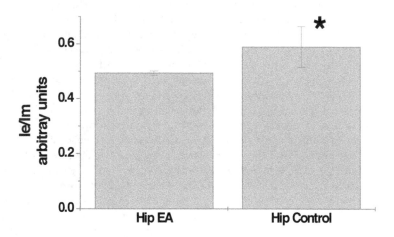

Figure 6. Excimer to monomer fluorescent ratio of dipirenylpropane on plasma membrane of hippocampus fom AD patients and aged-matched controls. The fluorescent probe was excited at 329 nm and emission of monomer (Ie) and excimer (Im) was read at 379 and 480 nm, respectively. Intramolecular excimer formation of this probe is related with the membrane fluidity. Therefore the ratio (Ie/Im) is directly proportional to membrane fluidity, which is reciprocal to membrane viscosity. The data shown are mean ± S.E.M. ∗p <0.01.

Some strategies for the preservation of membrane fluidity include the use of polyunsaturated fatty acid (PUFAs). The brain is particularly rich in PUFAs such as eicosapentaenoic (EPA) and docosahexaenoic acids (DHA). PUFAs play an essential role in the normal development and functioning of brain [91]. Diets enriched in n-3 PUFA increased membrane fluidity, affect signal transduction and modulate gene expression for brain function [92]. Furthermore, DHA have the following effects: maintains membrane fluidity, improved synaptic and neurotransmitter functioning, enhanced learning and memory performances and displayed neuroprotective properties [93], decreased the amount of vascular Aβ deposition [94] and reduced Aβ burden [22]. In AD mouse model, DHA modulated APP processing by decreasing both α- and β-APP C-terminal fragment products and full-length APP [22]. However, caution should be taken when PUFAs are used for dietary supplementation, since DHA could be increasing oxidative stress, resulting in lipid peroxidation [95,96].

Addition of cholesterol restored the membrane width to that of the age-matched control samples. Alterations in other membrane components of AD brains have also been reported. The cholesterol content in lipid rafts has been shown to contribute to the integrity of the raft structure and the functions of the rafts in signaling and membrane trafficking [97]. At this regard, it has been shown that cholesterol depletion leads to increased membrane fluidity [98] mainly in intracellular membranes [99] and reduced endocytosis, shifting sAPP shedding from β-cleavage towards α-cleavage [63]. In fact, the cleavage of APP by β-secretase [100], occurs mainly in highly ordered membrane microdomains dispersed at the cell surface. These microdomains known as lipid rafts are enriched in cholesterol, sphingolipids and saturated phospholipids. Lipid rafts appear to be a mechanism to compartmentalize various processes on the cell surface by bringing together various receptor-mediated and signal transduction processes. The cleavage of APP by α-secretase is done mostly in nonraft domains [101]. Furthermore, it has been shown *in vitro* that lowering cholesterol leads to decreased BACE-cleavage of APP [102,103] and increased α-cleavage of APP [102].

Increased membrane fluidity due to cholesterol depletion inhibits endocytosis which might explain the observed increase of sAPPα and shift towards α-secretase cleavage that happens on the cell surface. Cholesterol increase is associated with enhanced membrane stiffness possibly explaining the disrupted proximity of APP and BACE. Surprisingly this is associated with enhanced sAPPβ production, possibly explained by altered transport and endocytosis mechanisms [103]. Another explanation therefore is the direct impact of cholesterol environment upon BACE activity. In living cells, BACE seems to require intact rafts for activity, and BACE outside rafts seems to be inactive [104].

6. Role of dietary lipids in Alzheimer disease

Recent theories suggests that there would be an interaction between genetic predisposition and environmental factors that lead to cell death by amyloid toxicity or disruption of tau protein. Dietary lipids could be a determining factor in the difference in risk between developed and underdeveloped countries. Dietary lipids could be the primary risk factor in late-onset sporadic AD (LO-SAT). The critical factors seem to be the ratios of polyunsaturated fatty acids (PUFAs) to monounsaturated (MUFA), saturated fatty acids (SFA) to essential fatty acids (EFAs). These contents are modified by the APOE4 genotype [105].

Oxidation of neuronal lipid membranes could be the initiating event in the cascade of synergistic processes with subsequent expression of Aβ and helical filaments of hyper-phosphorylated tau protein. PUFAs are important in modulating the inflammatory bal-ance/systemic anti-inflammatory eicosanoids and fluidity and membrane function. Proinflammatory eicosanoids are derived from arachidonic acid (AA). The anti-inflamma-tory eicosanoids are derived from the via the n-3 EFA through DHA) and EPA. EFAs cannot be synthesized by animals and must be obtained from food. A diet rich in linole-ic acid promotes proinflammatory state, while a diet rich in linolenic acid promotes in-flammatory components. When lipids are exposed to free radicals begin an autoperoxidative process. This process is perpetual and changes the composition and rate of membrane lipids with loss of PUFA compared with MUFA and SFA. This causes the membrane to become less fluid and affecting the function of components, as well as of intracellular organelles and the vascular endothelium [106]. This seems to be the ini-tial process of the cascade that culminates in neuronal death and neuropathological se-quelae associated with LO-SAT. Antioxidant vitamins and vegetables may reduce the risk of AD. High levels of blood lipids are associated with atherosclerosis and diabetes, both risk factors for EA indirect. Recently it was found that the increase in LDL choles-terol, along with APOE epsilon4 genotype is associated with increased risk of AD [107].

The oxidative state of lipid membranes can have effects on neurons, at three levels:a) vascu-lar;b) endothelial cell membrane; and c) membrane organelles.At the level of cellular mem-branes lipid oxidation accelerates the aggregation of amyloid which consequently decreases membrane fluidity. This also is observed with decreases of the content of MUFA and PUFA esterified to phospholipid. Interestingly, these changes are seen in brain regions affected in AD, especially at the hippocampus. The decrease of the membrane fluidity affects the syn-aptic connections [108]. The EA may be preventable and treatable and possibly reversible to some extent, if the proposed hypothesis is correct. The changes in the fat composition of the diet are reflected in plasma lipids and phospholipids in the membrane of red blood cells, likewise in the neural cell membranes, especially in areas of rapid lipid turnover. A diet low of n-6 PUFA and MUFA, and an adequate amount of n-3 PUFA, but not too caloric, with antioxidants should protect neuronal damage, lipid oxidation and the inflammatory cascade and amyloid deposition.

Lipid lowering agents appear to have a protective effect, although studies are not conclu-sive. Statins decrease the oxidizability of LDL, with decreased levels of oxygen reactive spe-cies, anti-inflammatory effects and improve endothelial dysfunction, also increased alpha-secretase activity. Increase the synthesis of LDL receptors, with decreased circulating level and reduced production of PPA.

The histological changes seen in the initial stages of AD confirmed that membrane lipids and inflammation are involved in the disease (Figure 7). AGE n-3/n-6 rate has a major impact on the balance of eicosanoid metabolism inflammatory and anti-inflammatory, and the degree of saturation of membrane lipids and fluidity affects its function. The apoE4 genotype may influence the risk of AD, as it is unable to protect that transports lipids from oxidation [109].

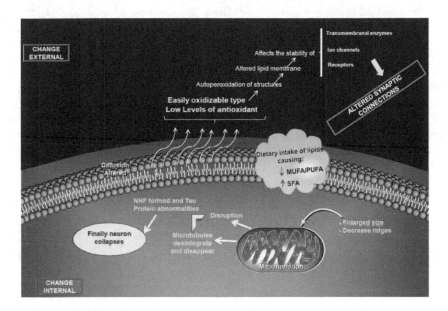

Figure 7. Cellular changes induced by lipid oxidation linked to dietary lipids. The change in dietary intake of lipids causing a low PUFA/MUFA (Polyunsaturated Fatty Acid/Monounsaturated Fatty Acids) ratio, which finally altered synaptic connections and neuron collapse [127].

7. Membrane phospholipid metabolism

The principal constituents of mammalian cell membranes are phospholipids, the most abundant of which is phosphatidylcholine (PC). PC biosynthesis is initiated by the phosphorylation of choline to form phosphocholine, which then combines with cytidine triphosphate (CTP) to form 5'-cytidine diphosphocholine (CDP-choline); this compound then reacts with diacylglycerol (DAG) to produce PC [110]. The rate at which cells form PC is affected by the availability of its precursors. Thus, uridine or cytidine increase CTP levels [111]; availability of CTP levels in turn can be rate-limiting in the syntheses of CDP-choline [112] and PC [113]; and DAG levels can control the conversion of CDP-choline to PC [114]. AD is also associated with abnormal metabolism of membrane phospholipids. Alterations in the metabolism of the phospholipids phosphatidylcholine (PC) have been detected in the cerebrospinal fluid of AD patients [115]. Neural membrane glycero-phospholipids, particularly ethanolamine plasmalogens, are markedly decreased in au-topsy samples from AD brain compared to age-matched control brain [116]. This decrease in glycerophospholipids is accompanied by a marked elevation in phospholipid degradation metabolites such as glycerophosphocholine, phosphocholine, and phosphoe-thanolamine [117]. Furthermore, marked increases have been reported in levels of prosta-glandins and lipid peroxides in AD brain [118,119]. The marked changes observed in phospholipids and their catabolic products may be coupled to the elevated activities of lipolytic enzymes in AD brain [120]. Moreover, cortices of AD patients have decreased levels of PC and phosphatidylethanolamine, compared with age-matched controls [116]. PC synthesis is regulated by levels of its precursors [113,114]; therefore, stimulation of PC synthesis by increasing precursor levels prevents the disruption in normal phospholi-pid metabolism caused by AD. Furthermore, increasing cell membrane synthesis may have morphological consequences for the cell. For instance, dendritic atrophy and loss occur in mouse models of AD [121,122] and dystrophic neurites are observed in human cases of AD [123]

8. Concluding remarks

Data from a series of biochemical, genetic, epidemiological studies and others exhibited that cholesterol is a key factor in APP processing and Aβ production. For instance, high cholesterol levels are linked to increased Aβ generation and deposition. It appears that there are many different ways in which abnormalities in cholesterol metabolism can af-fect the development of AD. Some polymorphisms in genes involved in cholesterol ca-tabolism and transport have been associated with an increased level of Aβ and are therefore potential risk factors for the disease. The best known of these genes is apoE4, which is the major genetic risk factor known for late-onset AD. Other genes implicated include cholesterol 24-hydroxylase (Cyp46), the LDL receptor related protein, the choles-terol transporter ABCA1, acyl-CoA:cholesterol acetyl transferase, and the LDL receptor. Then, we may conclude that what is bad for the heart is bad for the brain. We must pay attention to risk factors associated with heart disease to prevent Alzheimer's disease also. Considerable interest has also arisen regarding the effects of lifestyle interventions such as exercise and dietary/nutriceutical manipulations.

Acknowledgements

We dedicate this paper to Dr. Pedro Garzón de la Mora; who was for some of us a guide, and showed us to lose ourselves in the wonderful jungle of Biochemistry.

Author details

Genaro G. Ortiz[1]*, Fermín P. Pacheco-Moisés[2], Luis J. Flores-Alvarado[3], Miguel A. Macías-Islas[4], Irma E. Velázquez-Brizuela[5], Ana C. Ramírez-Anguiano[2], Erandis D. Tórres-Sánchez[1], Eddic W. Moráles-Sánchez[1], José A. Cruz-Ramos[1], Genaro E Ortiz-Velázquez[1] and Fernando Cortés-Enríquez[1]

*Address all correspondence to: genarogabriel@yahoo.com

1 Lab. Estrés Oxidativo-Mitocondria & Enfermedad, Centro de Investigación Biomédica de Occidente. Instituto Mexicano del Seguro Social (IMSS). Guadalajara, Jalisco, México

2 Dpto. de Química. CUCEI, Universidad de Guadalajara. Guadalajara, Jalisco, México

3 Dpto. de Bioquímica. CUCS, Universidad de Guadalajara. Guadalajara, Jalisco, México

4 Depto. de Neurología. UMAE,HE- IMSS. Guadalajara, Jalisco, México

5 OPD IJC-SSA- Jalisco. Guadalajara, Jalisco, México

References

[1] Reitz C, Carol Brayne & Richard Mayeux Epidemiology of Alzheimer disease. Nature Reviews Neurology 7, 137-152.

[2] Brookmeyer R, Johnson E, Ziegler-Graham K, Arrighi HM: Forecasting the global burden of Alzheimer's disease. Alzheimers Dement 2007, 3:186-191.

[3] Tiraboschi P, Hansen LA, Thal LJ, Corey-Bloom J (June 2004). The importance of neuritic plaques and tangles to the development and evolution of AD. Neurology 62 (11): pp. 1984–9

[4] L. Mosconi, Brain glucose metabolism in the early and specific diagnosis of Alzheimer's disease. FDG-PET studies in MCI and AD. Eur J Nucl Med Mol Imaging 2005: (32) 486-510.

[5] R. Peila, B.L. Rodriguez, L.J. Launer, Type 2 diabetes, APOE gene, and the risk for dementia and related pathologies: The Honolulu-Asia Aging Study. Diabetes 2002: (51) 1256-1262.

[6] Han W, Li C Linking type 2 diabetes and Alzheimer's disease. Proc Natl Acad Sci U S A. 2010 Apr 13;107(15):6557-8.

[7] T. Dyrks, A. Weidemann, G. Multhaup, J.M. Salbaum, H.G. Lemaire, J. Kang, B. Muller-Hill, C.L. Masters, K. Beyreuther, Identification, transmembrane orientation and

biogenesis of the amyloid A4 precursor of Alzheimer's disease. EMBO J 1988:(7) 949-957.

[8]   K. Kos, A.L. Harte, N.F. da Silva, A. Tonchev, G. Chaldakov, S. James, D.R. Snead, B. Hoggart, J.P. O'Hare, P.G. McTernan, S. Kumar, Adiponectin and resistin in human cerebrospinal fluid and expression of adiponectin receptors in the human hypothalamus. J Clin Endocrinol Metab 2007:(92) 1129-1136.

[9]   R.A. Whitmer, E.P. Gunderson, C.P. Quesenberry, Jr., J. Zhou, K. Yaffe, Body mass index in midlife and risk of Alzheimer disease and vascular dementia. Curr Alzheimer Res 2007:(4) 103-109. J Neurochem. 2005 Aug;94(4):1158-66.

[10] van der Heide LP, Kamal A, Artola A, Gispen WH, Ramakers GM. Insulin modulates hippocampal activity-dependent synaptic plasticity in a N-methyl-d-aspartate receptor and phosphatidyl-inositol-3-kinase-dependent manner.

[11] Son SM, Song H, Byun J, Park KS, Jang HC, Park YJ, Mook-Jung I. Altered APP Processing in Insulin-Resistant Conditions Is Mediated by Autophagosome Accumulation via the Inhibition of Mammalian Target of Rapamycin Pathway. Diabetes. 2012 Jul 24.

[12] Plum L, Belgardt BF, Brüning JC. Central insulin action in energy and glucose homeostasis. J Clin Invest 2006; 116(7): 1761-1766

[13] Pardini AW, Nguyen HT, Figlewicz DP, Baskin DG, Williams DL, Kim F, Schwartz MW. Distribution of insulin receptor substrate-2 in brain areas involved in energy homeostasis. Brain Res 2006; 1112(1): 169-178.

[14] Abbott MA, Wells DG, Fallon JR. The insulin receptor tyrosine kinase substrate p58/53 and the insulin receptor are components of CNS synapses. J Neurosci 1999; 19(17): 7300-7308.

[15] Gerozissis K. Brain insulin, energy and glucose homeostasis; genes, environment and metabolic pathologies. Eur J Pharmacol 2008; 585(1): 38-49.

[16] Gasparini L, Netzer WJ, Greengard P, Xu H. Does insulin dysfunction play a role in Alzheimer's disease? Trends Pharmacol Sci 2002; 23(6): 288-293.

[17] Wei Y, Williams JM, Dipace C, Sung U, Javitch JA, Galli A, Saunders C. Dopamine transporter activity mediates amphetamine-induced inhibition of Akt through a Ca2+/calmodulin-dependent kinase II-dependent mechanism. Mol Pharmacol 2007; 71(3): 835-842

[18] Man HY, Wang Q, Lu WY, Ju W, Ahmadian G, Liu L, D'Souza S, Wong TP, Taghibiglou C, Lu J, Becker LE, Pei L, Liu F, Wymann MP, MacDonald JF, Wang YT. Activation of PI3-Kinase is required for AMPA receptor insertion during LTP of mEPSCs in cultured hippocampal neurons. Neuron 2003; 38(4): 611-624.

[19] Zhao WQ, De Felice FG, Fernández S, Chen H, Lambert MP, Quon MJ, Krafft GA, Klein WL. Amyloid beta oligomers induce impairment of neuronal insulin receptors. FASEB J 2008; 22(1): 246-260.

[20] Nelson T, Alkon D. Insulin and cholesterol pathways in neuronal function, memory and neurodegeneration. Biochem Soc Trans 2005; 33(Pt 5): 1033-1036.

[21] Tang SJ, Reis G, Kang H, Gingras AC, Sonenberg N, Schuman EM. A rapamycin-sensitive signaling pathway contributes to long-term synaptic plasticity in the hippocampus. Proc Natl Acad Sci USA 2002; 99(1): 467-472.

[22] Lim GP, Calon F, Morihara T, Yang F, Teter B, Ubeda O, Salem N Jr, Frautschy SA, Cole GM. A diet enriched with the omega-3 fatty acid docosahexaenoic acid reduces amyloid burden in an aged Alzheimer mouse model. J Neurosci 2005; 25(12): 3032-3040.

[23] 2002; 22(22): 9785-9793. 45. Kern W, Peters A, Fruehwald-Schultes B, Deininger E, Born J, Fehm IIL. Improving influence of insulin on cognitive functions in humans. Neuroendocrinology 2001; 74(4): 270-280

[24] Park CR, Seeley RJ, Craft S, Woods SC. Intracerebroventricular insulin enhances memory in a passive-avoidance task. Physiol Behav 2000; 68(4): 509-514.

[25] Blennow K, de Leon MJ, Zetterberg H. Alzheimer's disease. Lancet 2006; 368(9533): 387-403.

[26] J.M. Dietschy, S.D. Turley, Cholesterol metabolism in the brain. Curr Opin Lipidol 2001:(12) 105-112.

[27] O. Levi, D. Lutjohann, A. Devir, K. von Bergmann, T. Hartmann, D.M. Michaelson, Regulation of hippocampal cholesterol metabolism by apoE and environmental stimulation. J Neurochem 2005:(95) 987-997.

[28] H. Jurevics, J. Hostettler, C. Barrett, P. Morell, A.D. Toews, Diurnal and dietary-induced changes in cholesterol synthesis correlate with levels of mRNA for HMG-CoA reductase. J Lipid Res 2000:(41) 1048-1054.

[29] C. Kirsch, G.P. Eckert, A.R. Koudinov, W.E. Muller, Brain cholesterol, statins and Alzheimer's Disease. Pharmacopsychiatry 2003:(36 Suppl 2) S113-119.

[30] I. Bjorkhem, D. Lutjohann, U. Diczfalusy, L. Stahle, G. Ahlborg, J. Wahren, Cholesterol homeostasis in human brain: turnover of 24S-hydroxycholesterol and evidence for a cerebral origin of most of this oxysterol in the circulation. J Lipid Res 1998:(39) 1594-1600.

[31] A. Papassotiropoulos, J.R. Streffer, M. Tsolaki, S. Schmid, D. Thal, F. Nicosia, V. Iakovidou, A. Maddalena, D. Lutjohann, E. Ghebremedhin, T. Hegi, T. Pasch, M. Traxler, A. Bruhl, L. Benussi, G. Binetti, H. Braak, R.M. Nitsch, C. Hock, Increased brain beta-amyloid load, phosphorylated tau, and risk of Alzheimer disease associated with an intronic CYP46 polymorphism. Arch Neurol 2003:(60) 29-35.

[32] G.W. Rebeck, S.D. Harr, D.K. Strickland, B.T. Hyman, Multiple, diverse senile pla-
      que-associated proteins are ligands of an apolipoprotein E receptor, the alpha 2-mac-
      roglobulin receptor/low-density-lipoprotein receptor-related protein. Ann Neurol
      1995:(37) 211-217.

[33] M. Shibata, S. Yamada, S.R. Kumar, M. Calero, J. Bading, B. Frangione, D.M. Holtz-
      man, C.A. Miller, D.K. Strickland, J. Ghiso, B.V. Zlokovic, Clearance of Alzheimer's
      amyloid-ss(1-40) peptide from brain by LDL receptor-related protein-1 at the blood-
      brain barrier. J Clin Invest 2000:(106) 1489-1499.

[34] Q. Liu, C.V. Zerbinatti, J. Zhang, H.S. Hoe, B. Wang, S.L. Cole, J. Herz, L. Muglia, G.
      Bu, Amyloid precursor protein regulates brain apolipoprotein E and cholesterol me-
      tabolism through lipoprotein receptor LRP1. Neuron 2007:(56) 66-78.

[35] M.D. Haag, A. Hofman, P.J. Koudstaal, B.H. Stricker, M.M. Breteler, Statins are asso-
      ciated with a reduced risk of Alzheimer disease regardless of lipophilicity. The Rot-
      terdam Study. J Neurol Neurosurg Psychiatry 2009:(80) 13-17.

[36] S.R. Hughes, O. Khorkova, S. Goyal, J. Knaeblein, J. Heroux, N.G. Riedel, S. Sahasra-
      budhe, Alpha2-macroglobulin associates with beta-amyloid peptide and prevents fi-
      bril formation. Proc Natl Acad Sci U S A 1998:(95) 3275-3280.

[37] J. Bauer, S. Strauss, U. Schreiter-Gasser, U. Ganter, P. Schlegel, I. Witt, B. Yolk, M.
      Berger, Interleukin-6 and alpha-2-macroglobulin indicate an acute-phase state in Alz-
      heimer's disease cortices. FEBS Lett 1991:(285) 111-114.

[38] W. Borth, Alpha 2-macroglobulin, a multifunctional binding protein with targeting
      characteristics. FASEB J 1992:(6) 3345-3353.

[39] D. Blacker, M.A. Wilcox, N.M. Laird, L. Rodes, S.M. Horvath, R.C. Go, R. Perry, B.
      Watson, Jr., S.S. Bassett, M.G. McInnis, M.S. Albert, B.T. Hyman, R.E. Tanzi, Alpha-2
      macroglobulin is genetically associated with Alzheimer disease. Nat Genet 1998:(19)
      357-360.

[40] E.A. Rogaeva, S. Premkumar, J. Grubber, L. Serneels, W.K. Scott, T. Kawarai, Y. Song,
      D.L. Hill, S.M. Abou-Donia, E.R. Martin, J.J. Vance, G. Yu, A. Orlacchio, Y. Pei, M.
      Nishimura, A. Supala, B. Roberge, A.M. Saunders, A.D. Roses, D. Schmechel, A.
      Crane-Gatherum, S. Sorbi, A. Bruni, G.W. Small, P.M. Conneally, J.L. Haines, F. Van
      Leuven, P.H. St George-Hyslop, L.A. Farrer, M.A. Pericak-Vance, An alpha-2-macro-
      globulin insertion-deletion polymorphism in Alzheimer disease. Nat Genet 1999:(22)
      19-22.

[41] M. Simons, P. Keller, B. De Strooper, K. Beyreuther, C.G. Dotti, K. Simons, Cholester-
      ol depletion inhibits the generation of beta-amyloid in hippocampal neurons. Proc
      Natl Acad Sci U S A 1998:(95) 6460-6464.

[42] D.S. Howland, S.P. Trusko, M.J. Savage, A.G. Reaume, D.M. Lang, J.D. Hirsch, N.
      Maeda, R. Siman, B.D. Greenberg, R.W. Scott, D.G. Flood, Modulation of secreted be-

ta-amyloid precursor protein and amyloid beta-peptide in brain by cholesterol. J Biol Chem 1998:(273) 16576-16582.

[43] L.M. Refolo, B. Malester, J. LaFrancois, T. Bryant-Thomas, R. Wang, G.S. Tint, K. Sambamurti, K. Duff, M.A. Pappolla, Hypercholesterolemia accelerates the Alzheimer's amyloid pathology in a transgenic mouse model. Neurobiol Dis 2000:(7) 321-331.

[44] D.L. Sparks, Y.M. Kuo, A. Roher, T. Martin, R.J. Lukas, Alterations of Alzheimer's disease in the cholesterol-fed rabbit, including vascular inflammation. Preliminary observations. Ann N Y Acad Sci 2000:(903) 335-344.

[45] A.G. Mainous, 3rd, S.L. Eschenbach, B.J. Wells, C.J. Everett, J.M. Gill, Cholesterol, transferrin saturation, and the development of dementia and Alzheimer's disease: results from an 18-year population-based cohort. Fam Med 2005:(37) 36-42.

[46] M.M. Mielke, P.P. Zandi, M. Sjogren, D. Gustafson, S. Ostling, B. Steen, I. Skoog, High total cholesterol levels in late life associated with a reduced risk of dementia. Neurology 2005:(64) 1689-1695.

[47] V. Leoni, C. Caccia, Oxysterols as biomarkers in neurodegenerative diseases. Chem Phys Lipids 2011:(164) 515-524.

[48] R.P. Koldamova, I.M. Lefterov, M. Staufenbiel, D. Wolfe, S. Huang, J.C. Glorioso, M. Walter, M.G. Roth, J.S. Lazo, The liver X receptor ligand T0901317 decreases amyloid beta production in vitro and in a mouse model of Alzheimer's disease. J Biol Chem 2005:(280) 4079-4088.

[49] D.R. Riddell, H. Zhou, T.A. Comery, E. Kouranova, C.F. Lo, H.K. Warwick, R.H. Ring, Y. Kirksey, S. Aschmies, J. Xu, K. Kubek, W.D. Hirst, C. Gonzales, Y. Chen, E. Murphy, S. Leonard, D. Vasylyev, A. Oganesian, R.L. Martone, M.N. Pangalos, P.H. Reinhart, J.S. Jacobsen, The LXR agonist TO901317 selectively lowers hippocampal Abeta42 and improves memory in the Tg2576 mouse model of Alzheimer's disease. Mol Cell Neurosci 2007:(34) 621-628.

[50] N. Zelcer, P. Tontonoz, Liver X receptors as integrators of metabolic and inflammatory signaling. J Clin Invest 2006:(116) 607-614.

[51] B.A. Hamelin, J. Turgeon, Hydrophilicity/lipophilicity: relevance for the pharmacology and clinical effects of HMG-CoA reductase inhibitors. Trends Pharmacol Sci 1998: (19) 26-37.

[52] K. Nezasa, K. Higaki, M. Takeuchi, M. Nakano, M. Koike, Uptake of rosuvastatin by isolated rat hepatocytes: comparison with pravastatin. Xenobiotica 2003:(33) 379-388.

[53] L.N. Johnson-Anuna, G.P. Eckert, J.H. Keller, U. Igbavboa, C. Franke, T. Fechner, M. Schubert-Zsilavecz, M. Karas, W.E. Muller, W.G. Wood, Chronic administration of statins alters multiple gene expression patterns in mouse cerebral cortex. J Pharmacol Exp Ther 2005:(312) 786-793.

[54] B. Wolozin, W. Kellman, P. Ruosseau, G.G. Celesia, G. Siegel, Decreased prevalence of Alzheimer disease associated with 3-hydroxy-3-methyglutaryl coenzyme A reductase inhibitors. Arch Neurol 2000:(57) 1439-1443.

[55] K. Rockwood, S. Kirkland, D.B. Hogan, C. MacKnight, H. Merry, R. Verreault, C. Wolfson, I. McDowell, Use of lipid-lowering agents, indication bias, and the risk of dementia in community-dwelling elderly people. Arch Neurol 2002:(59) 223-227.

[56] S. Pedrini, T.L. Carter, G. Prendergast, S. Petanceska, M.E. Ehrlich, S. Gandy, Modulation of statin-activated shedding of Alzheimer APP ectodomain by ROCK. PLoS Med 2005:(2) e18.

[57] X. Bi, M. Baudry, J. Liu, Y. Yao, L. Fu, F. Brucher, G. Lynch, Inhibition of geranylgeranylation mediates the effects of 3-hydroxy-3-methylglutaryl (HMG)-CoA reductase inhibitors on microglia. J Biol Chem 2004:(279) 48238-48245.

[58] A. Cordle, G. Landreth, 3-Hydroxy-3-methylglutaryl-coenzyme A reductase inhibitors attenuate beta-amyloid-induced microglial inflammatory responses. J Neurosci 2005:(25) 299-307.

[59] A. Sebok, N. Nusser, B. Debreceni, Z. Guo, M.F. Santos, J. Szeberenyi, G. Tigyi, Different roles for RhoA during neurite initiation, elongation, and regeneration in PC12 cells. J Neurochem 1999:(73) 949-960.

[60] A.M. Pooler, S.C. Xi, R.J. Wurtman, The 3-hydroxy-3-methylglutaryl co-enzyme A reductase inhibitor pravastatin enhances neurite outgrowth in hippocampal neurons. J Neurochem 2006:(97) 716-723.

[61] E. Zamrini, G. McGwin, J.M. Roseman, Association between statin use and Alzheimer's disease. Neuroepidemiology 2004:(23) 94-98.

[62] G.P. Eckert, Manipulation of lipid rafts in neuronal cells. The Open Biology Journal 2010:(3) 1874–1967.

[63] B. Wolozin, Cholesterol and the biology of Alzheimer's disease. Neuron 2004:(41) 7-10.

[64] W.G. Wood, F. Schroeder, U. Igbavboa, N.A. Avdulov, S.V. Chochina, Brain membrane cholesterol domains, aging and amyloid beta-peptides. Neurobiol Aging 2002: (23) 685-694.

[65] Y. Young-Xu, K.A. Chan, J.K. Liao, S. Ravid, C.M. Blatt, Long-term statin use and psychological well-being. J Am Coll Cardiol 2003:(42) 690-697.

[66] V.I. Zannis, J.L. Breslow, Human very low density lipoprotein apolipoprotein E isoprotein polymorphism is explained by genetic variation and posttranslational modification. Biochemistry 1981:(20) 1033-1041.

[67] Mahley RW, Rall SC: APOLIPOPROTEIN E: Far More Than a Lipid Transport Protein. Annu Rev Genomics Hum Genet 2000, 1:507-537.

[68] W.J. Strittmatter, A.D. Roses, Apolipoprotein E and Alzheimer disease. Proc Natl Acad Sci U S A 1995:(92) 4725-4727.

[69] E.H. Corder, A.M. Saunders, N.J. Risch, W.J. Strittmatter, D.E. Schmechel, P.C. Gaskell, Jr., J.B. Rimmler, P.A. Locke, P.M. Conneally, K.E. Schmader, et al., Protective effect of apolipoprotein E type 2 allele for late onset Alzheimer disease. Nat Genet 1994:(7) 180-184.

[70] Y. Song, M.J. Stampfer, S. Liu, Meta-analysis: apolipoprotein E genotypes and risk for coronary heart disease. Ann Intern Med 2004:(141) 137-147.

[71] A. Tammi, T. Ronnemaa, L. Rask-Nissila, T.A. Miettinen, H. Gylling, L. Valsta, J. Viikari, I. Valimaki, O. Simell, Apolipoprotein E phenotype regulates cholesterol absorption in healthy 13-month-old children--The STRIP Study. Pediatr Res 2001:(50) 688-691.

[72] A. Tammi, T. Ronnemaa, J. Viikari, E. Jokinen, H. Lapinleimu, C. Ehnholm, O. Simell, Apolipoprotein E4 phenotype increases non-fasting serum triglyceride concentration in infants - the STRIP study. Atherosclerosis 2000:(152) 135-141.

[73] P.A. Janmey, P.K. Kinnunen, Biophysical properties of lipids and dynamic membranes. Trends Cell Biol 2006:(16) 538-546.

[74] Eckert GP, Wood WG, Muller WE (2005) Statins: drugs for Alzheimer's disease? J Neural Transm.

[75] Y. Barenholz, Sphingomyelin and cholesterol: from membrane biophysics and rafts to potential medical applications. Subcell Biochem 2004:(37) 167-215.

[76] U. Igbavboa, N.A. Avdulov, F. Schroeder, W.G. Wood, Increasing age alters transbilayer fluidity and cholesterol asymmetry in synaptic plasma membranes of mice. J Neurochem 1996:(66) 1717-1725.

[77] Wood W, Eckert GP, Igbavboa U, Muller WE (2003) Amyloid beta-protein interactions with membranes and cholesterol: causes or casualties of Alzheimer's disease. Biochim Biophys Acta 1610:281-290.

[78] R.P. Mason, W.J. Shoemaker, L. Shajenko, T.E. Chambers, L.G. Herbette, Evidence for changes in the Alzheimer's disease brain cortical membrane structure mediated by cholesterol. Neurobiol Aging 1992:(13) 413-419.

[79] P. Mecocci, A. Cherubini, M.F. Beal, R. Cecchetti, F. Chionne, M.C. Polidori, G. Romano, U. Senin, Altered mitochondrial membrane fluidity in AD brain. Neurosci Lett 1996:(207) 129-132.

[80] G.G. Ortiz, F. Pacheco-Moises, M. El Hafidi, A. Jimenez-Delgado, M.A. Macias-Islas, S.A. Rosales Corral, A.C. de la Rosa, V.J. Sanchez-Gonzalez, E.D. Arias-Merino, I.E. Velazquez-Brizuela, Detection of membrane fluidity in submitochondrial particles of platelets and erythrocyte membranes from Mexican patients with Alzheimer disease

by intramolecular excimer formation of 1,3 dipyrenylpropane. Dis Markers 2008:(24) 151-156.

[81] E. Bonilla, K. Tanji, M. Hirano, T.H. Vu, S. DiMauro, E.A. Schon, Mitochondrial involvement in Alzheimer's disease. Biochim Biophys Acta 1999:(1410) 171-182.

[82] I. Hajimohammadreza, M.J. Brammer, S. Eagger, A. Burns, R. Levy, Platelet and erythrocyte membrane changes in Alzheimer's disease. Biochim Biophys Acta 1990: (1025) 208-214.

[83] G.S. Zubenko, U. Kopp, T. Seto, L.L. Firestone, Platelet membrane fluidity individuals at risk for Alzheimer's disease: a comparison of results from fluorescence spectroscopy and electron spin resonance spectroscopy. Psychopharmacology (Berl) 1999: (145) 175-180.

[84] G.S. Zubenko, I. Malinakova, B. Chojnacki, Proliferation of internal membranes in platelets from patients with Alzheimer's disease. J Neuropathol Exp Neurol 1987:(46) 407-418.

[85] M.H. Fukami, L. Salganicoff, Isolation and properties of human platelet mitochondria. Blood 1973:(42) 913-918.

[86] S.M. Cardoso, M.T. Proenca, S. Santos, I. Santana, C.R. Oliveira, Cytochrome c oxidase is decreased in Alzheimer's disease platelets. Neurobiol Aging 2004:(25) 105-110.

[87] M. Ameloot, H. Hendrickx, W. Herreman, H. Pottel, F. Van Cauwelaert, W. van der Meer, Effect of orientational order on the decay of the fluorescence anisotropy in membrane suspensions. Experimental verification on unilamellar vesicles and lipid/ alpha-lactalbumin complexes. Biophys J 1984:(46) 525-539.

[88] K.A. Zachariasse, W.L. Vaz, C. Sotomayor, W. Kuhnle, Investigation of human erythrocyte ghost membranes with intramolecular excimer probes. Biochim Biophys Acta 1982:(688) 323-332.

[89] R.D. Kaiser, E. London, Location of diphenylhexatriene (DPH) and its derivatives within membranes: comparison of different fluorescence quenching analyses of membrane depth. Biochemistry 1998:(37) 8180-8190.

[90] I.A. Zainaghi, O.V. Forlenza, W.F. Gattaz, Abnormal APP processing in platelets of patients with Alzheimer's disease: correlations with membrane fluidity and cognitive decline. Psychopharmacology (Berl) 2007:(192) 547-553.

[91] J.P. Schuchardt, M. Huss, M. Stauss-Grabo, A. Hahn, Significance of long-chain polyunsaturated fatty acids (PUFAs) for the development and behaviour of children. Eur J Pediatr 2010:(169) 149-164.

[92] L.A. Horrocks, A.A. Farooqui, Docosahexaenoic acid in the diet: its importance in maintenance and restoration of neural membrane function. Prostaglandins Leukot Essent Fatty Acids 2004:(70) 361-372.

[93] I. Carrie, G. Abellan Van Kan, Y. Rolland, S. Gillette-Guyonnet, B. Vellas, PUFA for prevention and treatment of dementia? Curr Pharm Des 2009:(15) 4173-4185.

[94] C.R. Hooijmans, A.J. Kiliaan, Fatty acids, lipid metabolism and Alzheimer pathology. Eur J Pharmacol 2008:(585) 176-196.

[95] J.H. Song, T. Miyazawa, Enhanced level of n-3 fatty acid in membrane phospholipids induces lipid peroxidation in rats fed dietary docosahexaenoic acid oil. Atherosclerosis 2001:(155) 9-18.

[96] H. Grundt, D.W. Nilsen, M.A. Mansoor, A. Nordoy, Increased lipid peroxidation during long-term intervention with high doses of n-3 fatty acids (PUFAs) following an acute myocardial infarction. Eur J Clin Nutr 2003:(57) 793-800.

[97] K. Simons, E. Ikonen, Functional rafts in cell membranes. Nature 1997:(387) 569-572.

[98] E. Kojro, G. Gimpl, S. Lammich, W. Marz, F. Fahrenholz, Low cholesterol stimulates the nonamyloidogenic pathway by its effect on the alpha -secretase ADAM 10. Proc Natl Acad Sci U S A 2001:(98) 5815-5820.

[99] P. Weber, M. Wagner, H. Schneckenburger, Microfluorometry of cell membrane dynamics. Cytometry A 2006:(69) 185-188.

[100] C. Haass, A.Y. Hung, M.G. Schlossmacher, D.B. Teplow, D.J. Selkoe, beta-Amyloid peptide and a 3-kDa fragment are derived by distinct cellular mechanisms. J Biol Chem 1993:(268) 3021-3024.

[101] P.C. Reid, Y. Urano, T. Kodama, T. Hamakubo, Alzheimer's disease: cholesterol, membrane rafts, isoprenoids and statins. J Cell Mol Med 2007:(11) 383-392.

[102] R. Ehehalt, P. Keller, C. Haass, C. Thiele, K. Simons, Amyloidogenic processing of the Alzheimer beta-amyloid precursor protein depends on lipid rafts. J Cell Biol 2003: (160) 113-123.

[103] K. Fassbender, M. Simons, C. Bergmann, M. Stroick, D. Lutjohann, P. Keller, H. Runz, S. Kuhl, T. Bertsch, K. von Bergmann, M. Hennerici, K. Beyreuther, T. Hartmann, Simvastatin strongly reduces levels of Alzheimer's disease beta -amyloid peptides Abeta 42 and Abeta 40 in vitro and in vivo. Proc Natl Acad Sci U S A 2001:(98) 5856-5861.

[104] C.A. von Arnim, B. von Einem, P. Weber, M. Wagner, D. Schwanzar, R. Spoelgen, W.L. Strauss, H. Schneckenburger, Impact of cholesterol level upon APP and BACE proximity and APP cleavage. Biochem Biophys Res Commun 2008:(370) 207-212.

[105] Paula RS, Souza VC, Benedet AL, Souza ER, Toledo JO, Moraes CF, Gomes L, Alho CS, Córdova C, Nóbrega OT. Dietary fat and apolipoprotein genotypes modulate plasma lipoprotein levels in Brazilian elderly women. Mol Cell Biochem. 2010 Apr; 337(1-2):307-15.

[106] Catalá A. Lipid peroxidation modifies the picture of membranes from the "Fluid Mosaic Model" to the "Lipid Whisker Model" Biochimie 94 (2012) 101e109.

[107] Hoshino T, Kamino K, Matsumoto M. Gene dose effect of the APOE-epsilon4 allele on plasma HDL cholesterol level in patients with Alzheimer's disease. Neurobiol Aging. 2002 Jan-Feb;23(1):41-5.

[108] Eckert GP, Wood WG, Müller WE. Effects of aging and beta-amyloid on the properties of brain synaptic and mitochondrial membranes. J Neural Transm. 2001;108(8-9): 1051-64.

[109] Axelsen PH, Komatsu H, Murray IV. Oxidative stress and cell membranes in the pathogenesis of Alzheimer's disease. Physiology (Bethesda). 2011 Feb;26(1):54-69.

[110] E.P. Kennedy, S.B. Weiss, The function of cytidine coenzymes in the biosynthesis of phospholipides. J Biol Chem 1956:(222) 193-214.

[111] U.I. Richardson, C.J. Watkins, C. Pierre, I.H. Ulus, R.J. Wurtman, Stimulation of CDP-choline synthesis by uridine or cytidine in PC12 rat pheochromocytoma cells. Brain Res 2003:(971) 161-167.

[112] P.C. Choy, H.B. Paddon, D.E. Vance, An increase in cytoplasmic CTP accelerates the reaction catalyzed by CTP:phosphocholine cytidylyltransferase in poliovirus-infected HeLa cells. J Biol Chem 1980:(255) 1070-1073.

[113] V. Savci, R.J. Wurtman, Effect of cytidine on membrane phospholipid synthesis in rat striatal slices. J Neurochem 1995:(64) 378-384.

[114] W. Araki, R.J. Wurtman, Control of membrane phosphatidylcholine biosynthesis by diacylglycerol levels in neuronal cells undergoing neurite outgrowth. Proc Natl Acad Sci U S A 1997:(94) 11946-11950.

[115] C. Mulder, L.O. Wahlund, T. Teerlink, M. Blomberg, R. Veerhuis, G.J. van Kamp, P. Scheltens, P.G. Scheffer, Decreased lysophosphatidylcholine/phosphatidylcholine ratio in cerebrospinal fluid in Alzheimer's disease. J Neural Transm 2003:(110) 949-955.

[116] R.M. Nitsch, B.E. Slack, R.J. Wurtman, J.H. Growdon, Release of Alzheimer amyloid precursor derivatives stimulated by activation of muscarinic acetylcholine receptors. Science 1992:(258) 304-307.

[117] Pettegrew, J. W. (1989). Molecular insights into Alzheimer disease. Ann. N. Y. Acad. Sci. 568:5–28.

[118] Subbarao, K. V., Richardson, J. S., and Ang, L. C. (1990). Autopsy samples of Alzheimer's cortex show increased peroxidation in vitro. J. Neurochem. 55:342–345.

[119] Palmer, A. M., and Burns, M. A. (1994). Selective increase in lipid peroxidation in the inferior temporal cortex in Alzheimer's disease. Brain Res. 645:338–342.

[120] Farooqui, A. A., and Horrocks, L. A. (1991). Excitatory amino acid receptors, neural membrane phospholipid metabolism and neurological disorders. Brain Res. Rev. 16:171–191.

[121] F. Calon, G.P. Lim, F. Yang, T. Morihara, B. Teter, O. Ubeda, P. Rostaing, A. Triller, N. Salem, Jr., K.H. Ashe, S.A. Frautschy, G.M. Cole, Docosahexaenoic acid protects

from dendritic pathology in an Alzheimer's disease mouse model. Neuron 2004:(43) 633-645.

[122] D.L. Moolman, O.V. Vitolo, J.P. Vonsattel, M.L. Shelanski, Dendrite and dendritic spine alterations in Alzheimer models. J Neurocytol 2004:(33) 377-387.

[123] A.C. McKee, K.S. Kosik, N.W. Kowall, Neuritic pathology and dementia in Alzheimer's disease. Ann Neurol 1991:(30) 156-165.

[124] Figure Modified Pathway central: CD40 Signaling (Fig 5), www.sabiosciences.com/pathway.php?sn=CD40_Signaling

[125] Figure Modified Pathway central: Insulin Receptor (Fig 2), www.sabiosciences.com/pathway.php?sn=Insulin_Receptor

[126] Figure Modified Pathway Central: CREB Pathway (Figure 3), www.sabiosciences.com/pathway.php?sn=CREB

[127] Figure Modified Pathway Central: Mito (Figure 7), www.sabiosciences.com/pathway.php?sn=Mitochondrial_Apoptosis

Diagnosis

Pre-Analytical and Analytical Critical Factors Influencing the High Variability of the Concentrations Levels of Alzheimer Disease Biomarkers in Cerebral Spinal Fluid

Armand Perret-Liaudet, Aline Dorey,
Yannick Tholance, Benoit Dumont and
Isabelle Quadrio

Additional information is available at the end of the chapter

1. Introduction

Alzheimer's disease (AD) is a fatal neurodegenerative disorder characterized by a progressive neuronal death and loss of cognitive functions. AD is the most common type of dementia and its incidence rise to 10% in people aged over 90 [1]. Due to Increased longevity, it has been estimated that the number of people suffering from this neurodegenerative disorder will rise from 26.6 million cases in 2006 to 106,8 million worldwide in 2050 [2].

Although clinical intervention to halt the disease is inefficient, the clinical and psychological cares are likely known to significantly improve the quality of life of the patient but also those of the family. At the prodromal stage of the disease (Mild cognitive Impairment linked to AD), there are no sufficient evidences that treating the patient improves the patient outcome. This lack of evidence poses in some cases an ethical problem that is to announce the diagnosis of AD at an autonomous patient who will shift irreversibly in the coming years to the dementia stages. However, as reported in new criteria established by the National Institute on Aging (NIA) and the Alzheimer's Association, core clinical criteria could be used by healthcare providers without access to advanced imaging techniques or cerebrospinal fluid analysis. Criteria including these last advanced tools still remain in the research field [3]. On the contrary, the diagnosis is highly aimed to be accurate at least at the clinical stage of mild dementia, to detect the AD pathology. Core clinical criteria seems to be enough to ensure the AD diagnosis and the use of biomarkers (imaging or CSF biomarkers) can only increase the certainty that the basis of the clinical dementia syndrome is the AD pathophysiological process in a patient presenting the core clinical diagnosis [4]. The CSF biomarker panel of AD is a picture of the neurodegeneration, the neuronal loss, the tangle formation and $A\beta$-amyloid$_{42}$ ($A\beta_{42}$) peptide accumulation in the brain. Indeed, the core CSF biomarkers for AD diagnosis are a decrease of $A\beta_{42}$ levels and more recently a decrease of the ratio of $A\beta$-amyloid$_{42}$ / $A\beta$-amyloid$_{40}$ ($A\beta_{42}/A\beta_{40}$) which reflect senile plaques pathology as well as an increase of total tau (T-tau) and phosphorylated tau (P-tau) which reflect axonal degeneration [5,6]. The use of AD biomarker tests for routine diagnostic purposes at the present time, is only proposed as optional for use in patients with dementia when deemed appropriate by the clinician. From the several reasons for this limitation, the workgroup with the task of revising the 1984 criteria for Alzheimer's disease (AD) dementia, highlighted the limited standardization of biomarkers from one locale to another [4]. Despite a decrease in the number of side effects associated with the puncture, lumbar puncture remains an invasive procedure that is clearly the main factor preventing the wide dissemination of these biomarkers in the routine. However, we cannot ignore that the significant variability in measured biomarkers levels found in various studies, resulting in a high variability of both the diagnostic accuracy [7] and of the clinical cut-off for the diagnostic of AD [8], is a hindrance to the spread of these markers and their integration in the diagnostic criteria [3]. The cut-offs obtained in Europe for CSF total tau and beta-amyloid measured by the ELISA assays from the same manufacturer, were reported highly diverse, with two to three fold differences between the highest and lowest reported values [8]. Three major explanations are proposed in this report: first, the inter-laboratory comparisons are very difficult, as some laboratories have adopted the cut-off values from the research literature whereas others have established their own controls, these last controls being likely different in neuropsychology evaluation, neuroimaging and the follow-up. Secondly, the lack of standardized material between the different assays but also the lack of standardized protocols, seem to be a major source of this variation. Finally, pre-analytical factors are those factors that contribute to the variation of the laboratory results before the analysis of the sample. One consensus report has already established the main pre-analytical factors that should be standardized for CSF AD biomarkers analysis [9]. However, the importance of some pre-analytical confounding factors highlighted in this report remained to be elucidated. The aim of this report is to discuss and focus on main critical points in the different preanalytical steps likely to be responsible of data variability. For analytical steps, the introduction since 2009 of an external quality control at a large scale gave an overview of the «desaster», in the same line that prior results. We will discuss rapidly the prior results reported in 2011 and we will underline the urgent need for standardization.

2. Influence of confounding factors in pre-analytical phases on the analysis of AD biomarkers

The confounding factors in pre-analytical phases have a great importance to biochemical analysis and can affect the reliability of the results. Specially in the context of biomarkers of AD in CSF, there are some experimental studies that support this proposition [10,11,12]. Those factors are classically dichotomized in two different groups, «in vivo» and «in vitro». The «in vivo» factors are those biological factors that are linked directly to the patient, the «in vitro» factors are linked to the procedure of sample handling and processing.

2.1. *In vivo* factors

2.1.1. *Is there a specific time of day needed to collect the CSF?*

Answering this issue needs to know if a nycthemeral cycle exists that could modify the concentrations levels of AD CSF biomarkers during the day. Although a lack of standardization in the diagnostic strategy of the patient still exists, in most cases, after a first examination including a clinical and a neuropsychological evaluation, if needed, the lumbar puncture is generally scheduled in a second visit with morphological brain imaging in the same time, with the aim to minimize the duration of the hospitalization. As the time of the lumbar puncture is highly dependent of the coordinated organization of the clinical memory centre, of the biological laboratory and of the imaging department associated with it (waiting homeostasis results, scheduling imaging...), this question is highly relevant.

Previous results have suggested the existence of a large diurnal variability in Aβ levels during a time period of 36 hours, but without significant differences between the hours all along the day period [13]. Following these amazing and unexplained data, recent studies were unable to demonstrate the existence of a temporal fluctuation in CSF biomarker levels, not only for Aβ, but also for T-tau and P-tau [10, 14, 15]. Therefore, there is no need to standardize a specific time interval during the day for CSF collection dedicated to the AD biomarkers assays.

2.1.2. *Is fasting able to modify the concentrations levels of AD biomarkers ?*

At our knowledge, there are no study that has analyzed the influence of fasting on AD CSF biomarkers. The comparison of patients with and without fasting would give a set of indirect and biased data without clear conclusion. Moreover, for ethical reasons, it seems to be impossible to start a research study focused on this topic, as this study would imply a protocol with the realization of successive lumbar punctures in a short delay. Therefore, it is not possible to answer scientifically this issue. Nevertheless, it has been shown that, independently of the patient food intake, Aβ levels in plasma are very stable [10]. As there is a lack of data concerning this topic, as those kind of data could probably never be obtained, and taking account of the large diversity in the locale organization, it is not logical to recommend fasting for the analysis of AD biomarkers in CSF.

2.2. *In vitro* factors

2.2.1. *Localization of the puncture*

Due to the possible decreased rostro-caudal concentration gradient, the site of CSF withdrawal must be also standardized. At our knowledge, there is no study reporting any difference between AD biomarkers concentrations obtained by a ventricular puncture and those obtained by lumbar puncture. Therefore, it is not recommended to analyse these markers in the ventricular punctures obtained during neurosurgical interventions. Nowadays, diagnostic CSF is usually obtained by LP between the L3/L4 and L4/L5 intervertebral space.

2.2.2. Does a CSF gradient of AD biomarkers exist ?

Most brain-derived proteins have a decreased rostro-caudal concentration gradient [16]. Therefore, the volume of CSF taken can influence protein concentration. Using unpublished data from Le Bastard et al., Vanderstichele et al reported the absence of a gradient effect in AD CSF biomarkers concentrations during [9]. It was confirmed by another experimental study analyzing the gradient effect in the spinal cord on $A\beta_{42}$ [10]. Therefore, there is no reason to recommend any specific fraction of CSF volume for the assay of AD biomarkers.

2.2.3. What kind of needle for the puncture ?

The type of needle is likely known to influence the percentage of side effects in patients and to be a factor leading to the presence of red cells [17, 18]. Therefore, the needle could influence the biomarkers concentrations. It has been shown that post-lumbar puncture headache (PLPH) severity was significantly decreased when a 22G needle was used instead of a 20G needle [18]. Moreover, using a 22G atraumatic needle it was also observed a remarkably decrease of PLPH in comparison with 22G traumatic needles [19]. Finally, as lumbar puncture is sometimes difficult with 25G needle in elderly people, a korean group has compared the prevalence of PLPH using 23G and 25G needles. They concluded that the choice of a 23 or 25 gauge Quincke needle has no significant influence on post-dural puncture headache for Korean patients greater than 60 years old. Therefore, the 23 gauge Quincke needle is an option for lumbar punctures in this patient population [20].

2.2.4. Types of sampling tubes

It was established that polypropylene (PP) tubes should be preferred to glass or polystyrene tubes for collection of the CSF since $A\beta$ peptides, but also T-tau and P-tau, bind in a non specifically manner to the polystyrene tubes and to the glass tubes [10, 21]. However, two independent studies reported significant differences on $A\beta_{42}$ levels (up to 50 % compared to basal values !) when CSF was collected in PP tubes from different suppliers [11, 22]. For $A\beta_{42}$, we found that adsorption was effective in a contact time less than 15 minutes, the loss of $A\beta_{42}$ levels being highly significant [11]. Moreover the adsorption intensity was highly dependent on the levels of total proteinorachia, since we abolished this phenomenon when we spiked the CSF with solutions of bovine serum albumin. Amazingly, we also shown that, whereas all the tubes that we studied were commercialized by the providers as tubes in PP, a calorimetry and a spectroscopy analysis revealed that just one out of 11 tubes was pure PP while the others were copolymers made of PP and polyethylene (PE) [11]. Moreover, we also shown that the pure PP causes more adsorption of amyloid peptides than tubes in copolymers of PE and PP, with or without treatment surface, and that some tubes in copolymers could be worst than classical polystyrene: these highly striking results were reproducible in the independent laboratories which have collaborated in this study [11]. Moreover, it was also observed that the tubes that performed better for $A\beta_{42}$ were the worst for P-tau suggesting that hydrophilic-hydrophobic balance is a important point in protein adsorption [11, 23]. The variability of adsorption intensity of proteins onto the plastic of the tube is the result of the incredible jungle of the manufacturing of different tubes called PP: difference in the nature and in the percentage of the copolymers in the plastic, presence of additives, surface treatments, modification of the surface by the sterilization process... The possibility of modifying the protein adsorption by additives or surface treatments was underlined by different reports. First, when Tween-20 was added in the tube containing the CSF, the adsorption of amyloid peptides was significantly reduced [22]. Secondly we recently reported similar results using various plasma treatments of the tube surface, able to modify the adsorption of different proteins like prion protein, Tau and alpha synuclein [23]. These data highlight the need to standardize also the type of test tube used since the great variability found could even lead to a possible AD misdiagnosis. In our laboratory, we shifted to the best tube that we found in this study. This shift has introduced an averaged increase of 25 % of $A\beta_{42}$ levels leading to a modification of our cut off diagnostic value from 500 ng/L to 700 ng/L (data submitted). Currently the members of the Joint Programming Neurodegenerative Disease research (JPND) are performing a study which includes the analysis of the most suitable type of tube for AD CSF biomarkers research. Therefore, it is not reasonable to follow the actual guidelines recommending the use of generic PP tubes. Since the data of the JPND collaboration will probably not be available before 2 or 3 years, the best compromise would be that each laboratory concerned by these markers, compares its local tube with the best tubes identified in our study, which are easily available in the commercial market.

2.2.5. Time delay between CSF collection and storage before assay

This is an issue difficult to standardize due the high variety of existing procedures and its probable dependance of confounding factors (hemorragic puncture, hemolyzed samples, high levels of total protein, one sampling tube for AD biomarkers and various markers of others pathologies...) which could modify the stability of the biomarkers during this critical period.

For that, we will discuss first the need to centrifuge and the protocol of centrifugation. This step is able to avoid the presumed influence of the blood cells introduced by the hemorragic puncture. These hemorragic punctures occur in 14-20% cases of lumbar puncture. Bjerke et al. were unable to detect any difference in $A\beta_{42}$ levels when up to 5000 erythrocytes/μl were spiked to the CSF. This value was found ten fold higher than those recommended in the regulation's document included in the Innogenetics kits. However, they found significant decreased $A\beta_{42}$ levels in CSF when plasma was added which was attributed to the binding of $A\beta_{42}$ to different plasma proteins [10]. We cannot also neglect the presence of plasmatic proteases able to digest the peptides since it has been shown that blood contamination of CSF can also lead to protein degradation [25]. The guidelines of Vanderstichele et al. pointed out the absence of difference on the levels of $A\beta_{42}$, T-tau and P-tau between centrifuged and non-centrifuged samples (N. Le Bastard, unpublished data) [9] which could be explained by the fact that they used clear CSF samples. In these guidelines, it was pointed out that spinning speed did not modify significantly the concentration levels of the biomarkers. More recently, it was reported that the sample temperature was always similar to the temperature set up in the centrifuge showing that temperature is not increased by spinning itself [26]. We can then recommend, that centrifugation should be performed at 2,000 g during 10 minutes at room temperature (RT) following the standardized protocol [26].

If several publications and recommendations are related to the delay between sampling and storage [27], it seems that there is a lack of conclusive data about the influence of the delay between sampling and centrifugation for AD biomarkers, mainly for hemorragic puncture. Nevertheless, it was reported significant changes of various metabolites, various amino acids and proteins in presence of white blood cells in the CSF, using a proteomics approach when the CSF were left at RT in the first 30 minutes [28].These data could explain the apparent discrepancy between the study of Kaiser et al, describing a significant increase of the levels of $A\beta_{42}$ after 24 hours [29] and those of Bjerke, describing that $A\beta_{42}$ concentrations remained stable up to 24 hours after the sampling (storage at RT) [10]. The lack of centrifugation prior incubation is likely the reason of the increase in $A\beta_{42}$ previously observed. Taken all together, all these data highlight the importance of centrifugation to be realized, as soon as possible after sampling, for CSF biomarker analysis.

Although the aspect of the CSF was not always indicated, we can imagine that the different studies which have reported a stability of the CSF levels of $A\beta_{42}$, $A\beta_{40}$, T-tau and P-tau over a period of 24 h at least, were done with clear CSF. Thus, the concentrations of $A\beta_{42}$ were found stable 24 h [10], 72 h when the sample was stored at 4°C [12] and up to 7 days after LP at RT [30]. It was the same for the concentrations of T-tau [10, 12, 29, 30]. Regarding the temperature during the time delay, no significant difference was found between the storage of the CSF samples at RT, 4°C or frozen in any of the studies performed [9, 10].

2.2.6. Freezing process

This process is complex since different factors could influence the biomarkers concentrations: although it seems clear that heterogeneity also exists for storage tubes, the temperature of freezing, the volume of the aliquots, the length of the storage and the possible effect of freezing / thawing cycles are potential factors to evaluate. Moreover, these factors can be synergistic: the adsorption of proteins onto the tube walls could be increased by the lower volume of the aliquot and mainly by the ratio volume / surface, or by the temperature of freezing (-20 versus -80°C).

The first step is to choose a storage tube. In parallel to the test realized with 11 sampling tubes [11], we selected 9 different commercially available polypropylene storage tubes (Table 1, tubes 13 to 21), some of them being used by different clinical teams in the AD field. The volume capacity was ranged from 0,5 to 1,5 mL. We performed an analysis of the surface polymer composition using differential scanning calorimetry and Fourier Transformed Infrared spectroscopy. This revealed the same surprising results than obtained with the sampling tubes [11]: only one tube was constituted by pure polypropylene, the others being copolymers with at least polyethylene, with or without surface treatment. Using the same protocol as described for the sampling tubes [11], biomarkers concentrations showed variations that were significantly different for $A\beta_{42}$ peptide. Median values for $A\beta_{42}$ peptide varied from 94 % to 127 %.

These data confirmed those obtained for sampling tubes, although the variability was lower than those found with these last tubes. The effect was present after 15 min, but increasing the incubation time to 24h at 2-8°C, the values did not significantly change compared to 15 minutes incubation.

The next step consists to standardize if needed the temperature, i.e. the speed, of freezing.

Freezing temperatures may affect CSF proteins concentrations as it has previously been reported for cystatin C, which undergoes a proteolysis at -20°C but not at -80°C [31]. Recently, the levels of T-tau and P-tau were reported significantly lower when CSF samples were immediately frozen at -20°C instead of -80°C (N. Le Bastard, unpublished data) [19]. However, this group did not find any difference for the $A\beta_{42}$ levels when the CSF were frozen at -20°C or -80°C, confirming previous results [10]. Therefore, freezing and storage at -80°C the CSF samples, seem to be logical.

Aliquoting the supernatant of CSF is absolutely necessary since it avoids different Freeze/thaw cycles (see below). Although we did not realize a study designed to evaluate the possible synergy between the ratio volume/surface and the speed of freezing onto the absorption phenomenon in these storage tubes (total volume less than 1.5 ml), some procedures issued from previous reported guidelines can be logically applied [27]. They pointed out the need to use small volumes (never more than 0.5 ml), which would allow: a/to realize at least the assay of the 3 classical AD biomarkers and if needed the assay of $A\beta_{40}$, b/ to prevent freeze/thaw cycles and c/ fill the tube up to 75% to minimize the adsorption and the evaporation effect, this last effect being negligible when the sample is stored frozen at -80°C [26].

As mentioned before, the guidelines recommend separating the supernatant in several fractions, that which will reduce the numbers of freeze/thaw cycles since freezing was shown able to affect protein stability [32]. Some studies have already analyzed the influence of freeze/thaw cycles on AD CSF biomarkers. Most studies using an ELISA format no have found any change on $A\beta_{42}$ and Tau CSF levels after one freeze/thaw cycle [10, 12, 30, 33], whereas a significant loss of $A\beta_{42}$ was found after one single cycle in one study using a semi-quantitative method [34]. Increasing the number of cycles was reported able to modify the stability of $A\beta_{42}$ CSF levels. However, about the exact numbers of cycles able to impact the levels, no real consensus was found between the different studies. If the Tau CSF levels seem to be unaffected by 3 or 6 freeze/thaw cycles [30, 12], the $A\beta_{42}$ CSF levels were found either stable after 3 cycles [30], either were significantly decreased after the third cycle [12]. In case of immunoassay analysis, it is logically recommended to limit the number of freeze/thaw cycles up to two as maximum [9].

Finally, the length of storage at -80°C does not seem to present a major influence on stability of CSF AD biomarkers, at least for 2 years [30] according to unpublished data from Blennow K. et al., referenced in the guideline published by Vanderstichele et al. [19]. Moreover, the levels of $A\beta_{42}$ and T-tau but not $A\beta_{40}$, remained stable up to 6 years [35]. In summary, we can conclude that CSF can be stored up to 2 years at -80°C as previously reported [19].

3. Variability introduced by the analytical step

There are several available assays for the determination of CSF $A\beta_{42}$, T-Tau and P-Tau, commercialized by different companies (Covance, Cusabio, IBL international, Innogenetics, Invitrogen, Millipore, Meso Scale Discovery, Wako... list not exhaustive). Large variation, in assay performance and outcomes of CSF $A\beta_{42}$, T-Tau and P-Tau levels was observed between laboratories also when the same assay format was used, reaching in some cases an inter-assay and inter-laboratory coefficient variations of 20 to 35% [7, 36]. As shown in conclusions of the first report of the external quality control (EQC) program started by the Alzheimer's association [37], ELISA techniques dominate the market while multiplex techniques are used less. In this program, for $A\beta_{42}$, T-Tau and P-Tau, most of laboratories [26 laboratories) used the INNOTEST enzyme-linked immunosorbent assays (ELISAs) (Innogenetics, Ghent, Belgium, www.innogenetics.com), whereas 14 laboratories used the bead-based Luminex xMAP platform with the INNO-BIA AlzBio3 (Innogenetics, Ghent, Belgium, www.innogenetics.com). Moreover, for $A\beta_{42}$ and T-Tau, 5 laboratories used Meso Scale Discovery (MSD, Gaithersburg, MD, www.mesoscale.com) technology [37].

3.1. Principles of assays

INNOTEST enzyme-linked immunosorbent assays (ELISAs) (Innogenetics) are classical ELISAs with colorimetric detection.

INNO-BIA AlzBio3 allows the simultaneous quantification of $A\beta_{42}$, T-Tau and P-Tau in CSF using xMAP® technology (xMAP is a registered trademark of Luminex Corp). The microsphere-based Luminex xMAP technology involves covalent coupling of a capture antibody to spectrally specific fluorescent microspheres [38]. Each microsphere number has a unique spectral identity. The classification of each bead is made by excitation at 635 nm. Each bead number is linked with only one antibody and the signals from analytes in the mixture are identified unequivocally. The quantification of the molecular reaction that has occurred at the microsphere surface, is done using a fluorochrome, the phycoerythrin coupled to streptavidin. The intensity of the fluorescence, derived after excitation of PE at 532 nm, is reported.

MSD offers the possibility to measure in simplex or multiplex format, depending on the biomarker analysed. Whereas t-Tau is measured in simplex format by the participants of the external control program, $A\beta_{42}$ can be measured in simplex or multiplex format in combination with $A\beta_{38}$ and $A\beta_{40}$. Multi-array plate formats include 96- and 384-well plates. The multi-spot plates are available with up to 100 spots per well. MSD uses electrochemiluminescence to detect binding events on patterned arrays. Electrochemiluminescence detection uses labels that emit light at ~620 nm when electrochemically stimulated, the stimulation mechanism (electricity) being decoupled from the signal (light). The signals are treated by the SECTOR Imager Instrument, which is medium throughput imaging detection systems (charge-coupled device camera), capable of multiplexing in all spot formats and reads 96- and 384-well plates.

3.2. Extent of the variability highlighted by this EQC program [37]

3.2.1. Total variability

In this report, results were grouped according to analytical techniques and samples [37]. The total CVs among centers were 16% to 28% for ELISA, 13% to 36% for xMAP, and 16% to 36% for MSD. CVs for MSD must be interpreted with caution, because they included 2 different Monoclonal antibodies (Mab) for $A\beta_{42}$ assays, binding to different epitopes on the amyloid peptide. These data were totally conformed to those reported earlier [7, 36]. There was no major modification of the CV in the longitudinal evaluation, except a decrease in variation for T-tau measured by ELISA. This was expected, since there was no active intervention between the 2 rounds [37].

3.2.2. Within-laboratory precision

Within-laboratory CVs were examined at the reference laboratories for ELISA and xMAP in two consecutive rounds. CVs were 3.2% to 24% for ELISA and 2.3% to 26% for xMAP, but differed between analytes within individual laboratories, indicating assay-dependent variations [37].

3.2.3. Differences in absolute values

The analytical techniques reported different absolute values for the biomarkers. ELISA values for $A\beta_{42}$, were about 2 fold higher than xMAP values. MSD values for $A\beta_{42}$, were dependent of the Mab used. ELISA values for T-Tau were about 3 fold higher than xMAP values. Finally for P-Tau, the differences inter techniques were clearly decreased in comparison to $A\beta_{42}$, and T-Tau. Considerable variability exists among the same manufacturer between mono and multiplex technology. For example, the decision threshold of clinical disease was reported to be at 86 pg / mL and 350 pg / mL for T-TAU measured by xMAP technology of Innogenetics on the platform Luminex and the conventional ELISA, respectively [39]. Factors of correction between values obtained by xMAP and ELISA, were used for global comparison of groups of patients, i.e. controls, Mild Cognitive Impairment and AD patients to predict incipient AD by CSF biomarkers [40]. In an other side, it was clearly shown that the use of factors of correction did not resolve the discrepancy in values observed between xMAP and ELISAs [41]. Although the observed biomarker concentrations may vary significantly between platforms, including MSD, xMAP and ELISA, these techniques seem to have similar diagnostic accuracy for patients with AD versus controls [39] or for detecting early AD [41, 42].

3.3. Possible sources of variability

In this study analysing the variability of results from only two rounds of an EQC program and from many different assay lots used, the authors limited their interpretation of the relative contributions from between-laboratory, within-laboratory, and between-lot components to the total variability [37]. Differences in within-laboratory CVs among the biomarkers within individual reference laboratories suggest that assay-related factors are important. Moreover, the high variability of the results of biomarkers measured by different commercial kits can be explained, by the use of different antibodies, the nature of the calibrator, the calibration method and many others factors as for example the nature of standard. Increasing data during years and by incorporation of new centers (since this first report concerning 40 laboratories, in summer of 2012, 64 laboratories were participating at this program) will permit to better identify the major sources of variability in analytical steps. Thus, we can just list the different points to be further investigated.

In the laboratory, the biologist will take care for:

a. Pipetting

The pipetting mode (inverse pipetting...) is not specified by the manufacturer. Using a single tip can influence the standard curve accuracy. However, the magnitude of this effect, if any, should be tested, to provide a better basis for recommendation [43].

b. Calibration

For lyophilised standard, accurate solubilization and accurate pipetting is critical. Moreover, since for INNOTEST Ab42, the first point of the curve calibration must be adjusted depending of the set value, accurate pipeting is absolutely needed. The type of curve fitting used and the software for data calculation were shown as possible factors of variability [43].

c. Reagent handling and adhesion of biologists to the manufacturer standard operating procedure (SOP)

The adhesion of routine laboratories to the manufacturer SOP is absolutely needed to reduce the part of the variability found in CSF biomarkers analysis. For that, a great effort must be done by the different manufacturers to limit individual interpretation of the technical instructions. The best example consists in the definition of the «room temperature» which can mainly vary from the north to the south of Europe. The maintenance of laboratory equipment is a crucial point to ensure the accuracy of pipeting volumes, the accuracy of temperatures, the accuracy of detection signals and the quality and reproducibility of washing steps.

d. Familiarization with the method and Competency Train

Implementing these techniques in the laboratory needs a training program ensured by the manufacturer. Moreover, habilitation and qualification of the laboratory staff must be done.

e. Validation criteria of runs for rejecting data

Different means are used to ensure validation of results. The definition of the criteria of acceptance of results must be strict. They include the calibration curve parameters, the CV of the duplicate samples and the use of an internal quality control program. For the CV criteria acceptance, in our experience, it seems that they are to be adequately defined since, the recommendation of CV < 20% done in the INNOTEST documentation, is not acceptable all along the dynamical range of the assay, in particular when the concentration level is near the clinical cut-off. Moreover, in the absence of QC samples in the kit, the biologist needs to implement its own QC program with different crucial points to resolve: the nature of the sample (native CSF pools, spiked CSF with standards, peptides...) how many QC samples, range of concentrations to cover, absence of reference material. This point is crucial for laboratories concerned by accreditation scheme based on the application of ISO15189 standard.

3.3.1. Issues to be solved by manufacturers

Many crucial points need to be solved as the poor quality of the test procedure instructions to decrease variability induced by misunderstanding of the protocols. This lacking information is often an indicator of minimal method optimization of the protocol (for example incubation steps, handling the reagents...). The reagents must be proposed in a manner that permits to decrease variability, for instance the «ready to use» calibrators. The absence of quality control included in the kit is a major problem. In fact, part of the discrepancy observed in the concentrations levels between the analytical techniques ELISA, xMAP, and MSD is caused by the lack of certified reference materials (CRMs). This could mainly impact the interlot variability and is at least, a brake to standardization. Antibody purification, coating of plates and beads are also factors of lot-lot variability.

4. Conclusion

The present chapter highlights two main issues responsible for the lack of harmonization of CSF AD biomarkers cut-offs values: the lack of standardization of the pre-analytical steps and the high variability of results linked to the analytical step. This latter issue can be explained by the absence of transferability of results between the different platforms but also by the high inter laboratory dispersion within the same assays. Previous consensus guidelines for pre-analytical factor standardization gave the way to resolve this issue, evidencing the need to standardize sampling and storage tubes, the type of the needle for the CSF puncture and the long term storage. Establishing SOPs for sample processing would allow to compare diagnostic conclusions between different laboratories. The implementation of those SOPs in the clinical community may reduce part of the variability found in the analysis of AD CSF biomarkers. Antibody purification, coating surfaces, preparation of standards, manufacturers instructions are also sources of variation, which need to be decreased and requires increased efforts by kit manufacturers. The optimal approach is a collaborative effort between commercial kit and instrument platform manufacturers, laboratories concerned by those methods, and reference standardization programs.

Acknowledgements

We wish to thank all our collaborators of the JPND BIOMARKPD program, those of the French Society of Clinical Biology (SFBC) and those of the NEUROSCREEN European project for their valuable assistance.

Author details

Armand Perret-Liaudet[1,2*], Aline Dorey[1], Yannick Tholance[1,3], Benoit Dumont[1,2] and
Isabelle Quadrio[1,2]

*Address all correspondence to: armand.perret-liaudet@chu-lyon.fr

1 Hospices Civils de Lyon, Neurobiologie, Centre Mémoire de Recherche et de Ressources;
Hôpitaux de Lyon, Lyon, France

2 Université Lyon 1, CNRS UMR5292, INSERM U1028, Equipe BioRan, Lyon, France

3 Université Lyon 1, CNRS UMR5292, INSERM U1028, Equipe WAKING, Lyon, France

References

[1] Qiu C, Kivipelto M (2009) Epidemiology of Alzheimer's disease: occurrence, determinants, and strategies toward intervention. *Dialogues in Clinical Neuroscience* 111-128.

[2] Brookmeyer R, Johnson E, Ziegler-Graham K, Arrighi HM (2007) Forecasting the global burden of Alzheimer's disease. *Alzheimer's & dementia: the journal of the Alzheimer's Association* 3, 186-91.

[3] Albert M.A. DeKosky S.T., Dickson D., Dubois B., Feldman H., Fox N.C., Gamst A., Holtzman D.M., Jagust W.J., Petersen R.C., Snyder P, Carrillo M.C., Thies B., Phelps C. (2011) "The diagnosis of mild cognitive impairment due to Alzheimer's disease: Recommendations from the National Institute on Aging – Alzheimer's Association workgroups on diagnostic guidelines for Alzheimer's disease" Alzheimer's & *Dementia: The Journal of the Alzheimer's Association*, 7(3), 270 – 279.

[4] McKhann G.M., Knopman D.C., Chertkow H., Hyman T.H., Jack C.R.Jr., Kawash C.J., Klunkk W.E., Koroshetzl W.J., Manlym, J.J., Mayeux R., Mohs R.M.,. Morris J.C., Rossorr M.N, Scheltens P., Carrillo M.C., Weintraub S., Thies B., Phelps C. (2011) The diagnosis of dementia due to Alzheimer's disease: Recommendations from the National Institute on Aging-Alzheimer's Association workgroups on diagnostic guidelines for Alzheimer's disease : *The Journal of the Alzheimer's Association*, 7(3), 263 – 269.

[5] Teunissen C (2002) Biochemical markers related to Alzheimer's dementia in serum and cerebrospinal fluid. *Neurobiology of Aging* 23, 485-508.

[6] Blennow K, Hampel H, Weiner M, Zetterberg H (2010) Cerebrospinal fluid and plasma biomarkers in Alzheimer disease. *Nature reviews. Neurology* 6, 131-44.

[7] Verwey NA, van der Flier WM, Blennow K, Clark C, Sokolow S, De Deyn PP, Galasko D, Hampel H, Hartmann T, Kapaki E, Lannfelt L, Mehta PD, Parnetti L, Petzold A, Pirttila T, Saleh L, Skinningsrud A, Swieten JCV, Verbeek MM, Wiltfang J, Youn-

kin S, Scheltens P, Blankenstein MA (2009) A worldwide multicentre comparison of assays for cerebrospinal fluid biomarkers in Alzheimer's disease. *Annals of clinical biochemistry* 46, 235-40.

[8] Hort J., Bartos A., Pirttila T. and Scheltens P. (2010) Use of cerebrospinal fluid biomarkers in diagnosis of dementia across Europe. *European Journal of Neurology*, 17, 90–96

[9] Vanderstichele H, Bibl M, Engelborghs S, Le Bastard N, Lewczuk P, Molinuevo JL, Parnetti L, Perret-Liaudet A, Shaw LM, Teunissen C, Wouters D, Blennow K (2012) Standardization of preanalytical aspects of cerebrospinal fluid biomarker testing for Alzheimer's disease diagnosis: A consensus paper from the Alzheimer's Biomarkers Standardization Initiative. *Alzheimer's & dementia: the journal of the Alzheimer's Association* 8, 65-73.

[10] Bjerke M, Portelius E, Minthon L, Wallin A, Anckarsäter H, Anckarsäter R, Andreasen N, Zetterberg H, Andreasson U, Blennow K (2010) Confounding factors influencing amyloid Beta concentration in cerebrospinal fluid. *International journal of Alzheimer's disease*, 2010, Article ID 986310, 11 pages.

[11] Perret-Liaudet A, Pelpel M, Tholance Y, Dumont B, Vanderstichele H, Zorzi W, Elmoualij B, Schraen S, Moreaud O, Gabelle A, Thouvenot E, Thomas-Anterion C, Touchon J, Krolak-Salmon P, Kovacs GG, Coudreuse A, Quadrio I, Lehmann S (2012) Risk of Alzheimer's Disease Biological Misdiagnosis Linked to Cerebrospinal Collection Tubes. *Journal of Alzheimer's disease: JAD* 30, 1-8.

[12] Schoonenboom NSM, Mulder C, Vanderstichele H, Van Elk E-J, Kok A, Van Kamp GJ, Scheltens P, Blankenstein M a (2005) Effects of processing and storage conditions on amyloid beta (1-42) and tau concentrations in cerebrospinal fluid: implications for use in clinical practice. *Clinical chemistry* 51, 189-95.

[13] Bateman RJ, Wen G, Morris JC, Holtzman DM (2007) Fluctuations of CSF amyloid-beta levels: implications for a diagnostic and therapeutic biomarker. *Neurology* 68, 666-9.

[14] Moghekar A, Goh J, Li M, Albert M, O'Brien RJ (2012) Cerebrospinal fluid aβ and tau level fluctuation in an older clinical cohort. *Archives of neurology* 69, 246-50.

[15] Slats D, Claassen JAHR, Spies PE, Borm G, Besse KTC, van Aalst W, Tseng J, Sjögren MJC, Olde Rikkert MGM, Verbeek MM (2012) Hourly variability of cerebrospinal fluid biomarkers in Alzheimer's disease subjects and healthy older volunteers. *Neurobiology of aging* 33, 831.e1-9.

[16] Reiber H (2001) Dynamics of brain-derived proteins in cerebrospinal fluid. *Clinica Chimica Acta* 310, 173-186.

[17] Chevallier S, Monti M, Michel P, Vollenweider P. (2008) Lumbar puncture. *Rev Med Suisse* 177, 2312-4, 2316-8.

[18] Dietrich M. Post-lumbar puncture headache syndrome. (1996) In : Neurologic disorders : Course and treatment, Brandt T, Caplan LR, Dichgans J (Eds). San Diego : Elsevier Academic Press,;59.

[19] Lavi R, Yarnitsky D, Rowe JM, Weissman A, Segal D, Avivi I. Standard vs atraumatic Whitacre needle for diagnostic lumbar puncture: a randomized trial (2006) *Neurology*. 67(8), 1492-4.

[20] Kim M, Yoon H. (2011) Comparison of post-dural puncture headache and low back pain between 23 and 25 gauge Quincke spinal needles in patients over 60 years: randomized, double-blind controlled trial. *Int J Nurs Stud.* 48(11), 1315-22.

[21] Lewczuk P, Beck G, Esselmann H, Bruckmoser R, Zimmermann R, Fiszer M, Bibl M, Maler JM, Kornhuber J, Wiltfang J (2006) Effect of sample collection tubes on cerebrospinal fluid concentrations of tau proteins and amyloid beta peptides. *Clinical chemistry* 52, 332-4.

[22] Pica-Mendez AM, Tanen M, Dallob A, Tanaka W, Laterza OF (2010) Nonspecific binding of Aβ42 to polypropylene tubes and the effect of Tween-20. *Clinica chimica acta; international journal of clinical chemistry* 411, 1833.

[23] Poncin-Epaillard F, Mille C, Debarnot D, Zorzi W, Moualij BE, Coudreuse A, Legeay G, Quadrio I, Perret-Liaudet A. Study of the adhesion of neurodegenerative proteins on plasma-modified and coated polypropylene surfaces. *J Biomater Sci Polym Ed* 2011 Sep 22.

[24] Petzold A, Sharpe LT, Keir G (2006) Spectrophotometry for cerebrospinal fluid pigment analysis. *Neurocritical care* 4, 153-62.

[25] You J-S, Gelfanova V, Knierman MD, Witzmann FA, Wang M, Hale JE (2005) The impact of blood contamination on the proteome of cerebrospinal fluid. *Proteomics* 5, 290-6.

[26] Del Campo M, Mollenhauer B, Bertolotto A, Engelborghs S, Hampel H, Simonsen AH, Kapaki E, Kruse N, Le Bastard N, Lehmann S, Molinuevo JL, Parnetti L, Perret-Liaudet A, Sáez-Valero J, Saka E, Urbani A, Vanmechelen E, Verbeek M, Visser PJ, Teunissen C. (2012) Recommendations to standardize preanalytical confounding factors in Alzheimer's and Parkinson's disease cerebrospinal fluid biomarkers: an update. *Biomark Med.* 6, 419-30.

[27] Teunissen CE, Petzold a, Bennett JL, Berven FS, Brundin L, Comabella M, Franciotta D, Frederiksen JL, Fleming JO, Furlan R, Hintzen RQ, Hughes SG, Johnson MH, Krasulova E, Kuhle J, Magnone MC, Rajda C, Rejdak K, Schmidt HK, van Pesch V, Waubant E, Wolf C, Giovannoni G, Hemmer B, Tumani H, Deisenhammer F (2009) A consensus protocol for the standardization of cerebrospinal fluid collection and biobanking. *Neurology* 73, 1914-22.

[28] Rosenling T, Slim CL, Christin C, Coulier L, Shi S, Stoop MP, Bosman J, Suits F, Horvatovich PL, Stockhofe-Zurwieden N, Vreeken R, Hankemeier T, van Gool AJ, Luid-

er TM, Bischoff R (2009) The effect of preanalytical factors on stability of the proteome and selected metabolites in cerebrospinal fluid (CSF). *Journal of proteome research* 8, 5511-22.

[29] Kaiser E, Schönknecht P, Thomann P a, Hunt A, Schröder J (2007) Influence of delayed CSF storage on concentrations of phospho-tau protein (181), total tau protein and beta-amyloid (1-42). *Neuroscience letters* 417, 193-5.

[30] Zimmermann R, Lelental N, Ganslandt O, Maler JM, Kornhuber J, Lewczuk P (2011) Preanalytical sample handling and sample stability testing for the neurochemical dementia diagnostics. *Journal of Alzheimer's disease: JAD* 25, 739-45.

[31] Carrette O, Burkhard PR, Hughes S, Hochstrasser DF, Sanchez J-C (2005) Truncated cystatin C in cerebrospiral fluid: Technical artefact or biological process? *Proteomics* 5, 3060-5.

[32] Bhatnagar BS, Bogner RH, Pikal MJ (2007) Protein stability during freezing: separation of stresses and mechanisms of protein stabilization. Pharmaceutical development and technology 12, 505-23.

[33] Sjögren M, Vanderstichele H, Agren H, Zachrisson O, Edsbagge M, Wikkelsø C, Skoog I, Wallin A, Wahlund LO, Marcusson J, Nägga K, Andreasen N, Davidsson P, Vanmechelen E, Blennow K (2001) Tau and Abeta42 in cerebrospinal fluid from healthy adults 21-93 years of age: establishment of reference values. Clinical chemistry 47, 1776-81.

[34] Bibl M, Esselmann H, Otto M, Lewczuk P, Cepek L, Rüther E, Kornhuber J, Wiltfang J (2004) Cerebrospinal fluid amyloid beta peptide patterns in Alzheimer's disease patients and nondemented controls depend on sample pretreatment: indication of carrier-mediated epitope masking of amyloid beta peptides. Electrophoresis 25, 2912-8.

[35] Schipke CG, Jessen F, Teipel S, Luckhaus C, Wiltfang J, Esselmann H, Frölich L, Maier W, Rüther E, Heppner FL, Prokop S, Heuser I, Peters O (2011) Long-term stability of Alzheimer's disease biomarker proteins in cerebrospinal fluid. *Journal of Alzheimer's disease: JAD* 26, 255-62.

[36] Lewczuk P, Beck G, Ganslandt O, Esselmann H, Deisenhammer F, Regeniter A, Petereit H-F, Tumani H, Gerritzen A, Oschmann P, Schröder J, Schönknecht P, Zimmermann K, Hampel H, Bürger K, Otto M, Haustein S, Herzog K, Dannenberg R, Wurster U, Bibl M, Maler JM, Reubach U, Kornhuber J, Wiltfang J. International quality control survey of neurochemical dementia diagnostics. *Neurosci Lett.* 2006;409:1–4

[37] Mattsson N, Andreasson U, Persson S, Arai H, Batish SD, Bernardini S, Bocchio-Chiavetto L, Blankenstein M a, Carrillo MC, Chalbot S, Coart E, Chiasserini D, Cutler N, Dahlfors G, Duller S, Fagan AM, Forlenza O, Frisoni GB, Galasko D, Galimberti D, Hampel H, Handberg A, Heneka MT, Herskovits AZ, Herukka S-K, Holtzman DM, Humpel C, Hyman BT, Iqbal K, Jucker M, Kaeser S a, Kaiser E, Kapaki E, Kidd D,

Klivenyi P, Knudsen CS, Kummer MP, Lui J, Lladó A, Lewczuk P, Li Q-X, Martins R, Masters C, McAuliffe J, Mercken M, Moghekar A, Molinuevo JL, Montine TJ, Nowatzke W, O'Brien R, Otto M, Paraskevas GP, Parnetti L, Petersen RC, Prvulovic D, de Reus HPM, Rissman R a, Scarpini E, Stefani A, Soininen H, Schröder J, Shaw LM, Skinningsrud A, Skrogstad B, Spreer A, Talib L, Teunissen C, Trojanowski JQ, Tumani H, Umek RM, Van Broeck B, Vanderstichele H, Vecsei L, Verbeek MM, Windisch M, Zhang J, Zetterberg H, Blennow K (2011) The Alzheimer's Association external quality control program for cerebrospinal fluid biomarkers. *Alzheimer's & dementia: the journal of the Alzheimer's Association* 7, 386-395..

[38] Oliver KG, Kettman JR, Fulton RJ. Multiplexed analysis of human cytokines by use of the FlowMetrix system. Clin Chem 1998;44: 2057–60.

[39] Olsson A, Vanderstichele H, Andreasen N, De Meyer G, Wallin A, Holmberg B, et al. Simultaneous measurement of beta-amyloid(1- 42), total tau, and phosphorylated tau (Thr181) in cerebrospinal fluid by the xMAP technology. Clin Chem 2005; 51:336–45.

[40] Mattsson N, Zetterberg H, Hansson O, Andreasen N, Parnetti L, Jonsson M, et al. CSF biomarkers and incipient Alzheimer disease in patients with mild cognitive impairment. JAMA 2009;302:385–93.

[41] Jongbloed W, Kester MI, van der Flier WM, Veerhuis R, Scheltens P, Blankenstein MA, Teunissen CE. Discriminatory and predictive capabilities of enzyme-linked immunosorbent assay and multiplex platforms in a longitudinal Alzheimer's disease study. Alzheimers Dement. 2012 Oct 27. (Epub ahead of print)

[42] Schipke CG, Prokop S, Heppner FL, Heuser I, Peters O. Comparison of immunosorbent assays for the quantification of biomarkers for Alzheimer's disease in human cerebrospinal fluid Dement Geriatr Cogn Disord. 2011;31(2):139-45.

[43] Teunissen CE, Verwey N a, Kester MI, van Uffelen K, Blankenstein M a (2010) Standardization of Assay Procedures for Analysis of the CSF Biomarkers Amyloid β((1-42)), Tau, and Phosphorylated Tau in Alzheimer's Disease: Report of an International Workshop. International journal of Alzheimer's disease 2010, Article ID 635053, 6 pages.

Chapter 9

Using Magnetic Resonance Imaging in the Early Detection of Alzheimer's Disease

Emily J. Mason, Manus J. Donahue and
Brandon A. Ally

Additional information is available at the end of the chapter

1. Introduction

Alzheimer's disease (AD) is the most common form of dementia. While many strides have been made in elucidating the underlying causes of AD, studying the disorder *in vivo* has faced several hurdles: First, the structures affected by AD lie deep within the brain where biopsy is not practical. Second, animal models do not develop AD naturally, and genetically engineered models designed to mimic AD do not fully reproduce the human phenotypes [1-3]. Third, while studies using Positron Emission Tomography (PET) have been very useful for examining plaques and metabolic changes, they involve the injection of radioactive contrast agents. Many of these materials have short half-lives and must be created on-site, making PET very expensive and difficult to be performed at non-specialized centers. Finally, studies which examine cerebrospinal fluid (CSF) require participants to undergo an invasive and sometimes painful lumbar puncture, potentially on multiple occasions [4-7]

In contrast to other techniques, Magnetic Resonance (MR) offers a non-invasive method for analyzing structural and functional brain characteristics without the need for ionizing radiation. In other words, it can be performed in longitudinal studies without significant health concerns. Multiple scans can be performed quickly in the same testing session to assess tissue response to tasks or pharmacological administration. The scans are generally 2-5 minutes each and many analyses can be done post-hoc. Conveniently, most hospitals and clinics already possess the MR scanners at field strengths of 1.5 and 3.0 Tesla (T).

Many MR techniques have been used to understand the underlying pathology in patient populations already diagnosed with AD. Because MR studies require absolute stillness for several minutes, and some functional scans require the patient to focus on performing a difficult task, performing MR work in advanced AD cases is quite challenging and as such, most studies are limited to mild and very mild cases. While these studies are typically performed at a time when pathology is irreversible, the results of this work point to changes that may be apparent before cognitive decline has become clinically apparent. For this reason, studies that examine differences between people who will eventually develop AD and people who will not develop AD provide insight into both the cause and the physiology of the disease.

It is impossible to predict with certainty who will develop AD, but there are several factors that increase the risk. These at-risk populations include individuals in the prodromal stage of AD, termed amnestic mild cognitive impairment (aMCI), and people at a genetic risk for developing AD. A diagnosis of aMCI indicates that there is more memory decline than would be expected based on the person's age and education level, however memory impairment is not interfering with daily activities. It is estimated that 10-20% of people 65 and older have aMCI, and out of those 10-15% will progress to develop AD in 3-4 years. [8,9] Because approximately 30% of people diagnosed with aMCI will remain stable or improve over time, it is important to find biomarkers that will identify those most likely to progress to AD.

This chapter will focus on the use of MR in the early detection of AD. Major advances have been made in structural imaging of both gray and white matter using proton density, T1- and T2- weighted imaging, and Diffusion Tensor Imaging (DTI). Functional imaging in AD will also be reviewed, and Blood Oxygenation Level-Dependent (BOLD) functional Magnetic Resonance Imaging (fMRI) will be broken down into its primary contributors: Cerebral Blood Flow (CBF), Cerebral Blood Volume (CBV), and the Cerebral Metabolic Rate of Oxygen ($CMRO_2$). Finally, hemodynamic fMRI contrast can be complemented using measures of neurochemistry, including measuring the balance between excitatory (glutamatergic) and inhibitory (γ-aminobutyric acid; GABAergic) neurotransmission. This can be achieved with new single-voxel chemical imaging techniques such as Magnetic Resonance Spectroscopy (MRS), or more recently using multi-voxel MRS imaging (MRSi)

2. Basics of MRI

Before reviewing the work that has been done with MR, a brief overview of the theory behind MR should be covered. MR physics can essentially be understood using principles of classical physics, however for a more comprehensive understanding the reader is directed to an excellent review by Plewes and Kucharzck [4,10]. Briefly, MR takes advantage of the behavior of a system of protons in the presence of a magnetic field and how this behavior changes based on the micro- and macroscopic environment. Magnetic strength is generally reported in units of Tesla (T), and MRI scanners have very high field strengths. In human research, 1.5T, 3T, and 7T scanners are commonly used, though 1.5T and 3T scanners predominate the clinical setting. The magnet's strength and direction is represented by the vector B0 (see Figure 1), and lies along the Z-axis (generally from foot to head).

Due to the large amount of water that constitutes tissue (~80-99% depending on tissue type), most MR is specifically focused on the protons on water molecules. Protons have an intrinsic spin that in nature is oriented randomly. In the presence of a magnetic field however, these spins align themselves on average parallel or antiparallel to the axis of the field (Figure 1a). The number of protons aligned parallel to the field is very slightly larger than the number of protons aligned antiparallel, and it is this difference that produces the net magnetization vector in a voxel. When a radiofrequency (RF) pulse is applied at the proper frequency (Larmor frequency), the longitudinal (z) component of the magnetization vector is tipped away from the axis of the main magnetic field, but continues to spin around the longitudinal axis or "precess" (Figure 1b). When the pulse is removed, the longitudinal component of the magnetization vector will realign itself with the field with a unique time constant that varies with the local environment.

Manipulating the timing of the RF pulses controls the magnetization and creates the desired contrast. The most fundamental timing parameters of relevance are repetition time (TR), echo time (TE), and in some cases inversion time (TI). TR is the time between consecutive acquisitions, and TE is the time from the onset of the excitation pulse that is used for preparing the signal for detection to the signal refocusing and in most cases acquisition. In an inversion recovery pulse sequence, TI refers to the time between the inversion pulse and the excitation pulse. Importantly, simply by manipulating the timing of the above parameters a range of MR contrasts can be obtained with varying sensitivity to different tissue types. A simple pulse sequence indicating RF and gradient timing is illustrated in Figure 1c.

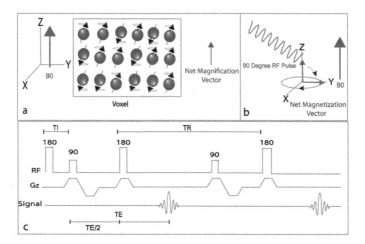

Figure 1. Physics underlying magnetic resonance. Hydrogen atoms align parallel and antiparallel to a strong magnetic field, producing a net magnification vector (a). When a radio frequency pulse is applied at the Larmor frequency, the net magnetization vector is tipped away from the main magnetic field (b). Example of a simple pulse sequence showing timing parameters of the application of radio frequency pulse (RF), the onset of gradients in the Z direction (Gz), and the timing of signal acquisition (Signal) (c).

In most cases, the detectible signal (S) that is measured in MRI is a combination of three primary factors: water proton density (C; ml tissue /100 ml water), magnetization in the longitudinal plane (M_Z) and magnetization in the transverse plane (M_{XY}):

$$S \propto C \bullet M_Z \bullet M_{XY} \qquad (1)$$

The two major methods or "weighting" that are used for generating contrast are T1 and T2. T1 and T2 are independent measures and reflect different properties of the tissue of interest, with T1 governing the M_z term and T2 the M_{xy} term in Eq. 1 above. The time it takes for the magnetization to realign itself longitudinally is measured using T1 weighting (Figure 2a), and is achieved with a short TR and a short TE sequence. T1 is a constant that is unique for each tissue type and is equal to the point when 63% of longitudinal magnetization is recovered (Figure 2b). At the times selected for T1 imaging, there is a high amount of contrast between gray and white matter and therefore T1 weighted imaging is useful for viewing structural changes in the brain (Figure 2c).

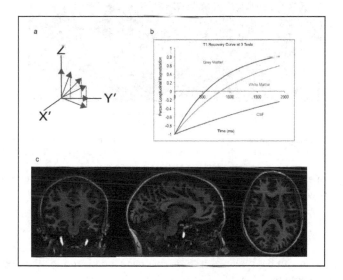

Figure 2. T1 weighted imaging. After removal of an RF pulse the magnetization vector recovers longitudinally (a). The recovery time is a constant for each tissue type based on the magnetic field strength that is applied (b). Example T1 weighted images (c).

The M_Z component of the magnetization vector is based on pulse timing as well as the T1 of tissue, and for magnetization following a pre-pulse with flip angle, α, is given by:

$$M_Z = \left(1 - \alpha e^{\frac{-TI}{T1}} + e^{\frac{-TR}{T1}}\right) \qquad (2)$$

Note that in the absence of a prepulse (α=0), the TR determines the T1-weighting. When the RF pulse is applied, individual protons will also precess in synchrony in the transverse plane. When the pulse is removed, the protons will lose that synchrony or dephase, which results in a reduced M_{XY} (Figure 3a). This is referred to as T2 decay. Like T1, the T2 time constant is unique for each tissue (Figure 3b). Unlike T1, T2 weighting is achieved with a long TE and long TR.

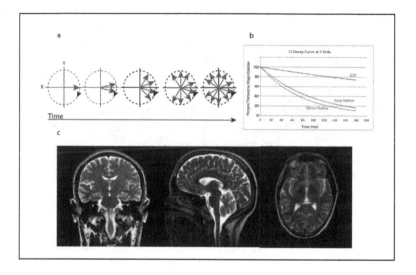

Figure 3. T2 weighted imaging. Protons lose synchrony after removal of an RF pulse (a). The amount of time it takes for protons to lose synchrony is a constant that is unique to each tissue type (b). Example of T2 weighted images (c).

The M_{XY} component of MRI is based on pulse timing as well as the T2 constant of the tissue area, and can be written:

$$M_{XY} = e^{-TE/T2} \tag{3}$$

The three equations can be combined to form one overall equation for the MR signal that takes into account both the T1 and the T2 properties of the tissue:

$$S \propto C \bullet \left(1 - \alpha e^{\frac{-TI}{T1}} + e^{\frac{-TR}{T1}}\right) \bullet e^{-TE/T2} \tag{4}$$

T1 and T2 components are each present whenever a proton is flipped out of alignment, but by manipulating the pulse sequences one can contribute to the signal more than the other. This is referred to as weighting. If neither the T1 nor the T2 signal contributes strongly to the signal, only the C component is left. These images are referred to as proton density images.

3. Structural imaging

By far, the most established use of MR is to examine the gross anatomy of the brain. With the right specifications, MR can provide a highly detailed three-dimensional image that allows for the examination of brain structures. Weighting is used to provide contrast for the tissue of interest.

3.1. Anatomical imaging

T1 weighted imaging is used to visualize structural changes in tissue. At a field strength of 3 Tesla, T1 weighted images can be acquired in about five minutes and have a resolution of approximately 1 mm^3.

The most significant differences reported in patients are atrophy of the structures in the medial temporal lobe (MTL) which typically follow the "Braak stages" of AD progression [11]. Briefly, pathology starts in the transentorhinal region (stages I and II), moves to the limbic region (stages III and IV) and ends in isocortical regions (stages V and VI). Studies that have been done in AD patients show that hippocampal and entorhinal cortex volume change, as well as temporal lobe morphology changes are the best measures to predict change over time [12]. A higher level of regional brain atrophy has also been associated with decreased levels of Aβ-42 and increased levels of phosphorylated tau in the CSF of AD patients [12].

In patients who have been diagnosed with aMCI, changes to the parahippocampal region are already apparent. It is up for debate whether the investigation of the entire brain or just volumes of interest (VOIs) are better at predicting conversion from aMCI to AD, but in a recent meta-analysis of work using data from the Alzheimer's Disease Neuroimaging Initiative (ADNI) only four methods were able to distinguish those who would convert more accurately than random chance. None of the four were more statistically reliable than the others, but three examined VOIs (Voxel-STAND, 57% sensitivity and 78% specificity; Voxel-COMPARE, 62% sensitivity and 67% specificity; Hippo-Volume, 62% sensitivity and 69% specificity) while only one examined the entire brain (Thickness-Direct, 32% sensitivity and 91% specificity) [11,13-15]. A protocol devised by Chincarini et al. to sample several VOIs has demonstrated a method of separating converters from non-converters with a sensitivity of 71% and a specificity of 65% [16,17]. Another method for predicting conversion is examining hippocampal shape, and Costafreda et. al. were able to develop a method with 77% sensitivity and 80% specificity. [18,19].

Patients that are at-risk for AD but have no cognitive deficit are much more difficult to identify. Most studies have been done in carriers of the ApoE ε4 allele, however it is important to remember that these studies have been cross sectional, and therefore may reflect a consequence of the gene that makes carriers more susceptible to AD, but not necessarily a stage of AD itself. There have been cortical thinning signatures identified in children, adolescent, and young adult carriers of the ε4 allele. These signatures reflect reductions in dorsolateral and medial prefrontal, lateral, temporal, and parietal cortices. [20-22]. Middle-aged carriers of the ε4 allele were found to have a thinning of the cortex in the entorhinal region, subiculum, and other MTL structures, although the results were stronger in those with a family history of AD than those that carried the ε4 allele alone [23,24].

The detectible changes are not limited to atrophy. There have been several studies that have discovered an increase in gray matter in young adult carriers of the ε4 ellele. Increases were found in bilateral cerebellar, occipital, and thalamic regions as well as in the fusiform and right lingual gyri [22,25]. Recent work has also suggested that changes in the basal cholinergic forebrain may be detectible decades before cognitive impairment, although this study did not take into account genetic status [26].

One of the significant weaknesses of analyzing structural changes is that the regions of interest can vary in size even across healthy individuals. Longitudinal studies are the only way to control for this variability. Secondly, the atrophy of brain regions likely occurs secondary to functional changes. The assessment of atrophy alone gives little information as to the underlying factors that led to neuronal loss.

3.2. White matter imaging

Unlike T1 weighted imaging, T2 imaging relies on the dephasing of the magnetization vector in the transverse plane. T2 weighting, specifically FLuid Attenuated Inversion Recovery (FLAIR) imaging, is used to identify White Matter Hyperintensities (WMH), which are increased in AD [27]. In contrast, diffusion tensor imaging (DTI) is able to indirectly measure the integrity of myelin sheaths surrounding white matter tracts, and Susceptibility weighted imaging (SWI) is able to distinguish tissues at a high resolution based on several properties.
FLuid Attenuated Inversion Recovery (FLAIR) and Diffusion Tensor Imaging (DTI)

If simply T2 weighted imaging was used, the signal from Cerebrospinal Fluid (CSF) is strong and therefore very bright (T2 of CSF ~ 600 ms at 3T). This makes it difficult to see subtle abnormalities in the white matter regions that partial volume with CSF. FLAIR imaging nulls the signal from CSF so that the image is focused solely on the white matter. The first RF pulse inverts the magnetization by 180 degrees. Then, when the longitudinal magnetization for the CSF = 0, an excitation pulse and readout is applied. Because T1 of CSF (~4000 ms at 3T) is much longer than that of tissue (T1~700-1200 ms at 3T), residual tissue signal remains at the time of the CSF nulling.

DTI measures fractional anisotropy (FA), a quantitative measure of the coordinated movement of water molecules. FA assumes that the stronger a white matter tract is, the more likely the water molecules will be to move along the tract rather than sideways within the myelin sheath. If the myelin sheath is damaged it becomes easier for water molecules to diffuse through it, and the FA value will decrease.

The loss of white matter integrity, either through WMH or FA differences, may correlate with increasing cognitive impairment [28,29]. In AD populations reduced FA values have been found in frontal and temporal lobes, the posterior cingulum, the corpus callosum, the superior longitudinal fasciculus and the uncinate fasciculus [30]. Both WMH and FA have been found to distinguish normal aging from aMCI[31] and predict conversion from aMCI to AD[32]. Results have differed in whether they correlate with ApoE ε4 status, with some studies saying they do not [33,34], while several others say they do [35-37]. Note that the studies that claim white matter integrity correlates with ApoE ε4 status are more recent, and their ability to detect differences are likely more sensitive. White matter integrity has also been found to correlate with a family history of AD regardless of ApoE status [38,39].

White matter hyperintensities are associated with vascular abnormalities and therefore highly correlated with cardiovascular disease. For this reason, many clinicians will exclude a diagnosis of AD if there are many apparent WMH and instead diagnose the patient with vascular dementia [32]. Many non-amnestic MCI patients tend to have a higher degree of cardiovascular disease than those with aMCI or AD, however aMCI and AD patients have increased WMH scores. For this reason, increased WMH scores in cognitively impaired individuals is likely associated with neurological disease rather than vascular disease [32].

Susceptibility Weighted Imaging (SWI)

Susceptibility weighted imaging is a method that can discriminate tissue content with a high level of resolution based on the tissue's intrinsic magnetic properties. SWI uses T2* weighting along with magnitude and phase information to enhance contrast, and when combined with traditional MR weighting it can be used to detect small differences in susceptibility between blood and tissue. It is particularly useful for detecting cerebral microbleeds because it can exploit the magnetic properties of blood since the susceptibility effects from fully oxygenated (arterial) and partially de-oxygenated (venous) blood water, and tissue, varies greatly – especially at high field strength. It can also be used to measure the iron content of a tissue.

Microbleeds are inversely correlated with performance during cognitive testing in healthy older adults, although this finding has never reached significance in an AD population [13,14]. SWI would allow for improved visualization of microbleeds so that if there is a relationship between microbleeds and susceptibility to AD pathology, it can be recognized. Techniques are being developed that semi-automatically detect cerebral microbleeds with little human interference. These would significantly reduce the processing time and standardize the quantification of microbleeds across patients and imaging centers.

In addition to microbleeds, one marker of oxidative stress is an increase in a tissue's iron content. Iron levels are highly elevated in AD patients as well as those with aMCI, and it is thought that changes in iron content may be detectible decades before the onset of the disease [16]. There is a theory that Aβ deposition may occur as a cellular response to an increased level of iron, and this is one of the underlying causes of amyloid plaque formation[40]. SWI has been shown to be a promising method to non-invasively assess iron distribution, and determine if there is a link between iron accumulation and the onset of AD pathology [18].

SWI has only been used as a technique since 2004, which makes it very new technology. Although it has not yet been used in an at-risk population, SWI studies will likely be important tools in assessing AD risk.

3.3. Future of structural imaging

There is still a lot of work to be done in structural imaging. Most clinical studies to date have used 1.5 Tesla (T) scanners, however many medical centers now have 3T scanners and there are approximately 50 7T scanners worldwide. These high-field scanners allow for increased resolution, and provide better spatial resolution for observing structural changes in the same scan time. Although 7T scanners are not yet FDA approved for clinical use, they are already being utilized in neuroimaging research, including in patients with AD.

Many atrophy measurements are made either through a trained radiologist's visual assessment, or by manually tracing the area of interest. As such, the measurement of atrophy can be subjective, and is not always reproducible across testing site. In fact, one study found that the ability of radiologists to diagnose subjects based on atrophy alone had a specificity of 85% and a sensitivity of only 27% [20]. The introduction of FDA-approved methods that can automatically detect atrophy will create standardization of the field, and decrease variability across medical centers [41].

4. Functional imaging

While structural imaging is important to assess brain atrophy, the hope is that AD pathology will be identified before neuronal death so that atrophy can be prevented. One current theory is that one of the major components leading to amyloid and tau pathologies could be vascular changes [42]. Two of the risk factors for AD are mutated forms of APP, and the ApoE ε4 isoform and both of these factors are involved in cholesterol processing. The inability of a neuron to clear amyloid plaques may be prognostic and indicate impaired blood flow as a risk factor for AD. While it is not immediately apparent how blood flow is contributing to AD, some vascular changes are being evaluated through the use of hemodynamic-based functional imaging techniques.

4.1. BOLD fMRI

Functional magnetic resonance imaging, or fMRI is a way to gain insight into the functional processes occurring in the brain. Most fMRI modalities are based on the blood oxygenation level-dependent (BOLD) effect. This is an indirect method of tracking the activation or inactivation of brain regions relative to a baseline state, and is based on the idea that an active area will need more energy and consume more glucose and oxygen and therefore more blood will need to be directed to that area. More specifically, oxygenated and deoxygenated blood water have different intrinsic magnetic properties (oxygenated blood is diamagnetic and deoxygenated blood is paramagnetic) and therefore affect the T2 and T2* relaxation times of surrounding water in blood and tissue in different ways. Deoxygenated blood has a strong enough magnetic affect (paramagnetic) that it will distort the local field and decrease the signal intensity (i.e. shorten T2) of surrounding water for that region. Oxygenated blood will not have the same effect, and therefore regions containing more oxygenated blood will have higher signal intensity (longer T2). Importantly, during functional activation the cerebral blood flow increases by a large amount (20-100%) relative to the cerebral metabolic rate of oxygen consumption (CMRO2), resulting in a relative decrease in the concentration of deoxyhemoglobin in capillaries and veins. By comparing the signal intensities of regions at baseline (Figure 4a) and during a task (Figure 4b), the regions that have an increase in capillary and venous oxygenation can be visualized.

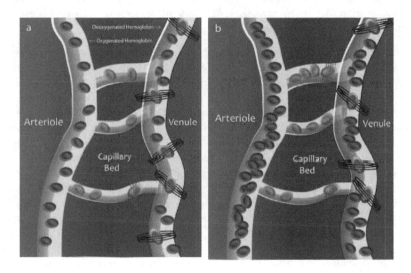

Figure 4. Blood flow at rest (a) and during activation (b)

BOLD imaging involves very fast sequences in order to visualize changes in functional activation on the timescale of the hemodynamic response. This rapid sequencing allows for a time resolution of approximately 2s. Total time required to perform a BOLD scan varies with the task being performed, but typically scans take 5-15 minutes.

There are two main types of fMRI: evoked (task-related) and spontaneous ("resting" state). Evoked fMRI is the more commonly performed test in which the same task is repeated many times with a baseline measurement taken between trials. Statistical tests (Z- and t-tests) are used to differentiate the regions activated during the task from those active at baseline. By contrast, spontaneous BOLD specifically measures synchrony of baseline signal fluctuations to determine how the brain is functionally connected.

Evoked BOLD fMRI

There are several established testing paradigms that have been designed to study memory. The most commonly used paradigms look specifically at either episodic or semantic memory. Episodic memories involve the recognition of autobiographical or cued information (e.g., faces, words, other visual stimuli) while semantic memory involves the recognition of a fact or information regardless of personal context (e.g., famous faces, geographical locations). Because episodic memory is highly affected by AD, many fMRI paradigms use an episodic memory task to elicit functional differences between patients and controls. While encoding a new memory, activation of the hippocampal and parahippocampal regions is decreased in mild AD patients compared to healthy controls [43]. In a block design face name paradigm, AD patients also show decreased hippocampal activation to novel stimuli compared to repeated comparisons [43].

A multitude of studies have been performed in asymptomatic carriers of ApoE ε4 with mixed results. In an extensive review of the literature by Trachtenberg et al, some claim that carriers have increased activation across brain structures while others claim the opposite[44]. Moreover, there have been reports of both increases and decreases of activation or that there is no significant effect at all of carrying the ApoE ε4 allele[44]. In each case, investigators have provided hypotheses to explain both increased and decreased activation in ApoE ε4 carriers: decreased activation can be easily explained by the fact that presymptomatic carriers are already accumulating AD pathology hallmarks before cognitive decline is experienced. These pathologies may be hindering the BOLD response in the specific areas that experience a decrease in activation, or they may be inhibiting areas that lie functionally upstream. In contrast, an increase in activation can be explained in two ways, which take into account AD pathology. For one, the accumulation of pathology may lead to the dedifferentiation of neural network such that many networks become involved in a specific process. This may in fact be a part of healthy aging [45] and could be found in young, presymptomatic carriers of ApoE ε4 because their brains are aging more rapidly. Alternatively, the brain may have a cognitive reserve that needs to "work harder" during a difficult task to perform at a normal level, and thus would have a higher amount of activation. Trachtenberg et al [44] argue that the populations tested in these studies are very young (20s and 30s) and have a great deal of time before they will begin to experience cognitive decline. He suggests instead that the possession of an ApoE ε4 allele leads to a fundamental difference in neurophysiology that could be contributing to this effect.

A growing body of evidence suggests that an episodic memory task may not be the best way to characterize memory loss because episodic memory declines as a part of healthy aging as well. Episodic memory tasks are also more difficult than semantic memory tasks, The work may therefore be experiencing a basement effect[45]. Semantic memory, in contrast, is affected very early in AD, but remains relatively untouched in the healthy aging process [45]. Most semantic memory tests involve the recognition of famous names and faces [45-47] or categorizing word lists [1,3]. These types of studies have shown an increase in activation and a decrease in deactivation the MTL regions of carriers of the ApoE ε4 allele.

Spontaneous BOLD fMRI

Resting state, or functional connectivity MRI (fcMRI) is a task-independent measurement of brain regions that fluctuate in their BOLD signal together, indicating that they are functionally connected. The Default Mode Network (DMN) is a collection of brain regions that seem to activate together while the brain is at rest, and are deactivated while the brain is engaged in a cognitive task. The DMN is composed of MTL and lateral frontal regions, particularly the posterior cingulate complex [4,6,7]. This network is altered in AD and is a potent biomarker for separating patients with AD from healthy controls [8], patients with aMCI from healthy controls [48], and genetically at-risk individuals from healthy controls [4].

Caveats to BOLD fMRI

Although BOLD fMRI is an important tool for research, there are some limitations to its clinical feasibility as a biomarker for future AD. To date, it has not successfully been used in predicting patient prognosis or trajectory. In terms of practicality, fMRI is expensive and requires extensive image processing, which will drive up the cost of any tests. It is also not completely reproducible across testing sites or days. Different equipment and software can create variables in data analysis across testing sites. Longitudinal studies can present difficulties because as they age, patients may develop comorbidities, or begin taking drugs that will interfere with the BOLD signal in a way unrelated to AD pathology. Even subtle changes can influence the BOLD signal such as recent alcohol [49] or caffeine [50] intake.

The biggest difficulty with BOLD fMRI is that it is generally not quantitative. Changes in blood oxygenation are based on three individual components: Cerebral Blood Flow (CBF), Cerebral Blood Volume (CBV), and the Cerebral Metabolic Rate of Oxygen ($CMRO_2$) [51]. Figure 5 represents the many ways that CBF, CBV, and $CMRO_2$ can contribute to the BOLD effect. It is impossible to determine which of these is contributing to a BOLD fluctuation with fMRI alone. For this reason, vascular imaging techniques are being developed that are able to quantitatively determine the physiological changes that are contributing to the BOLD signal. Techniques to quantify CBF and CBV have been validated and are gaining popularity. $CMRO_2$ methods are still in development and have not been used in an AD population and will therefore not be covered.

Positive BOLD Effect	↑ CBF	↑ CBV	↑ $CMRO_2$
	↑ CBF	↑ CBV	— $CMRO_2$
	↑ CBF	↑ CBV	↓ $CMRO_2$
Negative BOLD Effect	— CBF	↑ CBV	— $CMRO_2$
	— CBF	— CBV	↑ $CMRO_2$
	↓ CBF	— CBV	— $CMRO_2$
	↓ CBF	↑ CBV	↑ $CMRO_2$

Figure 5. Positive and negative BOLD effects are influenced by CBF, CBV, and CMRO2 and it is not possible to distinguish which factor is contributing by only measuring BOLD.

4.2. Cerebral blood flow

Cerebral blood flow is a measurement of the rate of tissue perfusion, usually measured by the amount of blood that reaches a tissue per unit time (mL blood per 100 g tissue per minute) [52]. CBF has been quantified by Positron Emission Tomography (PET) [53,54] and Single Photon Emission Computed Tomography (SPECT) [10,55,56] but today it can also be quantified noninvasively using a technique called Arterial Spin Labeling (ASL). ASL uses a radiofrequency pulse to label blood water in an area outside of the region of interest, usually in the neck. After 1-2s, the labeled blood water flows into the imaging region and exchanges with tissue water and a tagged image can be obtained [51,57]. This image is compared with an image where the blood water is not labeled, and the difference between the two images provides a map proportional to CBF. As can be seen, ASL is analogous to tracer-based approaches such as 15O PET and Gadolinium-MRI, however the tracer is endogenous blood water as opposed to an exogenous contrast agents. Whole-brain ASL scans can be performed in less than 5 minutes with a spatial resolution of 3-5 mm.

In AD patients, deficits in CBF have been seen in the temporoparietal cortex, posterior cingulate cortex, and frontal cortex [57-59]. CBF as measured by ASL has been shown to be increased in aMCI patients but decreased pre-symptomatic carriers of ApoE ε4 [11,60]. The increase that is seen in aMCI has been attributed to compensatory mechanisms [60].

Often, changes in blood flow precede structural changes, but reduced CBF is not necessarily an indicator of vascular dysfunction. For instance, CBF alterations may be due to a lower metabolic demand, cardiac output, or blood pressure [10,61,62]. Longitudinal analysis of CBF in at-risk populations should be developed for its potential as a method for tracking disease progress or recognizing it before cognitive symptoms begin.

4.3. Cerebral blood volume

Cerebral blood volume measures the amount of blood per 100 mL brain tissue. It is an indirect measurement of the vascularization of brain regions, and is less dependent on the subject's respiration than CBF[11,15,63,64]. There are currently two major techniques that measure CBV: Dynamic Susceptibility Contrast MRI (DSC-MRI) and Vascular Space Occupancy MRI (VASO). DSC-MRI involves the injection of gadolinium as a contrast agent, and is the best validated measure. Unfortunately, the injection of gadolinium is dose-restricted because of its toxic effect on kidneys which limits its potential for longitudinal studies and older patient populations [17,65]. VASO is a completely non-invasive method of measuring CBV changes and has been gaining popularity in recent years. Unlike DSC-MRI, VASO uses endogenous blood water as a contrast agent. VASO can be performed by measuring the tissue signal with and without blood water nulled, and subtracting one image from the other. Although VASO is correlated with DSC-MRI there are some minor variations in the two measurements, suggesting that the underlying physiology may be different [19,63].

VASO has been applied to a mixed group of patients with aMCI and AD and found that there are CBV reductions in the frontal and parietal lobes. These reductions were most striking in white matter which suggests that any vascular component of AD is especially damaging to white matter compared to gray matter [21,22,61]. In the future, longitudinal studies should be performed in carriers of ApoE ε4 to determine if these white matter vascular deficiencies can be recognized at a young age.

5. Chemical imaging

Structural and functional imaging are important for assessing the damage caused by AD, but for designing therapeutics the ability to view changes at the macromolecular level would be highly beneficial. New techniques are being developed that can do just that. Magnetic Resonance Spectroscopy (MRS) can be done in a single voxel or across multiple voxels (MRS imaging, MRSi) to assess macromolecular concentration. Both are new techniques that are still being optimized, but will be extremely useful in understanding AD.

5.1. Magnetic resonance spectroscopy

MR imaging primarily measures signal from water protons, but in MR spectroscopy protons of various metabolites can be assessed at one time. Quantification is achieved by exciting a single voxel with a combination of RF pulses, and obtaining a free induction decay (FID) spectrum. When this spectrum is Fourier transformed, metabolites can be visualized due to their variability in chemical shift (Figure 6). Because the chemical shift of a single metabolite is constant, it will always peak at the same frequency (measured in parts per million, ppm). By calculating the area under the peak, the concentration of a metabolite relative to an internal standard can be obtained.

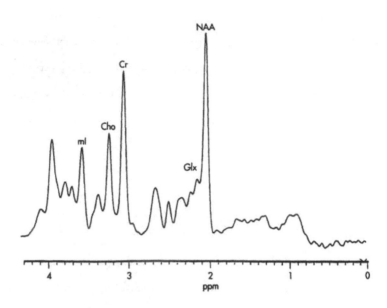

Figure 6. Example of chemical shift spectrum from a normal brain (from the University of Missouri-Kansas City Radiology Resident Resource Webpage

The most common macromolecules studied in neuroimaging are creatine (Cr) which is usually unaffected by disease and can act as an internal standard, N-acetyl-aspartate (NAA), a marker for neuronal health, myo-inositol (mI), a marker of gliosis [32,66], and choline (Cho). In AD, NAA is typically decreased in AD and mI is typically increased so NAA/Cr, mI/Cr and NAA/mI ratios are good markers of the disease with the ratio of NAA to mI being the strongest. The mI concentration has been found to be elevated in aMCI [33,34,67]. There is a trend that NAA is decreased in aMCI, however the effect is much more mild if it exists [35-37,68]. Glutamate (Glu) is the primary excitatory neurotransmitter, and is significantly reduced in AD [69] Gamma-amino butyric acid (GABA) is an inhibitory neurotransmitter, and its concentration may be decreased in AD [70]. It is possible to use MRS to estimate relative concentrations of both Glu and GABA *in vivo*, but due to their low concentrations compared to NAA and other metabolites, and the fact that signal from these metabolites is very close in frequency space to other metabolites of larger concentration, it is more difficult to identify them without suppressing or "editing" other signals. One of the common methods used to quantify GABA is a PRESS or MEGA-PRESS sequence which suppresses or edits signals from water, creatine, and other nearby metabolites so that the characteristic GABA peaks can be identified. For more information on the MEGA-PRESS sequence, see Waddell 2007 [71].

The importance of MRS research is clear, but there are some difficulties associated with it. To begin with, the scans take a long time to complete—more than ten minutes in some cases—and because the measurements are taken in a single voxel the subject must stay absolutely still throughout the scan. This is very difficult for young healthy subjects, and may be nearly impossible in older, demented subjects. Common sedation drugs such as propofol will change the levels of brain metabolites and should be avoided[72]. In premenopausal women GABA levels also vary depending on the stage of the menstrual cycle, and may introduce variability[73].

Typically, spectroscopy is done in the posterior cingulate or medial temporal cortices, but these are only affected by AD in late stages of the disease. It would be more helpful to study the smaller limbic areas that are affected sooner, but the voxel sizes typically used in spectroscopy are larger than many of these areas [66]. Falini et al developed a technique to perform spectroscopy across the entire brain and found that NAA levels are reduced in those with AD, however whole-brain spectroscopy is a non-specific marker [41,74]. These limitations will be overcome with higher field strength, advances in shimming algorithms, and improvements to computerized registration techniques [42,68].

5.2. Magnetic Resonance Spectroscopy imaging (MRSi)

MRSi is a technique that uses spectroscopy but applies it to voxels across the entire brain. The concentration of the chemical of interest corresponds to the brightness or color of the voxel in the image produced. It can achieve high spatial resolution (up to 0.25 cm^3), and when optimized can produce a wealth of information [44,75]. This technique has largely been developed for breast cancer imaging, and can identify chemical "hot spots" that are of use when categorizing a tumor. It has great potential as a technique for understanding AD.

6. Concluding remarks

There is still a long way to go before AD can be fully understood and treated. With magnetic resonance technologies, it is possible to observe changes before cognitive decline begins. A lot of work has been done with structural imaging of gray and white matter, and changes are detectible in ApoE ε4 carriers decades before the onset of symptoms. More longitudinal studies need to be performed to determine which of these changes will specifically lead to AD. Functional studies offer a window of the changes that occur before neuronal atrophy, but the specific vascular causes behind the BOLD effect need to be further studied. Finally, chemical imaging can provide a glimpse of the changes occurring at the molecular level, and by further developing and standardizing these measures there is much that can be learned.

Author details

Emily J. Mason[1*], Manus J. Donahue[2] and Brandon A. Ally[1]

*Address all correspondence to: emily.mason.1@vanderbilt.edu

1 Department of Neurology, Vanderbilt University, Nashville, TN, USA

2 Department of Radiology, Vanderbilt University, Nashville, TN, USA

References

[1] Lind J, Persson J, Ingvar M, Larsson A, Cruts M, Van Broeckhoven C, et al. Reduced functional brain activity response in cognitively intact apolipoprotein E epsilon4 carriers. Brain. 2006 May;129(Pt 5):1240–8.

[2] Wilcock DM. The usefulness and challenges of transgenic mouse models in the study of Alzheimer's disease. CNS Neurol Disord Drug Targets. 2010 Aug.;9(4):386–94.

[3] Persson J, Lind J, Larsson A, Ingvar M, Sleegers K, Van Broeckhoven C, et al. Altered deactivation in individuals with genetic risk for Alzheimer's disease. Neuropsychologia. 2008;46(6):1679–87.

[4] Fleisher AS, Sherzai A, Taylor C, Langbaum JBS, Chen K, Buxton RB. Resting-state BOLD networks versus task-associated functional MRI for distinguishing Alzheimer's disease risk groups. NeuroImage. 2009 Oct. 1;47(4):1678–90.

[5] Sinha G. Peering inside Alzheimer's brains. Nat. Biotechnol. 2011 May;:384–7.

[6] Filippini N, Macintosh BJ, Hough MG, Goodwin GM, Frisoni GB, Smith SM, et al. Distinct patterns of brain activity in young carriers of the APOE-epsilon4 allele. Proc Natl Acad Sci USA. 2009 Apr. 28;106(17):7209–14.

[7] Boly M, Phillips C, Tshibanda L, Vanhaudenhuyse A, Schabus M, Dang-Vu TT, et al. Intrinsic brain activity in altered states of consciousness: how conscious is the default mode of brain function? Ann N Y Acad Sci. 2008;1129:119–29.

[8] Greicius MD, Srivastava G, Reiss AL, Menon V. Default-mode network activity distinguishes Alzheimer's disease from healthy aging: evidence from functional MRI. Proc Natl Acad Sci USA. 2004 Mar. 30;101(13):4637–42.

[9] Alzheimer's Association. 2012 Alzheimer's disease facts and figures. Alzheimers Dement. 8th ed. 2012 Mar. 5;:131–68.

[10] Plewes DB, Kucharczyk W. Physics of MRI: a primer. J Magn Reson Imaging. 2012 May;35(5):1038–54.

[11] Braak H, Braak E. Neuropathological stageing of Alzheimer-related changes. Acta Neuropathol. 1991;82(4):239–59.

[12] Jack CR Jr., Bernstein MA, Borowski BJ, Gunter JL, Fox NC, Thompson PM, et al. Update on the Magnetic Resonance Imaging core of the Alzheimer's Disease Neuroimaging Initiative. Alzheimer's and Dementia. 2010 May;6(3):212–20.

[13] Poels MMF, Ikram MA, van der Lugt A, Hofman A, Niessen WJ, Krestin GP, et al. Cerebral microbleeds are associated with worse cognitive function: the Rotterdam Scan Study. Neurology. 2012 Jan. 31;78(5):326–33.

[14] Pettersen JA, Sathiyamoorthy G, Gao F-Q, Szilagyi G, Nadkarni NK, St George-Hyslop P, et al. Microbleed topography, leukoaraiosis, and cognition in probable Alzheimer disease from the Sunnybrook dementia study. Arch Neurol. 2008 Jun.;65(6): 790–5.

[15] Cuingnet R, Gerardin E, Tessieras J, Auzias G, Lehéricy S, Habert M-O, et al. Automatic classification of patients with Alzheimer's disease from structural MRI: a comparison of ten methods using the ADNI database. NeuroImage. 2011 May 15;56(2): 766–81.

[16] Smith MA, Zhu X, Tabaton M, Liu G, McKeel DW, Cohen ML, et al. Increased iron and free radical generation in preclinical Alzheimer disease and mild cognitive impairment. J Alzheimers Dis. 2010;19(1):363–72.

[17] Chincarini A, Bosco P, Calvini P, Gemme G, Esposito M, Olivieri C, et al. Local MRI analysis approach in the diagnosis of early and prodromal Alzheimer's disease. NeuroImage. 2011 Sep. 15;58(2):469–80.

[18] Hopp K, Popescu BFG, McCrea RPE, Harder SL, Robinson CA, Haacke ME, et al. Brain iron detected by SWI high pass filtered phase calibrated with synchrotron X-ray fluorescence. J Magn Reson Imaging. 2010 Jun.;31(6):1346–54.

[19] Costafreda SG, Dinov ID, Tu Z, Shi Y, Liu C-Y, Kloszewska I, et al. Automated hippocampal shape analysis predicts the onset of dementia in mild cognitive impairment. NeuroImage. 2011 May 1;56(1):212–9.

[20] Ringman JM, Pope W, Salamon N. Insensitivity of visual assessment of hippocampal atrophy in familial Alzheimer's disease. J Neurol. 2010 May 1;257(5):839–42.

[21] Shaw P, Lerch JP, Pruessner JC, Taylor KN, Rose AB, Greenstein D, et al. Cortical morphology in children and adolescents with different apolipoprotein E gene polymorphisms: an observational study. Lancet Neurol. 2007 Jun. 1;6(6):494–500.

[22] Alexander GE, Bergfield KL, Chen K, Reiman EM, Hanson KD, Lin L, et al. Gray matter network associated with risk for Alzheimer's disease in young to middle-aged adults. Neurobiology of aging. 2012 Dec.;33(12):2723–32.

[23] Donix M, Burggren AC, Suthana NA, Siddarth P, Ekstrom AD, Krupa AK, et al. Family history of Alzheimer's disease and hippocampal structure in healthy people. Am J Psychiatry. 2010 Nov. 1;167(11):1399–406.

[24] Donix M, Burggren AC, Suthana NA, Siddarth P, Ekstrom AD, Krupa AK, et al. Longitudinal changes in medial temporal cortical thickness in normal subjects with the APOE-4 polymorphism. NeuroImage. 2010 Oct. 15;53(1):37–43.

[25] Espeseth T, Westlye LT, Fjell AM, Walhovd KB, Rootwelt H, Reinvang I. Accelerated age-related cortical thinning in healthy carriers of apolipoprotein E epsilon 4. Neurobiology of aging. 2008 Mar. 1;29(3):329–40.

[26] Grothe M, Heinsen H, Teipel SJ. Atrophy of the cholinergic Basal forebrain over the adult age range and in early stages of Alzheimer's disease. Biol Psychiatry. 2012 May 1;71(9):805–13.

[27] Brickman AM, Honig LS, Scarmeas N, Tatarina O, Sanders L, Albert MS, et al. Measuring cerebral atrophy and white matter hyperintensity burden to predict the rate of cognitive decline in Alzheimer disease. Arch Neurol. 2008 Sep.;65(9):1202–8.

[28] Yoshita M, Fletcher E, Harvey D, Ortega M, Martinez O, Mungas DM, et al. Extent and distribution of white matter hyperintensities in normal aging, MCI, and AD. Neurology. 2006 Dec. 26;67(12):2192–8.

[29] Carmichael O, Schwarz C, Drucker D, Fletcher E, Harvey D, Beckett L, et al. Longitudinal changes in white matter disease and cognition in the first year of the Alzheimer disease neuroimaging initiative. Arch Neurol. 2010 Nov.;67(11):1370–8.

[30] Sexton CE, Kalu UG, Filippini N, Mackay CE, Ebmeier KP. A meta-analysis of diffusion tensor imaging in mild cognitive impairment and Alzheimer's disease. Neurobiology of aging. 2011 Dec.;32(12):2322.e5–18.

[31] Smith EE, Egorova S, Blacker D, Killiany RJ, Muzikansky A, Dickerson BC, et al. Magnetic resonance imaging white matter hyperintensities and brain volume in the prediction of mild cognitive impairment and dementia. Arch Neurol. 2008 Jan.;65(1): 94–100.

[32] Appel J, Potter E, Bhatia N, Shen Q, Zhao W, Greig MT, et al. Association of white matter hyperintensity measurements on brain MR imaging with cognitive status, medial temporal atrophy, and cardiovascular risk factors. American Journal of Neuroradiology. 2009 Nov.;30(10):1870–6.

[33] Hirono N, Yasuda M, Tanimukai S, Kitagaki H, Mori E. Effect of the apolipoprotein E epsilon4 allele on white matter hyperintensities in dementia. Stroke. 2000 Jun.;31(6): 1263–8.

[34] Sawada H, Udaka F, Izumi Y, Nishinaka K, Kawakami H, Nakamura S, et al. Cerebral white matter lesions are not associated with apoE genotype but with age and female sex in Alzheimer's disease. J. Neurol. Neurosurg. Psychiatr. 2000 May;68(5): 653–6.

[35] Persson J, Lind J, Larsson A, Ingvar M, Cruts M, Van Broeckhoven C, et al. Altered brain white matter integrity in healthy carriers of the APOE epsilon4 allele: a risk for AD? Neurology. 2006 Apr. 11;66(7):1029–33.

[36] Høgh P, Garde E, Mortensen EL, Jørgensen OS, Krabbe K, Waldemar G. The apolipoprotein E epsilon4-allele and antihypertensive treatment are associated with in-

creased risk of cerebral MRI white matter hyperintensities. Acta Neurol. Scand. 2007 Apr.;115(4):248–53.

[37] Ryan L, Walther K, Bendlin BB, Lue L-F, Walker DG, Glisky EL. Age-related differences in white matter integrity and cognitive function are related to APOE status. NeuroImage. 2011 Jan. 15;54(2):1565–77.

[38] Bendlin BB, Ries ML, Canu E, Sodhi A, Lazar M, Alexander AL, et al. White matter is altered with parental family history of Alzheimer's disease. Alzheimers Dement. 2010 Sep. 1;6(5):394–403.

[39] Smith CD, Chebrolu H, Andersen AH, Powell DA, Lovell MA, Xiong S, et al. White matter diffusion alterations in normal women at risk of Alzheimer's disease. Neurobiology of aging. 2010 Jul. 1;31(7):1122–31.

[40] Atwood CS, Obrenovich ME, Liu T, Chan H, Perry G, Smith MA, et al. Amyloid-beta: a chameleon walking in two worlds: a review of the trophic and toxic properties of amyloid-beta. Brain Res. Brain Res. Rev. 2003 Sep.;43(1):1–16.

[41] Brewer JB, Magda S, Airriess C, Smith ME. Fully-automated quantification of regional brain volumes for improved detection of focal atrophy in Alzheimer disease. American Journal of Neuroradiology. 2009 Mar. p. 578–80.

[42] la Torre de JC. Is Alzheimer's disease a neurodegenerative or a vascular disorder? Data, dogma, and dialectics. Lancet Neurol. 2004 Mar. 1;3(3):184–90.

[43] Sperling R. Functional MRI Studies of Associative Encoding in Normal Aging, Mild Cognitive Impairment, and Alzheimer's Disease. Ann N Y Acad Sci. 2007 Feb. 1;1097(1):146–55.

[44] Trachtenberg AJ, Filippini N, Mackay CE. The effects of APOE-ε4 on the BOLD response. NBA. Elsevier Inc; 2012 Feb. 1;33(2):323–34.

[45] Sugarman MA, Woodard JL, Nielson KA, Seidenberg M, Smith JC, Durgerian S, et al. Functional magnetic resonance imaging of semantic memory as a presymptomatic biomarker of Alzheimer's disease risk. Biochimica et Biophysica Acta (BBA) - Molecular Basis of Disease. 2012 Mar.;1822(3):442–56.

[46] Seidenberg M, Guidotti L, Nielson KA, Woodard JL, Durgerian S, Antuono P, et al. Semantic memory activation in individuals at risk for developing Alzheimer disease. Neurology. 2009 Aug. 25;73(8):612–20.

[47] Woodard JL, Seidenberg M, Nielson KA, Antuono P, Guidotti L, Durgerian S, et al. Semantic memory activation in amnestic mild cognitive impairment. Brain. 2009 Aug.;132(Pt 8):2068–78.

[48] Sorg C, Riedl V, Muhlau M, Calhoun VD, Eichele T, Laer L, et al. Selective changes of resting-state networks in individuals at risk for Alzheimer's disease. Proc Natl Acad Sci USA. 2007 Nov. 20;104(47):18760–5.

[49] Luchtmann M, Jachau K, Tempelmann C, Bernarding J. Alcohol induced region-dependent alterations of hemodynamic response: implications for the statistical interpretation of pharmacological fMRI studies. Exp Brain Res. 2010 Jul.;204(1):1–10.

[50] Koppelstaetter F, Poeppel TD, Siedentopf CM, Ischebeck A, Kolbitsch C, Mottaghy FM, et al. Caffeine and cognition in functional magnetic resonance imaging. J Alzheimers Dis. 2010;20 Suppl 1:S71–84.

[51] Donahue MJ, Blicher JU, Østergaard L, Feinberg DA, Macintosh BJ, Miller KL, et al. Cerebral blood flow, blood volume, and oxygen metabolism dynamics in human visual and motor cortex as measured by whole-brain multi-modal magnetic resonance imaging. J Cereb Blood Flow Metab. 2009 Nov.;29(11):1856–66.

[52] KETY SS, SCHMIDT CF. The nitrous oxide method for the quantitative determination of cerebral blood flow in man; theory, procedure and normal values. J. Clin. Invest. 1948 Jul.;27(4):476–83.

[53] Corder EH, Saunders AM, Strittmatter WJ, Schmechel DE, Gaskell PC, Small GW, et al. Gene dose of apolipoprotein E type 4 allele and the risk of Alzheimer's disease in late onset families. Science. 1993 Aug. 13;261(5123):921–3.

[54] Ishii K, Sasaki M, Yamaji S, Sakamoto S, Kitagaki H, Mori E. Demonstration of decreased posterior cingulate perfusion in mild Alzheimer's disease by means of H215O positron emission tomography. Eur J Nucl Med. 1997 Jun.;24(6):670–3.

[55] Bartenstein P, Minoshima S, Hirsch C, Buch K, Willoch F, Mösch D, et al. Quantitative assessment of cerebral blood flow in patients with Alzheimer's disease by SPECT. J. Nucl. Med. 1997 Jul.;38(7):1095–101.

[56] Kogure D, Matsuda H, Ohnishi T, Asada T, Uno M, Kunihiro T, et al. Longitudinal evaluation of early Alzheimer's disease using brain perfusion SPECT. J. Nucl. Med. 2000 Jul.;41(7):1155–62.

[57] Schmitz BL, Aschoff AJ, Hoffmann MHK, Grön G. Advantages and pitfalls in 3T MR brain imaging: a pictorial review. AJNR Am J Neuroradiol. 2005 Oct.;26(9):2229–37.

[58] Alsop DC, Detre JA, Grossman M. Assessment of cerebral blood flow in Alzheimer's disease by spin-labeled magnetic resonance imaging. Ann Neurol. 2000 Jan.;47(1):93–100.

[59] Johnson NA, Jahng G-H, Weiner MW, Miller BL, Chui HC, Jagust WJ, et al. Pattern of cerebral hypoperfusion in Alzheimer disease and mild cognitive impairment measured with arterial spin-labeling MR imaging: initial experience. Radiology. 2005 Mar.;234(3):851–9.

[60] Kim SM, Kim MJ, Rhee HY, Ryu C-W, Kim EJ, Petersen ET, et al. Regional cerebral perfusion in patients with Alzheimer's disease and mild cognitive impairment: effect of APOE Epsilon4 allele. Neuroradiology. 2012 Jul. 25.

[61] Uh J, Lewis-Amezcua K, Martin-Cook K, Cheng Y, Weiner M, Diaz-Arrastia R, et al. Cerebral blood volume in Alzheimer's disease and correlation with tissue structural integrity. Neurobiology of aging. 2010 Dec.;31(12):2038–46.

[62] Vernooij MD M, Smits MD M. Structural Neuroimaging in Aging and Alzheimer's Disease. Neuroimaging Clinics of NA. Elsevier Inc; 2012 Feb. 1;22(1):33–55.

[63] Lu H, Law M, Johnson G, Ge Y, Van Zijl PCM, Helpern JA. Novel approach to the measurement of absolute cerebral blood volume using vascular-space-occupancy magnetic resonance imaging. Magn Reson Med. 2005 Dec. 1;54(6):1403–11.

[64] Grubb RL, Raichle ME, Eichling JO, Ter-Pogossian MM. The effects of changes in Pa-CO2 on cerebral blood volume, blood flow, and vascular mean transit time. Stroke. 1974 Sep.;5(5):630–9.

[65] Donahue MJ, Strother MK, Hendrikse J. Novel MRI approaches for assessing cerebral hemodynamics in ischemic cerebrovascular disease. Stroke. 2012 Mar.;43(3):903–15.

[66] Kantarci K. 1H magnetic resonance spectroscopy in dementia. Br J Radiol. 2007 Dec.; 80 Spec No 2:S146–52.

[67] Kantarci K, Smith GE, Ivnik RJ, Petersen RC, Boeve BF, Knopman DS, et al. 1H magnetic resonance spectroscopy, cognitive function, and apolipoprotein E genotype in normal aging, mild cognitive impairment and Alzheimer's disease. J Int Neuropsychol Soc. 2002 Nov.;8(7):934–42.

[68] Schott JM, Frost C, Macmanus DG, Ibrahim F, Waldman AD, Fox NC. Short echo time proton magnetic resonance spectroscopy in Alzheimer's disease: a longitudinal multiple time point study. Brain. 2010 Nov. 1;133(11):3315–22.

[69] Selkoe DJ. Alzheimer's disease is a synaptic failure. Science. 2002 Oct. 25;298(5594): 789–91.

[70] Limon A, Reyes-Ruiz JM, Miledi R. Loss of functional GABAA receptors in the Alzheimer diseased brain. Proc Natl Acad Sci USA. 2012 Jun. 19;109(25):10071–6.

[71] Waddell KW, Avison MJ, Joers JM, Gore JC. A practical guide to robust detection of GABA in human brain by J-difference spectroscopy at 3 T using a standard volume coil. Magn Reson Imaging. 2007 Sep.;25(7):1032–8.

[72] Zhang H, Wang W, Gao W, Ge Y, Zhang J, Wu S, et al. Effect of propofol on the levels of neurotransmitters in normal human brain: A magnetic resonance spectroscopy study. Neurosci Lett. 2009 Dec.;467(3):247–51.

[73] Harada M, Kubo H, Nose A, Nishitani H, Matsuda T. Measurement of variation in the human cerebral GABA level by in vivo MEGA-editing proton MR spectroscopy using a clinical 3 T instrument and its dependence on brain region and the female menstrual cycle. Hum. Brain Mapp. 2011 May;32(5):828–33.

[74] Falini A, Bozzali M, Magnani G, Pero G, Gambini A, Benedetti B, et al. A whole brain MR spectroscopy study from patients with Alzheimer's disease and mild cognitive impairment. NeuroImage. 2005 Jul. 15;26(4):1159–63.

[75] Hu J, Feng W, Hua J, Jiang Q, Xuan Y, Li T, et al. A high spatial resolution in vivo 1H magnetic resonance spectroscopic imaging technique for the human breast at 3 T. Med Phys. 2009 Nov.;36(11):4870–7.

Chapter 10

Candidate Bio-Markers of Alzheimer's Disease

B.K. Binu Kumar and Harish C. Pant

Additional information is available at the end of the chapter

1. Introduction

Alzheimer's disease (AD) is a neurodegenerative disorder of the central nervous system characterized by a progressive loss of short-term memory accompanied by a gradual loss of cognitive functions (Ross et al., 2004). AD is among the most frequently encountered diseases in aging societies with an estimated 5million people in the United States and 17 million people worldwide suffering from the disease. It is expected that these numbers will quadruple by the year 2040, by which 1 out of 45 Americans will be affected, leading to a considerable public health burden (Fratiglioni et al., 1999). AD pathogenic mechanisms contributing to neuronal loss and brain dysfunction are still unclear. However, remarkable advances have taken place in understanding of both the genetics and molecular biological aspects of the intracellular processing of amyloid and tau and the changes leading to the pathologic formation of extracellular amyloid plaques and the intraneuronal aggregation of hyperphosphorylated tau into neurofibrillary tangles. This progress in our understanding of the molecular pathology has set the stage for clinically meaningful advances in the development of biomarkers.

Proper diagnosis is essential for instituting appropriate clinical management. While diagnostic accuracy for the disease has improved, the differential diagnosis of the disorder is still problematic. In the very early stages of the disease, frequently classified as mild cognitive impairment (MCI), delineating disease process from "normal ageing" may be difficult; in later stages of the disease, distinguishing AD from a number of neurodegenerative diseases associated with dementia may also be difficult. Furthermore, the disease progression is slow and there is variability of performance on clinical measures, making it difficult to monitor change effectively. Since disease modifying therapy is likely to be most effective early in the course of disease, early diagnosis is highly desirable before neurodegeneration becomes severe and widespread.

In clinical practice, the diagnosis of AD is still largely based on consensuscriteria combined with the exclusion of secondary causes of memory loss (Knopman et al., 2001; McKhann et al., 1984).Thus, there is an urgent and desperate need for a biomarker that can reliably prognose the disease. Biomarkers of AD occupy an essential place in recently formulated diagnostic criteria for AD, in which their role is to identify the pathophysiological processes underlying cognitive impairment or to help predict time to reach up to dementia. Criteria for a useful biomarker have been proposed by an international consensus group on molecular and biochemical markers of AD in 1998 (The Ronald and Nancy Reagan Research Institute of the Alzheimer's Association and the National Institute on Aging Working Group, 1998). According to these guidelines, a biomarker for AD should detect a manifestation of the fundamental neuropathology and be validated in neuropathologically-confirmed cases. Its sensitivity for detecting AD should exceed 80% and its specificity in differentiating between AD and other dementias should be higher than 80%. Ideally, a biomarker should also be reliable, reproducible, non-invasive, simple to perform, and inexpensive. One further role of particular interest to patients and clinicians dealing with AD is its ability to detect the disease at the earliest possible stage.

Based on growing body of evidence concerning the pathophysiology of AD, a number of putative biological markers of disease have been evaluated against clinical and neuropathological standards. Biomarkers are very useful for diagnosing and monitoring disease progression (Ward et al., 2007) and are important for patient selection, monitoring side-effects, aiding selection of appropriate patient treatment, and helping new drug discovery. For the clinical studies of AD therapeutics, there is an increasing need for diagnostic markers to ensure that therapies are targeted at the right patient population, to initiate early treatment when disease-modifying drugs will be available, and to monitor disease progression (Hye et al., 2006).

2. Biomarkers in CSF

One of the most promising sources of biomarkers in AD is the cerebrospinal fluid (CSF).The molecular changes in the brain extracellular and interstitial environments are reflected in CSF. The single-cell layer epithelium separating the two compartments allows a virtually unhindered flow of molecules from the brain towards the CSF. CSF biomarkers for AD should reflect the central pathogenic processes in the brain. Furthermore the CSF is accessible to trained clinicians using a relatively simple lumbar puncture (Fenton et al., 1994). Several studies have investigated CSF inflammatory markers, immunological mediators, neurotrophins, metalloproteinases or isoprostenes. Candidate CSF biomarkers include total tau (T-tau) as a marker for the neuronal degeneration (table 1), phosphorylated tau (P-tau) as a marker for tau hyperphosphorylation (table 2) and formation of tangles $A\beta42$ as a marker for $A\beta$ metabolism and plaque formation (table 3, Blennow et al.,2003).

Category	Reference	Sensitivity range (100%) for AD versus controls	Methods	Study Title	Study population
Tau	Arai et al., 1995	80-90	ELISA	Tau in cerebrospinal fluid: a potential diagnostic marker in Alzheimer's disease	AD (n=70), non-AD (n=96) control (n=19)
Tau	Riemenschneider et al., 1996	90-100	ELISA	Cerebrospinal protein tau is elevated in early Alzheimer's disease.	AD(n=22), dementia(n=3) Healthy controls(HC)(n=19)
Tau	Shoji et al., 1998	20-30	ELISA	Combination assay of CSF tau, A beta 1-40 and A beta 1-42(43) as a biochemical marker of Alzheimer's disease	sporadic AD(n=55), controls(n=34), non-AD dementia(n=23), other neurological diseases(n=45)
Tau	Kanai et al., 1998	30-40	ELISA	Longitudinal study of cerebrospinal fluid levels of tau, A beta1-40, and A beta1-42(43) in Alzheimer's disease: a study in Japan	AD(n=93), non-AD dementia(n=33) other neurological diseases (n=56), HC(n=54)
Tau	Tapiola et al., 1998	50-60	ELISA	CSF tau is related to apolipoprotein E genotype in early Alzheimer's disease.	Early AD(n=81), other dementia (n=43), non demented neurologic HC(n=33)
Tau	Kahle et al., 2000	50-60	ELISA	Combined assessment of tau and neuronal thread protein in Alzheimer's disease CSF	Probable AD(n=25), definite AD(n=5), non demented with PD (n=29), HC(n=16).
Tau	Sjögren et al., 2000	60-70	ELISA	Decreased CSF -amyloid42 in Alzheimer's disease and amyotrophic lateral sclerosis may reflect mismetabolism of -amyloid induced by separate mechanisms	AD (n = 19), FTD (n = 14), ALS (n = 11) PD(n = 15) HC(n = 17)
Tau	Shoji et al., 2002	50-60	ELISA	Cerebrospinal fluid tau in dementia disorders:a large scale multicenter study by a Japanese study group	AD(n=366), 168 non-AD dementia(n=168) HC(n=181).
Tau	Buerger et al., 2002	70-80	ELISA	Differential diagnosis of Alzheimer's disease with cerebrospinal fluid levels of tau protein phosphorylated at threonine 231	AD(n=82) FTD(n=26) VD(n=20) HC(n=21)
Tau	Riemenschneider et al., 2002	80-90	ELISA	Tau and Abeta42 protein in CSF of patients with frontotemporal degeneration	FTD(n=34), AD(n=74), HC(n=40),
Tau	Schönknecht et al., 2003	50-60	ELISA	Levels of total tau and tau protein phosphorylated at threonine 181 in patients with incipient and manifest Alzheimer's disease	manifest AD (n=43) Incipient AD(n=8) VD(n=16) HC(n=16)

Data from Blennow K, Hampel H (2003)

Table 1. CSF total tau (T-tau) as a diagnostic marker for AD

Catagory	Reference	Sensitivity (100%) for AD versus controls	Methods	Study Title	Study population
p- tau	Ishiguro etal., 1999	80-90	ELISA	Phosphorylated tau in human cerebrospinal fluid is a diagnostic marker for Alzheimer's disease.	AD (n=36) , Controls (n=30)
p- tau	Kohnken et al., 2000	80-90	ELISA	Detection of tau phosphorylated at threonine 231 in cerebrospinal fluid of Alzheimer's disease patients	AD(n=27), non-AD(n=31)
p- tau	Sjögren et al., 2001	40-50	ELISA	The cerebrospinal fluid levels of tau, growth-associated protein-43 and soluble amyloid precursor protein correlate in Alzheimer's disease, reflecting a common pathophysiological process	FTD(n = 14), AD(n = 47) VAD(n = 16), controls (n = 12)
p- tau	Itoh et al.,2001	90-100	ELISA	Large-scale, multicenter study of cerebrospinal fluid tau protein phosphorylated at serine 199 for the antemortem diagnosis of AD	AD(n = 236), non-AD (n = 239), controls (n = 95)
p- tau	Parnetti et al., 2001	80-90	ELISA	CSF phosphorylated tau is a possible marker for discriminating AD from dementiawith Lewy bodies. Phospho-Tau International Study Group	AD (n=80), DLB (n=43) Controls (n=40)
p-tau	Sjögren et al., 2002	50-60	ELISA	Decreased CSF -amyloid42 in Alzheimer's disease and amyotrophic lateral sclerosis may reflect mismetabolism of -amyloid induced by separate mechanisms.	AD (n = 19), FTD (n = 14), ALS (n = 11) PD(n = 15)
p- tau	Buerger et al., 2002	90-100	ELISA	CSF tau protein phosphorylated at threonine 231 correlates with cognitive decline in MCI subjects	MCI(n=77), probable AD (n=55) Control (n=30)
p-tau	Hu et al., 2002	90-100	ELISA	Levels of nonphosphorylated and phosphorylated tau in cerebrospinal fluid of Alzheimer's disease patients: an ultrasensitive bienzyme-substrate-recycle enzyme-linked immunosorbent assay.	AD (n = 30), VaD, (n = 18) non-AD (n = 13): depression (n = 3), malignant lymphoma (n = 2) control (n = 24)
p-tau	Schönknecht et al.,2003	60-70	ELISA	CSF phosphorylated tau is a possible marker for discriminating Alzheimer's disease from dementia with Lewy bodies. Phospho-Tau International Study Group	AD (n=80) DLB (n=43) Controls (n=40).

Data from Blennow K, Hampel H.(2003)

Table 2. CSF Phosphorylaterd tau (p-tau) as a diagnostic marker for AD

Catagory	Reference	Sensitivity (100%) for AD versus controls	Methods	Study Title	Study group
$A\beta_{1-42}$	Galasko et al ., 1998	70-80	ELISA	High cerebrospinal fluid tau and low amyloid beta42 levels in the clinical diagnosis of Alzheimer disease and relation to apolipoprotein E genotype	Probable AD(n=82), control (n=60) ND (n= 74)
$A\beta_{1-42}$	Andreasen et al., 1999	90-100	ELISA	Cerebrospinal fluid -amyloid(1-42) in Alzheimer's disease: differences between early- and late-onset Alzheimer disease and stability during the course of disease	AD (n=53) Control (n=21)
$A\beta_{1-42}$	Andreasen et al.,1999	90-100	ELISA	Sensitivity, specificity and stability of CSF t-tau in AD in a community-based patient sample.	AD (n= 407) Depression(n=28) control (n=65).
$A\beta_{1-42}$	Andreasen et al., 1999C	80-90	ELISA	Cerebrospinal fluid -amyloid(1-42) In Alzheimer's disease: differences between early- and late-onset Alzheimer disease and stability during the course of disease.	AD (n=53) Control (n= 21)
$A\beta_{1-42}$	Hulstaert et al., 1999	70-80	ELISA	Improved discrimination of AD patients using beta-amyloid(1-42) and tau levels in CSF.	AD (n=150) control (n= 100) ND (n=84),
$A\beta_{1-42}$	Otto et al., 2000	90-100	ELISA	Decreased beta-amyloid1-42 in cerebrospinal fluid of patients with Creutzfeldt-Jakob disease	CJD (n=27), AD(n=14), other dementia(n=19), NDC(n=20)
$A\beta_{1-42}$	Kapaki et al., 2001	70-80	ELISA	Highly increased CSF tau protein and decreased beta-amyloid (1-42) in sporadic CJD: a discrimination from Alzheimer's disease?	CJD (n=14), AD(n=38)controls (n=47).
$A\beta_{1-42}$	Sjögren et al., 2002	90-100	ELISA	Decreased CSF -amyloid42 in Alzheimer's disease and amyotrophic lateral sclerosis may reflect mismetabolism of -amyloid induced by separate mechanisms	AD (n = 19), FTD (n = 14), ALS (n = 11) PD (n = 15) controls (n = 17).

Data from Blennow K, Hampel H.(2003)

Table 3. CSF $A\beta_{1-42}$ as a diagnostic marker for AD

2.1. Tau protein

One of the major neuropathological hallmarks of AD are neurofibrillary tangles composed of paired helical filaments (PHF). The principal protein subunit of PHF is abnormally phosphorylated tau (p-tau) (Iqbal et al., 1998). Physiologically, tau protein is located in neuronal axons, in components of the cytoskeleton and in the intracellular transport systems. Total-tau (t-tau) and truncated forms of monomeric and p-tau can be traced in the CSF. Using antibodies that detect all isoforms of tau proteins independent of phosphorylation, or specific phosphorylation Core biomarker candidates of Alzheimer's disease 251 sites, ELISA have been developed to measure t-tau and p-tau concentrations (Vandermeeren et al., 1993; Blennow et al., 2002, 1995; Hampel et al., 2003). CSF total tau protein in the differentiation between AD and normal aging. Total tau protein, thought to be a general marker of neuronal destruction, has been intensely studied in more than 2200 AD patients and 1000 age-matched elderly controls over the last 10 years (Sunderland et al., 2003, table 1). The most consistent finding is a statistically significant increase of CSF t-tau protein in AD. The mean level of CSF t-tau protein concentration is about 3 times higher in AD compared to elderly controls. A sensitivity and specificity level varies between studies primarily due to the different control groups used. Specificity levels between 65% and 86% and sensitivity levels between 40% and 86% have been found (Blennow et al., 2001, table 1). In several studies, a significant elevation was also found in patients with early dementia (Galasko et al., 1997; Kurz et al., 1998; Riemenschneider et al., 1997). In these studies of early dementia, the potential of CSF t-tau protein to discriminate between AD and normal aging appeared high, with average 75% sensitivity and 85% specificity. An age-associated increase of t-tau protein has been shown in nondemented subjects (Buerger et al., 2003; Sjogren et al., 2001b). Therefore, the effect of age should be considered when t-tau protein levels are employed diagnostically.

2.2. Phosphorylated tau (p-tau)

Tau protein exists in six isoforms of 352–441 amino acids in length that are subject to a variety of posttranslational modifications (Hanger et al., 2007) and, presumably, function. Of the 79 serine and threonine phosphorylation sites on the longest isoform of tau, 4R/2N, approximately 40 have been verified (Iqbal et al., 2010) of which 25 have been identified as sites of "abnormal phosphorylation" (Mazanetz et al., 2007). The phosphorylation state of tau is the net result of a balance of kinase and phosphatase activity. Much of the activity in tau-based drug discovery has been focused on selective finding inhibitors of "tau kinase", a combination of the activity of two serine/threonine kinases that can phosphorylate tau – glycogen synthase kinase 3 (GSK3; tau protein kinase I), cyclin-dependent kinase 5 (CDK5; tau protein kinase II) and a third kinase, extracellular signal-regulated kinase 2 (ERK2), from the possible 518 member kinase family, as a possible therapeutic approach to treating AD (Hanger et al.,2009 Mazanetz et al.,2007, Brunden et al., 2009). Other kinases that are possible targets to prevent tau hyperphosphorylation are casein kinase 1 (Hanger et al.,2007), AMP-activated protein kinase (AMPK) (Greco et al.,2009) and DYRK1A and AKAP-13 (Azorsa et al., 2010). From a biomarker perspective, t-tau, a generic measure of cortical axon damage associated with AD, multiple sclerosis (Hernandez et al., 2007, Bartosik-Psujek et al.,2006), stroke and Creuzfeldt-

Jacob disease, and p-tau are increased by three fold in the CSF of confirmed AD patients (Shaw et al.,2009). Of the 40 or so phosphorylation sites on tau, pThr181 (phosphothreonine-181), pSer199, pSer202/pThr205 (AT8, epitopes site), pSer214/pSer212 (AT100, epitopessite), pThr231/ pSer235 (TG3 site) and pSer396/pSer396 (PHF1 site)–have been associated with tau hyperphosphorylation and to screen NCEs for potential "tau kinase" inhibitory activity. While pSer199 and pThr231 (p-tau231) have been evaluated as CSF biomarkers (Buerger et al., 2002; Engelborghs et al., 2008., table 2), pThr181 (also designated as p-tau181 or P-Tau181P) is the most widely used CSF biomarker to assess tau hyperphosphorylation (Lewczuk et al., 2002; Hampel et al., 2004) having similar diagnostic accuracy to p-tau231 (Fagan et al., 2009, table 2). Like Ab42, the diagnostic value of both t-tau and p-tau181 has been questioned in terms of their specificity as AD biomarkers (Mattsson et al., 2009).

2.3. β-Amyloid-protein

Extracellular senile plaques consisting of beta-amyloid-protein (Aβ) are one of the histopa-thological hallmarks of AD (Hyman and Trojanowski., 1997). They are the source of a patho-genic protein with 42 amino acids (Aβ1–42) (Selkoe et al., 1993). Several groups have developed and studied different bioassays specifically designed for Ab1–42 protein (Arai et al., 1997c, Sunderland et al., 2003). The reduction in CSF Ab1–42 found in AD has been hypothesized to indirectly reflect the amyloid deposition in senile plaques (SP), resulting in lower CSF levels in AD. A marked reduction in CSF Ab1–42, however, is also found in CJD, even in cases without Ab-positive plaques (Kapaki et al., 2001; Otto et al., 2000., table 3).

To date, at least 900 patients with clinical AD and 500 healthy individuals have been enrolled in independent research studies (Andreasen et al., 2001; Andreasen et al., 1999; Galasko et al., 1998; Sunderland et al., 2003., table 3). The most consistent finding is a marked de-crease in Aβ1–42 protein in AD (to approximately 50% of control levels). Using Ab1–42 protein alone yielded sensitivities varying from 78% to 100% (table 3) and specificities from 47% to 81% when distinguish AD from elderly controls. There is a pronounced overlap, however, between studiesfrom different groups. Based on recent data a cut-off-level of >500 pg=ml has been suggested to discriminate AD best from normal aging (Sjogren et al., 2001a). One study has documented a significant decrease in CSF Aβ1–42 protein in MCI subjects compared to controls, but this study had no follow-up measure (Andreasen et al., 1999a). A second study examined MCI patients who went on to develop AD. However, in this sample Aβ1–42 protein levels did not differ significantly from age-matched normal controls (Maruyama et al., 2001). Blennow et al (2003) found Ab1–42 protein to be an indicator of early identification of AD in MCI subjects taking potential confounding factors into account such as age, severity of cognitive decline, time of observation, apolipoprotein E epsilon (e) 4 (APOE e4) carrier status, and gender (Blennow et al., 2003).Studies correlating CSF Aβ1–42 protein concentrations with cognitive performance in AD have been contradictory. Cross-sectionally, the concentration of Aβ1–42 protein and cognitive measures were either inversely correlated (Kanai et al., 1998; Samuels et al., 1999) or no significant correlation was found (Andreasenet al., 1999b; Hulstaert et al., 1999; Okamura et al., 1999). In a rare longitudinal study, a decrease in CSF Aβ1–42 protein was documented overa three year follow-up period (Tapiola et al., 2000). A highly significant correlation between low CSF concentrations at baseline and follow up. In a separate study, no correlation was found between CSF levels and duration or severity of AD (Andreasen et al., 1999b).

2.4. Combination of CSF amyloid and tau phosphorylation

The current limitations of the predictive value of Aβ 42, t-tau and p-tau181 as AD biomarkers alone, these have been used together to develop a "CSF AD signature", again, with mixed results (Shaw et al., 2009;Mattsso et al., 2009;Kauwe et al., 2009;Mihaescu et al., 2010;Breno et al.,2008;De Meyer et al., 2010). While some studies indicate that the combination Aβ 42, t-tau and p-tau181 biomarker signature in CSF has high predictivity in identifying cases of prodromal AD in MCI patents (Shaw et al.,2009; Jack et al.,2010; Hansson et al., 2006), there is considerable intersite variability that can confound biomarker accuracy (Kauwe et al., 2009). Reduced CSF Aβ 42 and increased CSF p-tau181 concentrations – were used independently of a clinical diagnosis to stratify patient groups (De Meyer et al., 2010). This AD signature was found in 90%, 72%, and 36% of patients with AD, mild MCI, and cognitively normal groups respectively (De Meyer et al., 2010). The cognitively normal group with an AD signature were enriched in apolipoprotein E4 alleles. Validation of these findings in two further data sets showed that 64/68 (94% sensitivity) of autopsy-confirmed AD patients were classified with an AD signature while 57 MCI patients followed for 5 years had a sensitivity of 100% in progressing to AD based on their biomarker signature. The presence of a CSF AD signature in cognitively normal subjects was interpreted by the authors as an indication of AD pathology being present and detectable far earlier than previously envisioned in disease progression.

2.5. NF proteins

Neurofilaments (NFs) are neuron-specific intermediate filaments and serve as a major cytoskeletal component in neurons. In a mature mammalian neuron, NFs are co-assembled from three subunits, termed NF-H (high), NF-M (medium) and NF-L (low). As NFs are confined to the nervous system, they might be one of the best markers reflecting neuronal pathogenic changes seen in some neurological disorders, such as AD. In AD brain, the levels of phosphorylated NF-H/M (pNF-H/M) have been found to be markedly increased (Wang et al., 2001). Hu et al., (2002) found that, the levels of phosphorylated NF-H/M (pNF-H/M), non-phosphorylated NF-H/M (npNF-H/M) and NF-L were significantly higher (pNF-H/M,,12–24-fold; npNF-H/M,,3–4-fold) in neurologically healthy aged people than young individuals. In AD, the levels of npNF-H/M, and NF-L were similar to vascular dementia (VaD), and higher than in age-matched controls and the levels of pNF-H/M were significantly higher AD and ALS than in aged controls and VaD. Based on these findings, it is suggested that the increased level of total NF, p-NF proteins in CSF could be used as a marker for brain aging and neurodegenerative disorders in general, and the levels of pNF-H/M as a marker to discriminate AD from normal brain aging and as well as neurological conditions including VaD (Hu et al 2002).

Specific antibodies derived from aberrantly and hyperphosphorylated neuronal intermediate filament peptides from AD brain as bio markers for early AD detection

In addition to hyperphosphorylated- tau, recently we have demonstrated the direct evidence of aberrantly and hyperphosphorylated neuronal intermediated proteins (NF-M/H) as integral part of NFTs of AD brain using phosphoproteomics (Rudrabhatla et al., 2011., table 5). Although, NFs have been shown immunohistologically to be part of NFTs, there has been debate that the identity of NF proteins in NFTs is due to the cross-reactivity of phosphorylated NF antibodies with phospho-Tau. This study has provided a direct evidence on the identity of NFs in NFTs by immunochemical and mass spectrometric analysis. For these studies purified NFTs were used and liquid chromatography/tandem mass spectrometry of NFT tryptic digests were analysed (table 4-6). The phosphoproteomics of NFTs clearly identified NF-M phosphopeptides (table 5). Western blotting of purified tangles with SMI31 showed a 150-kDa band corresponding to phospho-NF-M, while RT97 antibodies detected phospho-NF-H. These observations suggest that expression of some of these genes is elevated in AD in addition to their phosphorylation. Apart from phosphor Tau, phosphopeptides corresponding to MAP1B to Ser1270, Ser1274, and Ser1779); and MAP2 (corresponding to Thr350, Ser1702, and Ser1706) were also identified (table 6). These studies independently demonstrate that NF and other microtubule proteins are part of NFTs in AD brains (Rudrabhatla et al., 2011). These promising findings call for further studies on the diagnostic potential of specific antibodies derived from aberrantly and hyperphosphorylated neuronal intermediate filament (NF-M/H) peptides from AD brain as bio markers for early AD detection

Phosphopeptide	Phosphorylation site
TPPAPKT*PPSSGEPPK	Thr181
TPPAPKTPPS*SGEPPK	Ser184
TPPAPKTPPSS*GEPPK	Ser185
VAVVRT*PPKS*PSSAK	Thr231, Ser235
SRT*PSLPT*PPTR	Thr212, Thr217
TPSLPT*PPTR	Thr217
TDHGAEIVYKS*PVVSGDTSPR	Ser396
TDHGAEIVYKSPVVS*GDTSPR	Ser400
TDHGAEIVYKS*PVVSGDT*SPR	Ser396, Thr403

Table 4. Phosphopeptides and phosphorylation sites identified in NFT Tau

Phosphopeptides	Phosphorylation sites
NF-M SPVPKS*PVEEAK	Ser685
NF-M KAES*PVKEEAVAEVVTITK	Ser736
NF-M VSGSPSS*GFRSQSWSR	Ser33
NF-H EPDDAKAKEPS*K	Ser942

Table 5. Phosphopeptides and phosphorylation sites identified in NF-M and NF-H

MAP	Sequence	Phosphorylation site
MAP1B	VLSPLRS*PPLIGSESAYESFLSADDK	Ser1274
MAP1B	VLSPLRS*PPLIGSESAYESFLSADDK	Ser1270
MAP1B	VLS*PLRSPPLIGSESAYESFLSADDK	Ser1270
MAP2	KIDLS*HVTS*KCGS*LK	Ser1702, Ser1706
MAP2	VAIIRT*PPKSPATPK	Thr350

Table 6. Phosphopeptides and phosphorylation sites identified in MAP1 and MAP2

2.6. Microtubule-associated proteins and vimentin

Microtubules are polymers of α- and β-tubulin dimers that mediate many functions in neurons, including organelle transport and cell shape establishment and maintenance as well as axonal elongation and growthcone steering in neurons. The polymerization, stabilization, and dynamic properties of microtubules are influenced by interactions with microtubule-associated proteins (MAPs). Members of this protein family are classified by size: high molecular mass proteins (MAP1A, MAP1B, MAP2a, and MAP2b) and intermediate molecular mass MAPs (MAP2c, MAP2d, and tau) (Gonzalez-Billault,C et al.,2004).

Increasing evidence highlights the critical outcome of MAP modification in cytoskeletal disorganization associated with the early stages of AD development. A decreased content of MAP1B and tau associated with cytoskeletal breakdown was found in the brains of AD patients compared with those of control individuals, suggesting a decreased capacity of microtubule assembly and stability (Nieto,A et.al 1989). These results are consistent with those of Iqbal et al. (1986) describing a decreased capacity in the in vitro microtubule assembly from brain extracts of AD patients. One study has shown an early decrease in MAP2 labeling within dendrites from AD brain (Adlard, P. A., and Vickers, J. C. 2002). Other studies have demonstrated that MAP1B and MAP2 co-localize with NFTs (Kosik et al., 1984; Takahashi, et al., 1991). Alonso et al. (1997) studied the associations of the Alzheimer-hyperphosphorylated tau (AD P-tau) with the high molecular weight MAPs (HMW-MAPs) MAP1 and MAP2. The author found that AD P aggregate with MAP1 and MAP2. The association of AD P-tau to the MAPs resulted in inhibition of MAP-promoted microtubule assembly. These studies suggested that the abnormally phosphorylated tau can sequester both normal tau and HMW-MAPs and disassemble microtubules.

Vimentin is a 57-kDa intermediate filament (IF) protein commonly found in mesodermally derived cells. In the healthy adult brain, vimentin is lacking in neurons and generally restricted to vascular endothelial cells and certain subpopulations of glial cells at specific brain locations. Eli et al (2009) found that Vimentin was localized to neuronal perikarya and dendrites in AD brain, with vimentin-immunopositive neurons prevalent in regions exhibiting intra- and extracellular beta-amyloid1-42 (Aβ42) deposition. Neuronal colocalization of vimentin and Aβ42 was common in the cerebral cortex, cerebellum and hippocampus (Eli et al., 2009). Our lab recently discovered that the protein tangles which are a hallmark of the disease involve at least three different proteins rather than just one (table 4-6). The discovery of these additional proteins, neurofilaments, MAP2 and Vimentin, should provide better understanding the biology and progression of the disease as well as provide additional biomarker at the early stage of the disease.

2.7. Other CSF biomarkers for AD

As the AD signature approach based on the amyloid and tau causality hypothesis of AD continues to evolve, other CSF biomarkers are also being assessed. These include CSF cytokines (Swardfager et al.,2010; Olson etal.,2010)– specifically TGFβ increases in AD CSF (Swardfager et al.,2010)– CSF proteomic profiles (Papassotiropoulos et al.,2006), clusterin (Thambisetty et al.,2010)and IgG antibodies from the adaptive immune system (Reddy et al.,2011) The latter is a field of intense research, despite the challenges in analyzing proteome profiles, and involves the study of differences in the CSF proteome in AD, MCI and control subject groups (Papassotiropoulos et al.,2006;Zhang et al.,2005; Castano et al 2006; Finehout et al.,2007; Marouf et al.,2009; Choi et al.,2010). One study (Maarouf et al.,2009) reported changes in a variety of CSF proteins including a-2-macroglobulin, α1-antichymotrypsin,a1-antitrypsin, complement and heat shock proteins, cathepsinD, enolase and creatine. The ADNI is also generating CSF proteomic profiles as part of its "Use of Targeted Multiplex Proteomic Strategies to Identify Plasma-Based Biomarkers in Alzheimer's Disease" (Miller et al., 2009).

3. Oxidized proteins: Potential candidate biomarkers in AD

Although the pathogenesis of AD is not yet fully known, it is clear that the disease is caused by a combination of risk factors. Among several hypotheses, oxidative stress is considered to play a significant role (Butterfield, 2007). Although CSF represents the most suitable biological fluid to study neurodegenerative diseases since it can reflect the biochemical changes occurring in brain, its analysis is not always easily feasible for a large scale screening, because the costs involved are enormous and procedures are invasive, uncomfortable and not without risk. For a full screening and early diagnosis, biomarkers easily detectable in biological samples, such as plasma, are needed. Up to now, the search for reliable biomarkers for AD in peripheral blood is very challenging because of difficulties with the standardization of the methods of analysis and the low reproducibility of the results. Although a set of plasma markers that differentiated AD from controls have been shown to be useful in predicting conversion from MCI to AD (Song., 2009), the study has not been yet verified by other researchers and the application of these candidate biomarkers have yet to achieve the diagnostic power, sensitivity, and reproducibility necessary for widespread use in a clinical setting. Oxidized proteins may represent potential candidate biomarkers for "oxidative stress diseases", such as AD.

The first report on protein oxidation in CSF samples was from Tohgi et al. (1999) who demonstrated that 3-nitrotyrosine moderately but significantly increased with advancing age, and showed a remarkable increase in patients with AD. As the free tyrosine concentration did not decrease, the increase in 3-nitrotyrosine with age or associated with AD did not appear to be directly related to an increase in free-nitrated tyrosines. Rather, the increased 3-nitrotyrosine was likely due to an increase in nitrated tyrosines in proteins or increased degradation of 3-nitrotyrosin containing proteins, which are highly vulnerable to degradation.The most reliable CSF markers in AD are Aβ42 and tau. Low CSF Aβ 42 is associated with amyloid pathology in the brain and high Tau is linked with neurofibrillary pathology (Frey etal. 2005). Most subjects with decreased CSF Aβ42 and high tau develop AD during the follow-up (Herukka et al., 2007). Therefore, these CSF markers may reflect brain pathology and identify preclinical AD. Interestingly, the levels of CSF Aβ42 showed a tendency to correlate positively with serum oxidative markers in the whole study population and with plasma nitrotyrosines in AD patients. Moreover, a negative correlation between CSF tau and serum nitrotyrosine levels was evidenced in controls (Korolainen et al., 2009). The correlation between CSF AD markers and blood oxidative markers may suggest that oxidative metabolism is changed in AD. This hypothesis is further supported by the finding of decreased CSF protein carbonylation in APOE ε4 carriers, which is considered an important risk factor for developing AD (Raber et al., 2004) and correlates with redox proteomics studies that identified metabolic proteins as oxidatively modified and dysfunctional (Choi et al., 2004).

Subsequently, Ahmed et al. (2005) measured in CSF the levels of protein glycation, oxidation and nitration. The authors found that the concentrations of 3-nitrotyrosine,Nε-carboxymethyl-lysine,3-deoxyglucosone-derived hydroimidazolone and N-formylkynurenine (as markers of protein glycation) were increased in subjects with AD. The Mini-Mental State Examination (MMSE) score correlated negatively with 3-nitrotyrosine residue concentration. These findings indicated that protein glycation, oxidation and nitration were increased in the CSF of subjects with AD. A combination of nitration and glycation adduct estimates of CSF may conceivably provide an indicator for the diagnosis of AD. Increased levels of protein aggregates in the form of fibrils together with increased lipid peroxidation have been shown, both in AD andMCI brain (Butterfield et al., 2010).

Advanced oxidation end products (AOEs,) during AD, colocalize with neurofibrillary tangles, senile plaques, microglia, and astrocytes and have been also measured in plasma. Advanced oxidation protein products (AOPPs), a relatively novel marker of oxidative damage, are considered as reliable markers to estimate the degree of oxidant-mediated protein damage. A significant increase in protein carbonyls in hippocampus (HP) and inferior parietal lobule (IPL) of AD subjects compared with age-matched controls was observed. Dityrosine and 3-NT total levels were reported to be elevated in the hippocampus, IPL, and neocortical regions of AD brain. Alterations in brain phospholipids pattern, a more specific assessment of lipid peroxidation, have been reported for AD brain (Lovell et al., 1995; Nitsch etal.,1992; Prasad etal., 1998). The levels of phosphatidylinositol (PI) and phosphatidylethanolamine (PE), rich in easily oxidizable PUFA, are decreased in AD brain. The levels of F(2)-isoprostanes [F(2)-IsoP], F(4)-neuroprostane[F(4)-NP], and isoprostane 8,12-iso-iPF2(α)-VI were also found to be increased in AD brain compared to controls (Montine et al.,2002; Mark et al,1999). An increase in free HNE has been demonstrated in amygdala, hippocampus, and parahippocampal gyrus of the AD brain compared with age matched controls (Markesbery.,1998). Several proteins mainly involved in energy metabolism pathways, pH regulation, and mitochondrial functionsamong others, were found carbonylated, HNE-bound or nitrated in AD brain (Sultana,

2006). Newman et al (2007) also reported that a number of proteins modified by glutathiony-lation in AD IPL.

Previous studies on CSF nitrite and nitrate levels in patients with AD have provided contra-dictory results, with some showing decreased nitrate levels (Kuiper.,1994), others showing unaltered nitrite/nitrate levels (Ikeda.,1995), and still others increased nitrate levels (Tohgi., 1998). However, another study from the same group showed that nitrite/nitrate levels in AD were stage-dependent, being elevated only in the early phase of AD and decreasing to control levels with disease progression (Tohgi., 1998). This finding was interpreted to reflect progres-sive reduction of neurons. In contrast, free 3-nitrotyrosine levels increased significantly in parallel with the severity of AD, suggesting that protein degradation increases with disease progression, resulting in increased release of free 3-nitrotyrosine from tyrosine residues that have been nitrated. 3-nitrotyrosine and the 3-nitrotyrosine/tyrosine ratios in the CSF, both of which are believed to reflect degradation of nitrated tyrosine-containing proteins, increased significantly with age and were remarkably higher in patients with AD than in controls.

A study by Choi et al. (2002) identified uniquely oxidized proteins in AD plasma. These authors applied two-dimensional gel electrophoresis (2DE) coupled with immunological staining of protein carbonyl and the oxidized proteins observed in the plasma of both AD subjects and non-AD controls were determined. However, the level of oxidation of these protein spots was markedly higher in the AD samples. They also found that the increased oxidation was not a generalized phenomenon. In the total protein stain profile, more than 300 spots were detected, but less than 20 spots were positive by immunostain-ing with anti-DNP antibody. Furthermore, of the seven proteins that were most intensive-ly oxidized, their relative levels of oxidation differed. These studies found that fibrinogen gamma chain precursor and alpha 1 antitrypsinprecursor showed increased levels of carbonyl groups in AD comparedwith controls (Stief et al., 1989).

4. Identification of a new plasma biomarker of AD using metabolomics technology

Current metabolomics research involves the identification and quantification of hundreds to thousands of small-molecular-mass metabolites (<1,500 Daltons) in cells, tissues, or biological fluids. The aims of such studies are typically to understand new diagnosis biomarkers, to understand the mechanism of action of therapeutic compounds, and to uncover the pharma-codynamics and kinetic markers of drugs in patients and in preclinical in vivo and in vitro models (Wilcoxen et al., 2010). Lipidomics is one of the metabolomics approaches used to analyze lipid species in biological systems (Hu et al., 2009; Han et al., 2005; Han and Gross, 2003). Investigating lipid biochemistry using a lipidomics approach will not only provide insights into the specific roles of lipid molecular species in healthy individuals and patients but will also assist in identifying potential biomarkers for establishing preventive or thera-peutic approaches for human health (Hu et al., 2009,Wenk.,2005; Rosenson.,2010). Lipidomics has recently captured attention, owing to the well-recognized roles of lipids in numerous human diseases such as diabetes, obesity, atherosclerosis, and AD (Wenk et al., 2005; Watson., 2006; Steinberg,. 2005; Sato et al., 2010). In support of the hypothesis that lipid dysfunction plays an important role in AD pathogenesis, previous studies with post-mortem brain tissue samples have demonstrated altered lipidomes at the different stage of AD pathogenesis. For example, multiple classes of sphingolipids are altered not only at the late stage of the disease but also at the earliest clinically recognizable stage of AD. All major classes of phospholipids are ubiquitously decreased at the late stage of AD. Among these, the levels of plasmalogen (a major component in nerve tissue membranes counting for up to 85% of ethanolamine glycerophospholipid, or ~30% of total phospholipids of these membranes) are gradually reduced as progress of AD severity (Han et al., 2011). Sato et al (2011) established a lipidomics method for comprehensive phospholipids evaluation that identified 31 phospholipids as AD biomarker candidates in human plasma using LC/MS (Satoet al., 2010). Moreover, additional studies have suggested that AD associates with other lipid metabolism pathways and lipid carrier proteins such as apoE (Bertram et al., 2008; Corder et al., 1993; Farrer et al., 1997; Strittmatter et al., 1993).

A very recent study by Sato et al (2011) were able to find a biomarker desmosterol that changes in AD compared with plasma from healthy elderly controls. They have shown that desmosterol plasma level and the desmosterol/cholesterol ratio in the same patients was significantly decreased. This study is the first report that plasma desmosterol levels are decreased in AD and MCI. And future studies are needed to confirm whether desmosterol could become an attractive plasma AD biomarker that could perhaps also be utilized for diagnosis and as well as for monitoring noninvasively the effect of future AD drugs on disease progression.

5. MicroRNAs as biomarkers for AD

MicroRNAs (miRNAs) are a class of small, endogenous, noncoding RNA molecules that serve as posttranscriptional regulators of gene expression (Lee etal.,1993;Giannakakis etal.,2007). miRNAs are acquiring important and determinant roles in the regulation of brain gene transcription in health and disease: the fact that approximately 80% of the human brain genome is transcribed into RNA, but only about 2% of the genome is transcribed into protein, underscores the potential of various levels of RNA signaling and epigenetic mechanisms to contribute to physiological gene control (Makeyevetal., 2008). In the last few years, miRNAs have been emerging as important regulators of various aspects of neuronal development and dysfunction (Gao.,2007; Lukiw.,2007). The role of miRNAs in neurodegenerative diseases has been investigated using miRNA microarray profiling in brain tissue samples derived from patients and controls. Using miRNA expression profiling in cortex samples from a well-characterized clinicopathological series of elderly controls, MCI subjects and AD patients, Wang et al (2008) identified miR-107 to be specifically decreased early in the course of AD. Computational analyses predicted BACE1 mRNA as a target of miR-107 and correlative mRNA expression studies confirmed its role in regulating BACE1 expression. An independent miRNA profiling study by Hebert et al (2008) confirmed the importance of BACE1 regulation by miRNAs. The presence of a modulation of miRNA in regions of brain targeted by AD neuropathology was further demonstrated (Lukiw et al., 2008; Lukiw., 2009), thus suggesting a specific involvement of miRNAs in pathogenetic signaling pathways associated with the AD process. Recent findings suggest that neuronal miRNA deregulation in response to an insult by Aβ may be an important factor contributing to the cascade of events leading to AD (Schonrock, et al., 2010). Of note, the upregulation of peripheral miRNAs in AD could contribute to the diminished plasma proteins reported to be predictive biomarkers for AD (Ray Set al., 2007). In addition, it has recently been reported that miRNAs can be detected in CSF: an altered regulation of miRNA expression in AD brains was paralleled by a modulation of miRNA levels in the CSF (Cogswell et al., 2008). These studies provide an initial hope that miRNAs could represent accessible biomarkers to support clinical diagnosis in the near future.

6. Timing and other influencing factors of biomarker use

Disease modifying drugs are likely to be most effective in the earlier stages of AD, before neurodegeneration is too severe and widespread, so trials for this type of drug will need to include AD cases in the earlier stages of the disease. Validated biomarkers that could enable accurate identification of AD pathology at an early stage would be of great use (Hampel et al., 2011). Alternatively, baseline biomarker measurements can be used for enrichment and stratification in proof-of concept studies, as well as for supporting go/no-go decision making of phase III trials. Biomarkers should be used in all stages of drug development including phase I, phase II and phase III. They can be used to enhance inclusion and exclusion criteria, for stratification. Biomarkers can also be used as outcome markers to detect treatment effects. Particularly, if biomarkers are intended to be used as surrogate endpoints in pivotal studies, they must have been qualified to be a substitute for a clinical standard of truth and as such reasonably predict a clinical meaningful outcome. Finally, biomarkers can be used to identify adverse effects. Nevertheless there are several pitfalls to be faced in the interpretation of biomarker data in AD drug development, such as the fact that biomarkers may be non-specific to AD, it may not be feasible to measure them in the appropriate system (i.e. the central nervous system) and the risk of over-interpreting biomarker data in phase II trials if statistical significance levels are not adjusted for multiple comparisons (Aisen, 2009). Failure to consider these issues could contribute to false conclusions and costly errors (Hampel et al., 2011; Hampel et al., 2004)

7. Conclusion and future directions

Several promising drug candidates with disease-modifying effect, such as Aβ immunother-apy, secretase modulators, and tau aggregation inhibitors, have now reached the stage of being tested in clinical trials. The promise of disease-modifying therapy has created a need for biomarkers to enable the clinical identification of the disease at an early stage. Early diagnosis will be of great importance since disease-modifying drugs are likely to be most effective in the earlier stages of the disease, before neurodegeneration is too severe and widespread. A large number of studies have demonstrated that tests based on

CSF t-tau protein, p-tau and CSF beta-amyloid1–42 have reasonable specificity and sensitivity when differentiating AD from normal aging. A smaller number of studies show similar accuracy when distinguishing AD from major depression. These tests may also be useful in detecting MCI patients who go on to develop AD.

Unfortunately, the value of these biomarkers to clinicians is limited, because they are not specific enough to accurately separate AD from other common forms of dementia, such as VaD and LBD. Sometimes the combination of both CSF t-tau protein and CSF Aβ1–42 markers does not markedly improve on their individual sensitivity. CSF p-tau, based on different phosphorylation epitopes of tau protein, has now been examined in a number of independent studies. Initial results are extremely promising, showing that different p-tau protein epitopes may substantially contribute to improved diagnostic accuracy of AD in comparison with healthy aged controls, elderly depressed patients and those with other types of dementia. Compared with CSF t-tau protein and CSF Ab1–42 markers, CSF p-tau is more specific and less influenced by age or degree of cognitive decline (Hampel et al., 2004). This has an important implication for the value of CSF p-tau to clinicians. If the marker becomes abnormal very early in the course of disease relatively independent from the degree of cognitive decline than the marker may be ideal as a diagnostic test. If, however, the marker is closely linked to current or future cognitive decline, then it may be better suited as a prognostic tool. Studies of all possible biomarkers to date in AD, suggest p-tau comes the closest to the ideal diagnostic marker. However, different epitopes of p-tau may have different strengths and weaknesses. CSF p-tau231 may be most useful in distinguishing AD from frontotemporal dementia (FTD). CSF p-tau181 may improve separation between AD and LBD. In addition, CSF p-tau231 may be the most useful prognostic marker candidates that predicts cognitive decline to AD in MCI subjects.Further studies are needed to decide whether detection of multiple phosphoepitopes may allow a distinct representation of AD related pathology at different stages of the disease (Augustinack et al., 2002).

NFTs contain aberrantly hyperphosphorylated Tau as paired helical filaments. Although NFs have been shown immunohistologically to be part of NFTs, there has been debate that the identity of NF proteins in NFTs is due to the cross-reactivity of phosphorylated NF antibodies with phospho-Tau. Our laboratory recently reported (Rudrabhatla et al., 2010, 2011) the direct evidence of NFs in NFTs. Moreover, neuronal death and degeneration may release fragments of these proteins into body fluids at sufficient levels to be easily detected by specific antibodies at early, preclinical stages of AD. A battery of antibodies to NF-specific phosphoepitopes and Tau in NFTs may offer a unique approach to the design of effective early biomarkers.

The rapidly developing fields of large-scale and massive-scale genomics, proteomics, and metabolomics are now joining functional neuroimaging, structural neuroimaging, and neuropsychometric contenders in the race to establish useful biomarkers of AD and other dementing illnesses. Redox proteomics studies have provided insights into the role of oxidative stress in AD pathology. Posttranslational modifications of brain proteins, induced by oxidative damage, lead to impairment and dysfunction of several cellular functions thus providing clues about important molecular basis of neurodegeneration associated to AD. In addition, these studies have identified specific therapeutic targets in this disorder. In recent years, growing studies have been focused to establish a direct link between tissue specific oxidation and systemic oxidative damage (Blennow et al., 2010; Korolainen et al 2010; Ahmed et al., 2005; Aksenov et al., 2001). Correlations between total levels of oxidation markers in the brain and in the periphery have been shown. Although some of the reported results in AD are controversial, most of them support the presence of peripheral oxidative damage and of a characteristic panel of systemic oxidation that correlates with the occurrence of the disease. Studies investigating oxidative stress outside of the CNS, particularly in blood, while prove the occurrence of oxidative reactions, are not fully elucidating the complex cascade of events. Thus, one hypothesis is that oxidative stress first develops in the periphery as a result of different causes, and then it will contribute to perturb neuronal homeostasis, either by increasing the production of ROS or by depleting antioxidant defense, which will eventually lead to oxidative damage of the brain and neurodegeneration. The development of new plasma biomarkers could facilitate early detection, risk assessment and therapeutic monitoring in AD. On the other hand, it is also possible to imagine that oxidative stress starts in the CNS where several different metabolic end-products are formed and released into the blood stream. In this context, an important issue is to perform further studies in order to investigate the timing of appearance of oxidative damage signatures at systemic level during the onset of AD early stages and the progression to late stages.

Recently, important steps have been accomplished but there is still a lot of work to be directed towards the discovery, testing and validation of a panel of novel and old assays that could serve all the requirements for ideal biomarkers. However, the emerging trend which results from the collection of multiple data from different source is the wide variability among different studies that led to contrasting results. Thus, there is an urgent need to standardize protocols for replicate experiments on large population, which may allow to better under-standing the effect of systemic oxidative damage in the pathogenesis and progression of AD. Indeed, this is also evident by the lack of redox proteomics and microRNA studies applied to biological fluids. This approach has the power to search for specific microRNA and protein oxidative modification thus allowing the identification of altered miroRNA and protein in complex matrices such as body fluids, which may discriminate AD vs healthy condition.

There are several different reasons to support the development of more sensitive method to detect a biochemical marker in AD: to increase diagnostic accuracy; to identify MCI subjects who will progress to clinical AD; to monitor pharmacological and biological effects of drugs. There is an urgent need to add further peripheral markers of oxidative stress as useful diagnostic biomarker. There is clearly a growing interest among clinicians and basic scientists to tap on each other's expertise in the area of ageing neurobiology research. Such collaborations between geriatricians, neuroimaging specialists, neuropsychiatrists as well as molecular and cellular neurobiologists are being fostered. Further research is necessary to improve especially the early/differential biochemical diagnosis of AD. Some considerations need to be taken into account when designing future studies. These should include high numbers of relevant AD of different origin, a combination of biomarkers and other risk factors, long-term follow- up of patients and if possible neuropathological verification of the diagnosis. Standardization of methods seems critical to reducing inconsistency and increasing reliability. It is necessary to implement common protocols for sample preparation, experimental design and generation of proteomics data. Thus, global initiatives of standardization are of critical importance and large multicenter studies are needed to further define the added diagnostic value when multiple biomarker modalities are combined.

The essential goal in biomarker discovery studies is the identification of preclinical marker, which facilitates disease diagnosis at earlystages, is hoped that markers of prognosis will enable clinicians to monitor whether new candidate treatments of AD are working, effectively and inexpensively and assesses the response to treatments by the time that disease-modifying treatments become available in clinical practice.

Acknowledgement

This work is supported by NINDS/NIH intramural funds.

Author details

B.K. Binukumar and Harish C. Pant

Laboratory of Neurochemistry, NINDS, National Institutes of Health, Bethesda, Maryland, USA

References

[1] Adlard, P. A, & Vickers, J. C. (2002). Morphologically distinct plaque types differentially affect dendritic structure and organisation in the early and late stages ofAlzheimer's disease.ActaNeuropathol., 103, 377-383.

[2] Andreasen, N, Hesse, C, Davidsson, P, et al. Cerebrospinal fluid-amyloid(1-42) in Alzheimer's disease: differences between early- and late-onset Alzheimer disease and stability during the course of disease. Arch Neurol (1999). , 56, 673-80.

[3] Andreasen, N, Hesse, C, Davidsson, P, Minthon, L, & Wallin, . (1999b) Cerebrospinal fluid beta-amyloid (1-42) in Alzheimer disease: differences between early- and late-onset Alzheimer disease and stability during the course of disease. Arch Neurol 56: 673-680.

[4] Andreasen, N, Minthon, L, Clarberg, A, Davidsson, P, Gottfries, J, Vanmechelen, E, & Vanderstichele, . , specificity, and stability of CSF-tau in AD in a community-based patient sample. Neurology 53: 1488-1494

[5] Andreasen, N, Minthon, L, Clarberg, A, et al. Sensitivity, specificity and stability of CSF t-tau in AD in a community-based patient sample. Neurology (1999). , 53, 1488-94.

[6] Andreasen, N, Minthon, L, Davidsson, P, Vanmechelen, E, & Vanderstichele, . (2001) Evaluation of CSF-tau and CSF-A-beta-42 as diagnostic markers for Alzheimer disease in clinical practice. Arch Neurol 58: 373-379.

[7] Andreasen, N, Minthon, L, Vanmechelen, E, Vanderstichele, H, & Davidsson, . (1999a) Cerebrospinal fluid tau and A-beta42 as predictors of development of Alzheimer's disease in patients with mild cognitive impairment. NeurosciLett 273: 5-8.

[8] Arai, H, Higuchi, S, & Sasaki, H. and cerebrospinal fluid tau protein: implications for the clinical diagnosis of Alzheimer's disease. Gerontology , 43, 2-10.

[9] Arai, H, Terajima, M, Miura, M, et al. Tau in cerebrospinal fluid: a potential diagnostic marker in Alzheimer's disease. Ann Neurol (1995). , 38, 649-52.

[10] Azorsa, DO, Robeson, RH, Frost, D, Meechoovet, B, Brautigam, GR, & Dickey, . . 2008 . Genome-wide association analysis reveals putative Alzheimer's disease susceptibility loci in addition to APOE. Am. J. Hum. Genet.83 :623- 632.

[11] Blennow, K, & Hampel, H. (2003). Cerebrospinal fluid markers for incipient Alzheimer's disease.LancetNeurol 2003, 2(10): 605-613.

[12] Blennow, K, Vanmechelen, E, & Hampel, H. CSF total tau, A-beta42 and phosphorylated tau protein as biomarkers for Alzheimer's disease. MolNeurobiol(2002). , 24, 87-97.

[13] Blennow, K, Wallin, A, Ågren, H, Spenger, C, Siegfried, J, & Vanmechelen, E. Tau protein in cerebrospinal fluid: a biochemical diagnostic marker for axonal degeneration in Alzheimer's disease? Mol Chem Neuropathol (1995). , 26, 231-45.

[14] Blennow, K, Wallin, A, & Häger, O. Low frequency of post-lumbar puncture headache in demented patients. Acta Neurol Scand (1993). , 88, 221-23.

[15] Breno, S. O. Diniz, Jony A, Pinto Jr, Orestes Vicente Forlenz.Do CSF total tau,phosphorylated tau, and b-amyloid 42 help to predict progression of mild cognitive impairment to Alzheimer's disease? A systematic review and metaanalysis of the literature. World J Biol Psychiatry (2008). , 9, 172-82.

[16] Brunden, K. R, & Trojanowski, J. Q. Lee VMY. Advances in tau-focused drug discovery for Alzheimer's disease and related tauopathies. Nat Rev Drug Discov (2009). , 8, 783-93.

[17] Buerger, K, Teipel, S. J, Zinkowski, R, et al. CSF tau protein phosphorylated at threonine 231 correlates with cognitive decline in MCI subjects. Neurology (2002). , 59, 627-29.

[18] Buerger, K, Zinkowski, R, Teipel, S. J, Arai, H, Debernardis, J, Padberg, F, Faltraco, F, Goernitz, A, Tapiola, T, Rapoport, S. I, & Hampel, H. Differentiation of geriatric ma-

jor depression from Alzheimer's disease with CSF tau protein phosphorylated at threonine 231. Am J Psychiatry (2003). , 160, 376-379.

[19] Buerger, K, Zinkowski, R, Teipel, SJ, Tapiola, T, Arai, H, & Blennow, . .Differential-Castano EM, Roher AE, Esh CL, Kokjohn TA, Beach T. Comparative proteomics of cerebrospinal fluid in neuropathologically-confirmed Alzheimer's disease and nondemented elderly subjects. Neurol Res 2006;28:155-63.

[20] Choi, Y. S, Choe, L. H, & Lee, K. H. Recent cerebrospinal fluid biomarker studies of Alzheimer's disease.Exp Rev Proteome (2010). , 7, 919-29.

[21] Cogswell, JP, Ward, J, Taylor, IA, Waters, M, Shi, Y, Cannon, B, Kelnar, K, & Kemppainen, . .Identification of miRNA changes in Alzheimer's disease brain and CSF yields putative biomarkers and insights into disease pathways. J Alzheimers Dis 2008; 14: 27-41.

[22] Corder, E. H, Saunders, A. M, Strittmatter, W. J, Schmechel, D. E, Gaskell, P. C, Small, G. W, Roses, A. D, Haines, J. L, & Pericak-vance, M. A. (1993). Gene dose of apolipoprotein E type 4 allele and the risk of Alzheimer's disease in late onset families. Science ., 261, 921-923.

[23] Butterfield, D. A, & Bader, M. L. Lange, R. Sultana, Involvements of the lipid peroxidation product, HNE, in the pathogenesis and progression of Alzheimer's disease,Biochim. Biophys.Acta (2010). , 1801(2010), 924-929.

[24] Butterfield, D. A, Reed, T, Newman, S. F, & Sultana, R. Roles of amyloid beta-peptideassociated oxidative stress and brain protein modifications in the pathogenesis of Alzheimer's disease and mild cognitive impairment, Free Radic. Biol. Med. (2007). , 43(2007), 658-677.

[25] De Meyer, G, Shapiro, F, Vanderstichele, H, Vanmechelen, E, Engelborghs, S, De Deyn, P. P, et al. For the Alzheimer's disease neuroimaging initiative.Diagnosis-independent Alzheimer disease biomarker signature in cognitively normalelderly people. Arch Neurol (2010). , 67, 949-56.

[26] Engelborghs, S, & De Vreese, K. Van de Casteele T, Vanderstichele H, Van Everbroeck B, Cras P, Martin J-J, Vanmechelen E, De Deyn PP. Diagnostic performance of a CSF-biomarker panel in autopsy-confirmed dementia. Neurobiol Aging (2008). , 29, 1143-59.

[27] Song, F, Poljak, A, Smythe, G. A, & Sachdev, P. Plasma biomarkers for mild cognitive impairment and Alzheimer's disease, Brain Res. Rev. (2009). , 61(2009), 69-80.

[28] Fagan, A. M, Mintun, M. A, Shah, A. R, Alde, P, & Roe, C. M. Cerebrospinal fluid tau and ptau181 increase with cortical amyloid deposition in cognitively normal individuals: implications for future clinical trials of Alzheimer's disease.EMBOMol Med (2009). , 1, 371-80.

[29] Farrer, L. A, Cupples, L. A, Haines, J. L, Hyman, B, Kukull, W. A, Mayeux, R, Myers, R. H, & Pericak-vance, M. A. (1997). Effects of age, sex, and ethnicity on the associa-

tion betweenapolipoprotein E genotype and Alzheimer disease.A meta-analysis.APOE and Alzheimer Disease Meta AnalysisConsortium.J. Am. Med. Assoc., 278, 1349-1356.

[30] Fenton, G, Steffen, M, Sugarbaker, E, Miller, K, Swit, B, Green, P, & Charlton, R. (1994). The lumbar puncture- factors affecting success rate. Ann Neurol , 36(3), 544-545.

[31] Finehout, E. J, Franck, Z, Choe, L. H, Relkin, N, & Lee, K. H. Cerebrospinal fluid proteomic biomarkers for Alzheimer's disease. Ann Neurol (2007). , 61, 120-9.

[32] Fink, J. K, Jones, S. M, Esposito, C, & Wilkowski, J. (1996). Human microtubule-associated protein 1a (MAP1A) gene: genomic organization, cDNA sequence, anddevelopmental- andtissue-specific expression. Genomics , 35, 577-585.

[33] Fratiglioni, L, De Ronchi, D, & Agüero-torres, H. (1999). Worldwide prevalence and incidence of dementia.Drugs Aging. , 15(5), 365-75.

[34] Galasko, D, Chang, L, Motter, R, Clark, CM, Kaye, J, Knopman, D, Thomas, R, & Kholodenko, . . High cerebrospinal fluid tau and low amyloid-beta-42 levels in the clinical diagnosisof Alzheimer disease and relation to apolipoprotein E genotype. Arch Neurol 1998; 55: 937-945.

[35] Galasko, D, Clark, C, Chang, L, Miller, B, Green, R. C, Rotter, R, & Seubert, O. Assessment of CSF levels of tau protein in mildly demented patients with Alzheimer's disease. Neurology(1997). , 48, 632-635.

[36] Giannakakis, A, Coukos, G, Hatzigeorgiou, A, & Sandaltzopoulos, R. Zhang L: miRNA genetic alterations in human cancers. Expert OpinBiolTher (2007). , 7, 1375-1386.

[37] Gonzalez-billault, C, Jimenez-mateos, E. M, Caceres, A, Diaz-nido, J, & Avila, J. (2004). Microtubule-associated protein 1B function during normal development, regeneration, and pathological conditions in the nervous system. J Neurobiol. , 58(1), 48-59.

[38] Greco, S. J, Sarkar, S, Johnston, J. M, & Tezapsidis, N. Leptin regulates tau phosphorylation and amyloid through AMPK in neuronal cells. BiochemBiophys Res Commun (2009). , 380, 98-104.

[39] Tohgi, H, Abe, T, Yamazaki, K, Murata, T, Isobe, C, & Ishizaki, E. The cerebrospinal fluid oxidized NO metabolites, nitrite and nitrate, in Alzheimer's disease and vasculardementia of Binswanger type and multiple small infarct type, J. Neural Transm. (1998). , 105(1998), 1283-1291.

[40] Tohgi, H, Abe, T, Yamazaki, K, Murata, T, Ishizaki, E, & Isobe, C. Alterations of 3-nitrotyrosine concentration in the cerebrospinal fluid during aging and in patients with Alzheimer's disease, Neurosci. Lett. (1999). , 269(1999), 52-54.

[41] Frey, H. J, Mattila, K. M, Korolainen, M. A, & Pirttila, T. Problems associated with biological markers of Alzheimer's disease, Neurochem. Res. (2005). , 30(2005), 1501-1510.

[42] Hampel, H, Buerger, K, Zinkowski, R, Teipel, S. J, Goernitz, A, Andreasen, N, et al. Measurement of phosphorylated tau epitopes in the differential diagnosis of Alzheimer disease: a comparative cerebrospinal fluid study. Arch Gen Psychiatry (2004). , 61, 95-102.

[43] Hampel, H, Ornitz, G, & Urger, A, B. K ((2003). Advances in the development of biomarkers for Alzheimer's disease: from CSF total tau and Ab1-42 proteins to phosphorylated tau protein. Brain Res Bull , 61(3), 243-253.

[44] Hampel, H, Mitchell, A, Blennow, K, Frank, R. A, Brettschneider, S, Weller, L, & Möller, H. J. Core biological marker candidates of Alzheimer's disease- perspectives for diagnosis, predictionof outcome and reflection of biological activity.J Neural Transm. (2004). , 2004(111), 3-247.

[45] Han, X, & Gross, R. W. (2003). Global analyses of cellular lipidomes directly from crude extracts of biological samples by ESI mass spectrometry: a bridge to lipidomics.J. Lipid Res. , 44, 1071-1079.

[46] Han, X, & Gross, R. W. (2005). Shotgun lipidomics: electrospray ionization mass spectrometric analysis and quantitation of cellular lipidomes directly from crude extracts of biological samples. Mass Spectrom. Rev. , 24, 367-412.

[47] Han, X, Rozen, S, Boyle, S. H, Hellegers, C, Cheng, H, & Burke, J. R. Kaddurah-Daouk RMetabolomics in early Alzheimer's disease: identification of altered plasma sphingolipidome usingshotgun lipidomics. PLoS One. (2011). e21643.

[48] Hanger, D. P, Anderton, B. H, & Noble, W. Tau phosphorylation: the therapeutic challenge for neurodegenerative disease. Trends Mol Med (2009). , 15, 112-9.

[49] Hanger, D. P, Byers, H. L, Wray, S, Leung, K. Y, Saxton, M. J, Seereeram, A, et al. Novel phosphorylation sites in tau from Alzheimer brain support a role for casein kinase 1 in disease pathogenesis. J BiolChem (2007). , 282, 23645-54.

[50] Hansson, O, Zetterberg, H, Buchhave, P, Londos, E, Blennow, K, & Minthon, . .Association between CSF biomarkers and incipient Alzheimer's disease in patients with mild cognitive impairment: a follow-up study. Lancet Neurol 2006;5:228-34.

[51] HaraldHampelGordon Wilcock , Sandrine Andrieu , Paul Aisen f, KajBlennow , K. Broich Maria Carrillo , Nick C. Foxj, Giovanni B. Frisoni. Biomarkers for Alzheimer's disease therapeutic trials. Progress in Neurobiology 95 ((2011).

[52] Hébert, SS, Horré, K, Nicolaï, L, Papadopoulou, AS, Mandemakers, W, & Silahtaroglu, . , De Strooper B: Loss of microRNA cluster miR-29a/b-1 insporadic Alzheimer's disease correlates with increased BACE1/beta-secretaseexpressionProcNatlAcadSci USA 2008; 105: 6415-6420.

[53] Hernandez, F, & Avila, J. Tauopathies.Mol Life Sci (2007). Bartosik-Psujek H, Stelma-
      siak Z. The CSF levels of total-tau and phosphotau in patients with relapsing-remit-
      ting multiple sclerosis. J Neural Trans 2006;113:339-45., 64, 2219-33.

[54] Hu, C R, Van Der Heijden, M, Wang, J, Van Der Greef, T, & Hankemeier, G. Xu .
      (2009). Analytical strategies in lipidomics and applications in disease biomarker dis-
      covery.J. Chromatogr. B Analyt.Technol. Biomed. Life Sci. , 877, 2836-2846.

[55] Hu, Y. Y, He, S. S, Wang, X, et al. Levels of nonphosphorylated and phosphorylated
      tau in cerebrospinal fluid of Alzheimer's disease patients: an ultrasensitive bien-
      zyme-substrate-recycle enzyme-linked immunosorbent assay. Am J Pathol (2002). ,
      160, 1269-78.

[56] Hulstaert, F, Blennow, K, Ivanoiu, A, Schoonderwaldt, HC, Riemenschneider, M, &
      De Deyn, . (1999) Improved discrimination of AD patients using beta-amyloid (1-42)
      and tau levels in CSF. Neurology 52: 1555-1562.

[57] Hye, A, Lynham, S, Thambisetty, M, Causevic, M, Campbell, J, Byers, H. L, Hooper,
      C, Rijsdijk, F, Tabrizi, S. J, Banner, S, et al. (2006). Proteome-based plasma biomarkers
      for Alzheimer's disease.Brain ., 129, 3042-3050.

[58] Hyman, B. T, & Trojanowski, J. Q. Consensus recommendations for the postmortem
      diagnosis of Alzheimer disease from the National Institute on Aging and the Reagan
      InstituteWorking Group on diagnostic criteria for the neuropathological assessment
      of Alzheimer disease. J NeuropatholExpNeurol.(1997). , 56, 1095-1097.

[59] Iqbal, K, Alonso, A. C, Gong, C. X, Khatoon, S, Pei, J. J, Wang, J. Z, & Grundke-iqbal,
      I. (1998). Mechanisms of neurofibrillary degeneration and the formation of neurofi-
      brillary tangles. J Neural Transm [Suppl] , 53, 169-180.

[60] Iqbal, K, Liu, F, Gong, C-X, Alonso, A. D, & Grundke-iqbal, I. Mechanisms of tauin-
      ducedneurodegeneration. ActaNeuopathol (2010). , 118, 53-69.

[61] Iqbal, K, Grundke-iqbal, I, Zaidi, T, Merz, P. A, Wen, G. Y, & Shaikh, S. S. (1986). De-
      fetive brain microtubule assembly in Alzheimer's diseases.. Lancet , 2, 421-426.

[62] Ishiguro, K, Ohno, H, Arai, H, et al. Phosphorylated tau in human cerebrospinal flu-
      id is a diagnostic marker for Alzheimer's disease. Neurosci Lett (1999). , 270, 91-94.

[63] Itoh, N, Arai, H, Urakami, K, et al. Large-scale, multicenter study of cerebrospinal
      fluid tau protein phosphorylated at serine 199 for the antemortem diagnosis of Alz-
      heimer's disease. Ann Neurol (2001). , 50, 150-56.

[64] Choi, J, Malakowsky, C. A, Talent, J. M, Conrad, C. C, & Gracy, R. W. Identification
      of oxidized plasma proteins in Alzheimer's disease, Biochem. Biophys. Res. Com-
      mun.(2002). , 293(2002), 1566-1570.

[65] Choi, J, Forster, M. J, Mcdonald, S. R, Weintraub, S. T, Carroll, C. A, & Gracy, R. W. Proteomic identification of specific oxidized proteins in ApoE-knockout mice: relevance to Alzheimer's disease, Free Radic. Biol. Med. (2004). , 36(2004), 1155-1162.

[66] Raber, J, Huang, Y, & Ashford, J. W. ApoE genotype accounts for the vast majority of AD risk and AD pathology, Neurobiol. Aging (2004). , 25(2004), 641-650.

[67] Jack Jr CRWiste HJ, Vemuri P, Weigand SD, Senjem ML, Zeng G, et al. Brain beta-amyloid measures and magnetic resonance imaging atrophy both predict time-to-progression from mild cognitive impairment to Alzheimer's disease. Brain (2010). , 133, 3336-48.

[68] Blennow, K, Hampel, H, Weiner, M, & Zetterberg, H. Cerebrospinal fluid and plasma biomarkers in Alzheimer disease, Nat. Rev. Neurol. (2010). , 6(2010), 131-144.

[69] Kahle, P. J, Jakowec, M, Teipel, S. J, et al. Combined assessment of tau and neuronal thread protein in Alzheimer's disease CSF. Neurology (2000). , 54, 1498-504.

[70] Kanai, M, Matsubara, E, Isoe, K, et al. Longitudinal study of cerebrospinal fluid levels of tau, A beta1-40, and A beta1-42(43) in Alzheimer's disease: a study in Japan. Ann Neurol (1998). , 44, 17-26.

[71] Kanai, M, Matsubara, E, Isoe, K, Urakami, K, Nakashima, K, Arai, H, Sasaki, H, Abe, K, & Iwatsubo, . , (1998) Longitudinal study of cerebrospinal fluid levels of tau, A-beta1-40,and A-beta1-42(43) in Alzheimer's disease: a study in Japan. Ann Neurol 44: 17-26.

[72] Kapaki, E K. K, Paraskevas, G. P, Michalopoulou, M, & Patsouris, E. (2001). Highly increased CSFtau protein and decreased beta-amyloid (1-42) in sporadic CJD: a discrimination from Alzheimer's disease? J NeurolNeurosurg Psychiatry , 71, 401-403.

[73] Kauwe JSKWang J, Mayo K, Morris JC, Anne M, Fagan AM, et al. Alzheimer's disease risk variants show association with cerebrospinal fluid amyloid beta. Neurogenetics (2009). , 10, 13-7.

[74] Knopman, D. S, Dekosky, S. T, Cummings, J. L, Chui, H, Corey-bloom, J, Relkin, N, Small, G. W, Miller, B, & Stevens, J. C. (2001). Practice parameter: diagnosis of dementia (an evidence-based review)- Report of the Quality Standards Subcommittee of the American Academy of Neurology. Neurology , 56(9), 1143-1153.

[75] Kochanek, P. M, Berger, R. P, Bayir, H, Wagner, A. K, Jenkins, L. W, & Clark, R. S. (2008). Biomarkers of primary and evolving damage in traumatic and ischemic brain injury: diagnosis, prognosis, probing mechanisms, and therapeutic decision making. Curr.Opin.Crit. Care ., 14, 135-141.

[76] Kohnken, R, Buerger, K, Zinkowski, R, et al. Detection of tau phosphorylated at threonine 231 in cerebrospinal fluid of Alzheimer's disease patients. Neurosci Lett (2000). , 287, 187-90.

[77] Kosik, K. S, Duffy, L. K, Dowling, M. M, Abraham, C, Mccluskey, A, & Selkoe, D. J. (1984). Microtubule-associated protein 2: monoclonal antibodies demonstrate the selective incorporation of certain epitopes into Alzheimer neurofibrillary tangles.Proc-NatlAcad:, 7941-7945.

[78] Kurz, A, Riemenschneider, M, Buch, K, Willoch, F, Bartenstein, P, Muller, U, & Guder, W. (1998). Tau protein in cerebrospinal fluid is significantly increased at the earliest clinical stage of Alzheimer disease. Alzheimer Dis AssocDisord , 12, 372-377.

[79] Lee, R. C, & Feinbaum, R. L. Ambros V: The C. elegansheterochronic gene lin-4 encodes small RNAs with antisense complementarity to lin-14. Cell (1993). , 75, 843-854.

[80] Lewczuk, P, Esselmann, H, Bibl, M, Beck, G, Maler, J. M, Otto, M, et al. Tau protein phosphorylated at threonine 181 in CSF as a neurochemical biomarker in Alzheimer's disease. Original data and review of the literature.JMolNeurosci (2004). , 23, 115-22.

[81] Lukiw, W. J, & Zhao, Y. Cui JG: An NF-kB-sensitive micro RNA-146a-mediated inflammatory circuit in Alzheimer disease and in stressed human brain cells. J Biol-Chem (2008). , 283, 31315-31322.

[82] Lukiw WJ: Micro-RNA speciation in fetaladult and Alzheimer's disease hippocampus.Neuroreport (2007). , 18, 297-300.

[83] Ikeda, M, Sato, I, Yuasa, T, Miyatake, T, & Murota, S. Nitrite, nitrate and cGMP in the cerebrospinal fluid in degenerative neurologic diseases, J. Neural Transm. Gen. Sect. (1995). , 100(1995), 263-267.

[84] Korolainen, M. A, & Pirttila, T. Cerebrospinal fluid, serum and plasma protein oxidation in Alzheimer's disease, Acta Neurol. Scand. (2009). , 119(2009), 32-38.

[85] Korolainen, M. A, Nyman, T. A, Aittokallio, T, & Pirttila, T. An update on clinical proteomics in Alzheimer's research, J. Neurochem. (2010). , 112(2010), 1386-1414.

[86] Kuiper, M. A, Visser, J. J, Bergmans, P. L, Scheltens, P, & Wolters, E. C. Decreased cerebrospinal fluid nitrate levels in Parkinson's disease, Alzheimer's disease and multiple system atrophy patients, J. Neurol. Sci. (1994). , 121(1994), 46-49.

[87] Lovell, M. A, Ehmann, W. D, Butler, S. M, & Markesbery, W. R. Elevated thiobarbituric acid-reactive substances and antioxidant enzyme activity in the brain in Alzheimer's disease, Neurology (1995). , 45(1995), 1594-1601.

[88] Prasad, M. R, Lovell, M. A, Yatin, M, Dhillon, H, & Markesbery, W. R. Regional membrane phospholipid alterations in Alzheimer's disease, Neurochem. Res. (1998). , 23(1998), 81-88.

[89] Aksenov, M. Y, Aksenova, M. V, Butterfield, D. A, Geddes, J. W, & Markesbery, W. R. Protein oxidation in the brain in Alzheimer's disease, Neuroscience (2001). , 103(2001), 373-383.

[90] Maarouf, C. L, Andacht, T. M, Kokjohn, T. A, Castan, o E. M, Sue, L. I, Beach, T. G, et al. Proteomic analysis of Alzheimer's disease cerebrospinal fluid from neuropathologically diagnosed subjects.Curr Alzheimer Res (2009). , 6, 399-406.

[91] Makeyev, E. V. Maniatis T: Multilevel regulation of gene expression by microRNAs. Science (2008). Gao FB: Posttranscriptional control of neuronal development by microRNA networks. Nat Med 2007; 13: 1359-1362., 319, 1789-1790.

[92] Maruyama, M, Arai, H, Sugita, M, Tanji, H, Higuchi, M, Okamura, N, Matsui, T, Higuchi, S, Matsushita, S, Yoshida, H, & Sasaki, H. (2001). Cerebrospinal fluid amyloid beta(1-42) levelsin the mild cognitive impairment stage of Alzheimer's disease. ExpNeurol , 172, 433-436.

[93] Mattsson, N, Zetterberg, H, Hansson, O, Andreasen, N, Parnetti, L, Jonsson, M, et al. CSF biomarkers and incipient Alzheimer disease in patients with mild cognitive impairment. J Am Med Assoc (2009). , 302, 385-93.

[94] Mazanetz, M. P, & Fischer, P. M. Untangling tau hyperphosphorylation in drug design for neurodegenerative diseases. Nat Rev Drug Discov (2007). , 6, 464-79.

[95] Mckhann, G, Drachman, D, Folstein, M, Katzman, R, Price, D, & Stadlan, E. M. (1984). Clinical diagnosis of Alzheimer's disease: report of the NINCDS-ADRDA Work Group under the auspices of the Department of Health and Human Services Task Force on Alzheimer's disease. Neurology , 34, 939-944.

[96] Mihaescu, R, Detmar, S. B, Cornel, M. C, Van Der Flier, W. M, Heutink, P, Hol, E. M, et al. Translational research in genomics of Alzheimer's disease: a review of current practice and future perspectives. J Alzheimer Dis (2010). , 20, 967-80.

[97] Miller, G. Alzheimer's biomarker initiative hits its stride. Science (2009). , 326, 386-9.

[98] Ahmed, N, Ahmed, U, Thornalley, P. J, Hager, K, Fleischer, G, & Munch, G. Protein glycation, oxidation and nitration adduct residues and free adducts of cerebrospinal fluid in Alzheimer's disease and link to cognitive impairment, J. Neurochem.(2005). , 92(2005), 255-263.

[99] Nieto, A. Montejo de Garcini, E., and Avila, J. ((1989). Altered levels of microtubule-proteins in brains of Alzheimer's disease patients.ActaNeuropathol., 78, 47-51.

[100] Nishimura, T, Takeda, M, Nakamura, Y, et al. Basic and clinical studies on the measurement of tau protein in cerebrospinal fluid as a biological marker for Alzheimer's disease and related disorders: multicenter study in Japan. Methods Find Exp Clin Pharmacol (1998). , 20, 227-35.

[101] Okamura, N, Arai, H, Higuchi, M, Tashiro, M, Matsui, T, Itoh, M, Iwatsubo, T, Tomita, T, & Sasaki, H. (1999). Cerebrospinal fluid levels of amyloid beta-peptide 1-42, but not tau have positive correlation with brain glucose metabolism in humans. NeurosciLett , 273, 203-207.

[102] Olson, L, & Humpel, C. Growth factors and cytokines/chemokines as surrogate bio-markers in cerebrospinal fluid and blood for diagnosing Alzheimer's disease and mild cognitive impairment. ExpGerentol (2010). , 45, 41-6.

[103] Otto, M, Esselmann, H, Schulz-Shaeffer, W, Neumann, M, Schroter, A, Ratzka, P, Cepek, L, & Zerr, . (2000) Decreased beta-amyloid 1-42 in cerebrospinal fluid of patients with Creutzfeldt-Jakob disease. Neurology 54: 1099-1102

[104] Papassotiropoulos, A, Fountoulakis, M, Dunckley, T, & Stephan, D. A. Reiman EM Genetics, transcriptomics, and proteomics of Alzheimer's disease. J Clin Psychiatry (2006). , 67, 652-70.

[105] Parnetti, L, Lanari, A, Amici, S, Gallai, V, Vanmechelen, E, & Hulstaert, F. CSF phosphorylated tau is a possible marker for discriminating Alzheimer's disease from dementia with Lewy bodies. Phospho-Tau International Study Group. Neurol Sci (2001). , 22, 77-78.

[106] Sultana, R, Perluigi, M, & Butterfield, D. A. Protein oxidation and lipid peroxidation in brain of subjects with Alzheimer's disease: insights into mechanism of neurodegeneration from redox proteomics, Antioxid. Redox Signal. (2006). , 8(2006), 2021-2037.

[107] Mark, R. J, Fuson, K. S, & May, P. C. Characterization of 8-epiprostaglandin F2alpha as a marker of amyloid beta-peptide-induced oxidative damage, J. Neurochem. (1999). , 72(1999), 1146-1153.

[108] Nitsch, R. M, Blusztajn, J. K, Pittas, A. G, Slack, B. E, Growdon, J. H, & Wurtman, R. J. Evidence for a membrane defect in Alzheimer disease brain, Proc. Natl. Acad. Sci. U.S. A. (1992). , 89(1992), 1671-1675.

[109] Ray, S, Britschgi, M, Herbert, C, Takeda-uchimura, Y, Boxer, A, Blennow, K, Friedman, L. F, Galasko, D. R, Jutel, M, Karydas, A, Kaye, J. A, Leszek, J, Miller, B. L, Minthon, L, Quinn, J. F, Rabinovici, G. D, & Robinson, W. H. Classification and prediction of clinical Alzheimer's diagnosis based on plasma signaling proteins. Nat Med (2007). , 13, 1359-1362.

[110] Reddy, M. M, Wilson, R, Wilson, J, Connell, S, Gocke, A, Hynan, L, et al. Identification of candidate IgG biomarkers for Alzheimer's disease via combinatorial library screening. Cell (2011). , 144, 132-42.

[111] Riemenschneider, M, Buch, K, Schmolke, M, Kurz, A, & Guder, . (1997) Diagnosis of Alzheimer's disease with cerebrospinal fluid tau protein and aspartate aminotransferase. Lancet 350: 784.

[112] Riemenschneider, M, Buch, K, Schmolke, M, Kurz, A, & Guder, W. G. Cerebrospinal protein tau is elevated in early Alzheimer's disease. Neurosci Lett (1996). , 212, 209-11.

[113] Riemenschneider, M, Wagenpfeil, S, Diehl, J, et al. Tau and Abeta42 protein in CSF of patients with frontotemporal degeneration. Neurology (2002). , 58, 1622-28.

[114] Rosenson, R. S. (2010). New technologies personalize diagnostics and therapeutics. Curr.Atheroscler. Rep. , 12, 184-186.

[115] Ross, C. A, & Poirier, M. A. (2004). Protein aggregation and neurodegenerative disease.Nat. Med. 10 (Suppl.): , 10-17.

[116] Rudrabhatla, P, Grant, P, Jaffe, H, & Strong, M. J. Pant HCQuantitativephosphoproteomic analysis of neuronal intermediate filament proteins (NF-M/H) in Alzheimer's disease by iTRAQ.FASEB J. (2010). , 2010(11), 4396-407.

[117] Rudrabhatla, P, & Pant, H. C. Phosphorylation-specific peptidyl-prolyl isomerization of neuronal cytoskeletal proteins by Pin1: implications for therapeutics in neurodegeneration.JAlzheimers Dis. (2010). , 19(2), 389-403.

[118] Newman, S. F, Sultana, R, Perluigi, M, Coccia, R, Cai, J, Pierce, W. M, Klein, J. B, Turner, D. M, & Butterfield, D. A. An increase in S-glutathionylated proteins in the Alzheimer'sdisease inferior parietal lobule, a proteomics approach, J. Neurosci. Res. (2007). , 85(2007), 1506-1514.

[119] Herukka, S. K, Helisalmi, S, Hallikainen, M, Tervo, S, Soininen, H, & Pirttila, T. CSF Abeta42, Tau and phosphorylated Tau, APOE epsilon4 allele and MCI type in progressive MCI, Neurobiol. Aging (2007). , 28(2007), 507-514.

[120] Samuels, S. C S. J, Marin, D. B, Peskind, E. R, Younki, S. G, Greenberg, D. A, Schnur, E, Santoro, J, & Davis, K. L. (1999). CSF beta-amyloid, cognition, and APOE genotype in Alzheimer's disease.Neurology , 52, 547-551.

[121] Sanchez, C, Diaz-nido, J, & Avila, J. (2000). Phosphorylation of microtubule-associated protein 2 (MAP2) and its relevance for the regulation of the neuronal cytoskeleton function.ProgNeurobiol.;, 61(2), 133-68.

[122] Sato, Y, Nakamura, T, Aoshima, K, & Oda, Y. (2010). Quantitative and wide-ranging profi ling of phospholipids in human plasma by two-dimensional liquid hromatography/mass spectrometry. Anal. Chem. , 82, 9858-9864.

[123] Sato, Y, Suzuki, I, Nakamura, T, Bernier, F, Aoshima, K, & Oda, Y. Identification of a new plasma biomarker of Alzheimer's disease using metabolomics technology.J Lipid Res. (2012). Mar;, 53(3), 567-76.

[124] Schönknecht, P, Pantel, J, Hunt, A, et al. Levels of total tau and tau protein phosphorylated at threonine 181 in patients with incipient and manifest Alzheimer's disease. Neurosci Lett (2003). , 339, 172-74.

[125] Schonrock, N, Ke, Y. D, Humphreys, D, Staufenbiel, M, Ittner, L. M, & Preiss, T. Götz J: Neuronal microRNA deregulation in response to Alzheimer's disease amyloid-beta. PLoS One (2010). e11070.

[126] Sethi, P. Lukiw WJ: Micro-RNA abundance and stability in human brain: specific alterations in Alzheimer's disease temporal lobe neocortex. NeurosciLett (2009). , 459, 100-104.

[127] Shaw, L. M, Vanderstichele, H, Knapik-czajka, M, Clark, C. M, Aisen, P. S, Petersen, R. C, et al. Cerebrospinal fluid biomarker signature in Alzheimer's disease neuroimaging initiative studies. Ann Neurol (2009). , 65, 403-13.

[128] Shoji, M, Matsubara, E, Kanai, M, et al. Combination assay of CSF tau, A beta 1-40 and A beta 1-42(43) as a biochemical marker of Alzheimer's disease. J Neurol Sci (1998). , 158, 134-40.

[129] Shoji, M, Matsubara, E, Murakami, T, et al. Cerebrospinal fluid tau in dementia disorders: a large scale multicenter study by a Japanese study group. Neurobiol Aging (2002). , 23, 363-70.

[130] Sjögren, M, Davidsson, P, Gottfries, J, et al. The cerebrospinal fluid levels of tau, growth-associated protein-43 and soluble amyloid precursor protein correlate in Alzheimer's disease, reflecting a common pathophysiological process. Dement Geriatr Cogn Disord (2001). , 12, 257-64.

[131] Sjogren, M, Davidsson, P, Tullberg, M, Minthon, L, Wallin, A, Wikkelso, C, & Granerus, . (2001b) Both total and phosphorylated tau are increased in Alzheimer's disease. J NeurolNeurosurg Psychiatry 70: 624-630.

[132] Sjögren, M, Davidsson, P, Wallin, A, et al. Decreased CSF-amyloid42 in Alzheimer's disease and amyotrophic lateral sclerosis may reflect mismetabolism of-amyloid induced by separate mechanisms. Dementia Geriatr Cogn Disord (2002). , 13, 112-18.

[133] Sjogren, M, Minthon, L, Davidsson, P, Granerus, A. K, Clarberg, A, Vanderstichele, H, Vanmechelen, E, Wallin, A, & Blennow, K. (2000a). CSF levels of tau, beta-amyloid(1-42) and GAP-43 in frontotemporal dementia, other types of dementia and normal aging. J Neural Transm , 107, 563-579.

[134] Steinberg, D. (2005). Thematic review series: the pathogenesis of atherosclerosis.An interpretive history of the cholesterol controversy: part II: the early evidence linking hypercholesterolemia to coronary disease in humans. J. Lipid Res. , 46, 179-190.

[135] Strittmatter, W. J, Saunders, A. M, Schmechel, D, Pericak-vance, M, Enghild, J, Salvesen, G. S, & Roses, A. D. (1993). Apolipoprotein E: high-avidity binding to beta-amyloid and increased frequency of type 4 allele in late-onset familial Alzheimer disease. Proc. Natl.Acad. Sci. USA ., 90, 1977-1981.

[136] Sunderland, T, Linker, G, Mirza, N, Putnam, K. T, Friedman, D. L, Kimmel, L. H, Bergeson, J, Manetti, G. J, Zimmermann, M, Tang, B, Bartko, J. J, & Cohen, R. M. and increased Tau levels in cerebrospinal fluid of patients with Alzheimer disease. JAMA , 289(16), 2094-2103.

[137] Swardfager, W, Lanctot, K, Rothenburg, L, Wong, A, Cappell, J, & Hermann, N. A met-analysis of cytokines in Alzheimer's disease.Biol Psychiatry (2010). , 68, 930-41.

[138] Montine, T. J, Neely, M. D, Quinn, J. F, Beal, M. F, Markesbery, W. R, Roberts, L. J, & Morrow, J. D. Lipid peroxidation in aging brain and Alzheimer's disease, Free Rad-ic.Biol. Med. (2002). , 33(2002), 620-626.

[139] Stief, T. W, Marx, R, & Heimburger, N. Oxidized fibrin(ogen) derivatives enhance the activity of tissue type plasminogen activator, Thromb. Res. (1989). , 56(1989), 221-228.

[140] Takahashi, H, Hirokawa, K, Ando, S, & Obata, K. (1991). Immunohistological study on brains of Alzheimer's disease using antibodies to fetal antigens, C-series ganglio-sides and microtubule-associated protein 5.ActaNeuropathol., 81, 626-631.

[141] Tapiola, T, Lehtovirta, M, Ramberg, J, et al. CSF tau is related to apolipoprotein E genotype in early Alzheimer's disease. Neurology (1998). , 50, 169-74.

[142] Tapiola, T, Pirttil, a T, Mehta, P. D, Alafuzoff, I, Lehtovirta, M, & Soininen, H. (2000). Relationship between apoE genotype and CSF beta-amyloid (1-42) and tau in pa-tients with probable and definite Alzheimer's disease. Neurobiol Aging , 21, 735-740.

[143] Thambisetty, M, Simmons, A, Velayudhan, L, Hye, A, Campbell, J, Zhang, Y, et al. Association of plasma clusterin concentration with severity, pathology, and progres-sion in Alzheimer disease. Arch Gen Psychiatry (2010). , 67, 739-48.

[144] The Ronald and Nancy Reagan Research Institute of the Alzheimer's Association and the National Institute on Aging Working Group ((1998). Consensus report of the Working Group on: Molecular and Biochemical Markers of Alzheimer's Disease-Neurobiol Aging , 19, 109-116.

[145] Vandermeeren, M, Mercken, M, Vanmechelen, E, & Six, J. van de Voorde A, Martin JJ, Cras P. Detection of tau proteins in normal and Alzheimer's disease cerebrospinal fluid with a sensitive sandwich enzyme-linked immunosorbent assay. J Neurochem (1993). , 61, 1828-1834.

[146] Markesbery, W. R, & Lovell, M. A. Four-hydroxynonenal, a product of lipid peroxi-dation, is increased in the brain in Alzheimer's disease, Neurobiol. Aging (1998). , 19(1998), 33-36.

[147] Wang, W. X, Rajeev, B. W, Stromberg, A. J, Ren, N, Tang, G, Huang, Q, & Rigoutsos, I. Nelson PT:The expression of microRNA miR-107 decreases early in Alzheimer's disease and may accelerate disease progression through regulation of beta-site amy-loid precursor protein-cleaving enzyme 1. J Neurosci (2008). , 28, 1213-1223.

[148] Ward, M. Biomarkers for Alzheimer's disease. Expert Rev. Mol. Diagn.(2007). , 7, 635-646.

[149] Watson, A. D. Thematic review series: systems biology approaches to metabolic and cardiovascular disorders. Lipidomics: a global approach to lipid analysis in biological systems. J. Lipid Res.(2006)., 47, 2101-2111.

[150] Wenk, M. R. The emerging fi eld of lipidomics.Nat. Rev. Drug Discov(2005)., 4, 594-610.

[151] Wilcoxen, K. M, Uehara, T, Myint, T. T, Sato, Y, & Oda, Y. Practical metabolomics in drug discovery.Expert Opinion on Drug Discovery(2010)., 5, 249-263.

[152] Zhang, J, Goodlett, D. R, Quinn, J. F, Peskind, E, Kaye, J. A, Zhou, Y, et al. Quantitative proteomics of cerebrospinal fluid from patients with Alzheimer disease. J Alzheimers Dis (2005)., 7, 125-33.

Permissions

The contributors of this book come from diverse backgrounds, making this book a truly international effort. This book will bring forth new frontiers with its revolutionizing research information and detailed analysis of the nascent developments around the world.

We would like to thank Inga Zerr, MD, for lending her expertise to make the book truly unique. She has played a crucial role in the development of this book. Without her invaluable contribution this book wouldn't have been possible. She has made vital efforts to compile up to date information on the varied aspects of this subject to make this book a valuable addition to the collection of many professionals and students.

This book was conceptualized with the vision of imparting up-to-date information and advanced data in this field. To ensure the same, a matchless editorial board was set up. Every individual on the board went through rigorous rounds of assessment to prove their worth. After which they invested a large part of their time researching and compiling the most relevant data for our readers. Conferences and sessions were held from time to time between the editorial board and the contributing authors to present the data in the most comprehensible form. The editorial team has worked tirelessly to provide valuable and valid information to help people across the globe.

Every chapter published in this book has been scrutinized by our experts. Their significance has been extensively debated. The topics covered herein carry significant findings which will fuel the growth of the discipline. They may even be implemented as practical applications or may be referred to as a beginning point for another development. Chapters in this book were first published by InTech; hereby published with permission under the Creative Commons Attribution License or equivalent.

The editorial board has been involved in producing this book since its inception. They have spent rigorous hours researching and exploring the diverse topics which have resulted in the successful publishing of this book. They have passed on their knowledge of decades through this book. To expedite this challenging task, the publisher supported the team at every step. A small team of assistant editors was also appointed to further simplify the editing procedure and attain best results for the readers.

Our editorial team has been hand-picked from every corner of the world. Their multi-ethnicity adds dynamic inputs to the discussions which result in innovative outcomes. These outcomes are then further discussed with the researchers and contributors who give their valuable feedback and opinion regarding the same. The feedback is then collaborated with the researches and they are edited in a comprehensive manner to aid the understanding of the subject.

Apart from the editorial board, the designing team has also invested a significant amount of their time in understanding the subject and creating the most relevant covers. They scrutinized every image to scout for the most suitable representation of the subject and create an appropriate cover for the book.

The publishing team has been involved in this book since its early stages. They were actively engaged in every process, be it collecting the data, connecting with the contributors or procuring relevant information. The team has been an ardent support to the editorial, designing and production team. Their endless efforts to recruit the best for this project, has resulted in the accomplishment of this book. They are a veteran in the field of academics and their pool of knowledge is as vast as their experience in printing. Their expertise and guidance has proved useful at every step. Their uncompromising quality standards have made this book an exceptional effort. Their encouragement from time to time has been an inspiration for everyone.

The publisher and the editorial board hope that this book will prove to be a valuable piece of knowledge for researchers, students, practitioners and scholars across the globe.

List of Contributors

Ulrike Müller
Institut für Pharmazie und Molekulare Biotechnologie, Universität Heidelberg, Germany

Klemens Wild
Biochemiezentrum der Universität Heidelberg (BZH), Universität Heidelberg, Germany

Daniel A. Bórquez, Ismael Palacios and Christian González-Billault
Cell and Neuronal Dynamics Laboratory, Faculty of Sciences, Universidad de Chile, Santiago, Chile

Yuhki Saito, Takahide Matsushima and Toshiharu Suzuki
Laboratory of Neuroscience, Graduate School of Pharmaceutical Sciences, Hokkaido University, Sapporo, Japan

Kohzo Nakayama
Department of Anatomy, Shinshu University, School of Medicine, Matsumoto, Nagano, Japan
Department of Developmental and Regenerative Medicine, Mie University, Graduate School of Medicine, Tsu, Mie, Japan

Hisashi Nagase
Department of Immunology and Infectious Diseases, Shinshu University, School of Medicine, Japan

Chang-Sung Koh
Department of Biomedical Sciences, Shinshu University, School of Health Sciences, Matsumoto, Nagano, Japan

Takeshi Ohkawara
Department of Anatomy, Shinshu University, School of Medicine, Matsumoto, Nagano, Japan

Lucia Pastorino, Asami Kondo, Xiao Zhen Zhou and Kun Ping Lu
Department of Medicine, Beth Israel Deaconess Medical Center, Harvard Medical School, Boston, USA

José Luna-Muñoz, Paola Flores-Rodríguez, Raúl Mena Benjamin and Floran-Garduño
Departments of Physiology, Biophysics and Neurosciences, National Laboratory of experimental services (LaNSE), CINVESTAV-IPN, Mexico

Charles R. Harrington, Claude M. Wischik
Division of Applied Health Sciences, School of Medicine and Dentistry, University of Aberdeen, USA

Jesús Avila
Centro de Biología Molecular "Severo Ochoa", CSIC/UAM, Universidad Autónoma de Madrid, Madrid, Spain

Sergio R. Zamudio, Fidel De la Cruz
Department of Physiology, ENCB-IPN, Mexico

Marco A. Meraz-Ríos
Molecular Biomedicine, CINVESTAV-IPN, Mexico

Genaro G. Ortiz, Erandis D. Tórres-Sánchez, Eddic W. Moráles-Sánchez, José A. Cruz-Ramos,
Genaro E Ortiz-Velázquez and Fernando Cortés-Enríquez
Lab. Estrés Oxidativo-Mitocondria & Enfermedad, Centro de Investigación Biomédica de Occidente, Instituto Mexicano del Seguro Social (IMSS). Guadalajara, Jalisco, México

Fermín P. Pacheco-Moisés and Ana C. Ramírez-Anguiano
Dpto. de Química, CUCEI, Universidad de Guadalajara. Guadalajara, Jalisco, México

Luis J. Flores-Alvarado
Dpto. de Bioquímica, CUCS, Universidad de Guadalajara. Guadalajara, Jalisco, México

Miguel A. Macías-Islas
Depto. de Neurología, UMAE,HE- IMSS. Guadalajara, Jalisco, México

Irma E. Velázquez-Brizuela
OPD-IJC-SSA- Jalisco, Guadalajara, Jalisco, México

Armand Perret-Liaudet, Benoit Dumont and Isabelle Quadrio
Hospices Civils de Lyon, Neurobiologie, Centre Mémoire de Recherche et de Ressources, Hôpitaux de Lyon, Lyon, France
Université Lyon 1, CNRS UMR5292, INSERM U1028, Equipe BioRan, Lyon, France

Aline Dorey
Hospices Civils de Lyon, Neurobiologie, Centre Mémoire de Recherche et de Ressources, Hôpitaux de Lyon, Lyon, France

Yannick Tholance
Hospices Civils de Lyon, Neurobiologie, Centre Mémoire de Recherche et de Ressources, Hôpitaux de Lyon, Lyon, France
Université Lyon 1, CNRS UMR5292, INSERM U1028, Equipe WAKING, Lyon, France

Emily J. Mason and Brandon A. Ally
Department of Neurology, Vanderbilt University, Nashville, TN, USA

Manus J. Donahue
Department of Radiology, Vanderbilt University, Nashville, TN, USA

B.K. Binukumar and Harish C. Pant
Laboratory of Neurochemistry, NINDS, National Institutes of Health, Bethesda, Maryland, USA

Printed in the USA
CPSIA information can be obtained
at www.ICGtesting.com
JSHW011435221024
72173JS00004B/815

9 781632 420398